Study Guide

Clinical Procedures
for Medical Assistants

Tenth Edition

Kathy Bonewit-West, BS, MEd
Coordinator and Instructor
Medical Assistant Technology
Hocking College
Nelsonville, Ohio

Former Member, Curriculum Review Board of the
American Association of Medical Assistants

ELSEVIER

ELSEVIER

3251 Riverport Lane
St. Louis, Missouri 63043

Notices

Knowledge and best practice in this field are constantly changing. As new research and experience broaden
our understanding, changes in research methods, professional practices, or medical treatment may become
necessary.

Practitioners and researchers must always rely on their own experience and knowledge in evaluating and
using any information, methods, compounds, or experiments described herein. In using such information or
methods, they should be mindful of their own safety and the safety of others, including parties for whom they
have a professional responsibility.

With respect to any drug or pharmaceutical products identified, readers are advised to check the most
current information provided (i) on procedures featured or (ii) by the manufacturer of each product to be
administered and to verify the recommended dose or formula, the method and duration of administration, and
contraindications. It is the responsibility of practitioners, relying on their own experience and knowledge of
their patients, to make diagnoses, to determine dosages and the best treatment for each individual patient, and
to take all appropriate safety precautions.

To the fullest extent of the law, neither the Publisher nor the authors, contributors, or editors assume any
liability for any injury and/or damage to persons or property as a matter of products liability, negligence or
otherwise, or from any use or operation of any methods, products, instructions, or ideas contained in the
material herein.

Executive Content Strategist: Jennifer Janson
Content Development Manager: Ellen Wurm-Cutter
Senior Content Development Specialist: Rebecca Leenhouts
Publishing Services Manager: Deepthi Unni
Project Manager: Apoorva V
Design Direction: Muthukumaran Thangaraj

Printed in United States of America

Last digit is the print number: 9 8 7 6 5 4 3 2

Working together
to grow libraries in
developing countries

www.elsevier.com • www.bookaid.org

Contents

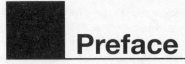

Preface

Outcome-based education prepares individuals to perform the prespecified tasks of an occupation under real-world conditions at a level of accuracy and speed required of the entry-level practitioner of that profession. Outcome-based education plays an important role in medical assisting programs in preparing qualified individuals for careers in medical offices, clinics, and related health care facilities. The *Study Guide for Clinical Procedures for Medical Assistants* has been developed using a thorough outcome-based approach. It meets the criteria stipulated by the Commission on Accreditation of Allied Health Education (CAAHEP)* Standards and Guidelines for the Medical Assisting Educational Programs and the Accrediting Bureau of Health Education Schools (ABHES) Programmatic Evaluation Standards for Medical Assisting. Instructors should find this Study Guide a valuable teaching aid for training students who are able to think critically and to perform competently in the clinical setting.

Each study guide chapter is organized into the following sections:

1. *ASSIGNMENT SHEETS*: The Study Guide Assignment Sheets indicate the assignments required for each chapter, along with a space provided for the student to document the following: the date each assignment is due, completion of the assignment, and points earned for each assignment. The Laboratory Assignment Sheet indicates the procedures required for each chapter, along with the textbook and Study Guide reference pages, the number of practices required to attain competency, and a space for documenting the score earned on the Performance Evaluation Checklist.

2. *PRETEST AND POSTTEST*: These tests have been included for each chapter using true/false questions that allow the student to test his or her acquisition of knowledge for each chapter before and after completing the chapter. These tests can be used as a study guide to prepare for chapter tests.

3. *KEY TERM ASSESSMENT*: This section provides the student with an assessment of his or her knowledge of the medical terms covered in each chapter. This section also includes an assessment of the word parts of the medical terms (prefixes, suffixes, and combining forms) to evaluate the student's knowledge of the meaning of the medical term through its word parts.

4. *EVALUATION OF LEARNING*: These questions help the student evaluate his or her progress throughout each chapter. After the student has completed these questions and checked them for accuracy, they provide an ongoing review of the textbook material. Individuals preparing for a certification examination will find the completed Evaluation of Learning sections useful study aids for the clinical aspect of the examination.

5. *CRITICAL THINKING ACTIVITIES*: In this section, the student performs activities that enhance his or her ability to think critically. Some situations require the student to become involved in a game or play a role; others require the student to use independent study to answer questions posed by a patient. Independent study helps the student become familiar with resources available to acquire additional knowledge and skills outside the classroom. By learning techniques of self-development, the medical assisting student may become aware of the necessity for continuing education after graduation and entrance into the medical assisting profession.

6. *PRACTICE FOR COMPETENCY*: This section consists of worksheets that provide the student with a guide for the practice of each clinical skill presented in the textbook.

7. *EVALUATION OF COMPETENCY*: This section has two parts. The first part is the Performance Objective, which provides an exact description of what the learner must be able to demonstrate to attain competency and has been developed to correspond to the procedures presented in the textbook. A performance objective consists of the (1) outcome, (2) conditions, and (3) standards. The second part is the Performance Evaluation Checklist, which provides quality control by comparing the student's performance against an established set of performance standards.

---

*The CAAHEP competencies used for the Evaluation of Competency sheets were used with permission from the American Association of Medical Assistants, Chicago, Illinois, and the Commission on Accreditation of Allied Health Education Programs, Clearwater, Florida.

8. *SUPPLEMENTAL EDUCATION*: Several medical assisting content areas are more difficult than others for the student to comprehend and perform. Because students have special difficulty in taking patients' symptoms and in calculating drug dosage, two supplemental education sections have been incorporated into this manual. The section "Taking Patients' Symptoms" provides supplemental education for Chapter 1 (The Medical Record) in the textbook; the section "Drug Dosage Calculation" provides supplemental education for Chapter 11 (Administration of Medication). In these two sections, a step-by-step, self-directed approach has been used, beginning with basic concepts and advancing to more difficult ones. The student should find that this type of approach facilitates the process of becoming proficient in these areas.

9. *EVOLVE SITE*: The Evolve site (http://evolve.elsevier.com/Bonewit) offers many opportunities for students to apply the theory and skills learned throughout the textbook. Organized by chapter, the Evolve site includes several games (e.g., Quiz Show, Road to Recovery) to provide entertainment while the student is learning important concepts related to selected chapters, matching exercises, labeling exercises, identification exercises, and other helpful activities. Of particular importance on the Evolve site are the following:
   a. *Apply Your Knowledge*: These multiple-choice questions allow the student to test his or her acquisition of practical knowledge for each chapter. These test questions can be used as a study guide to prepare for chapter tests and for a national certification examination.
   b. *Practicum Activity worksheets*: Practicum Activity worksheets are completed by the student at his or her practicum site. These worksheets assist the student in relating classroom knowledge to the real-world setting of the medical office.
   c. *Procedural Videos*: These step-by-step procedural videos directly correlate to procedures found in the textbook. They give students a visual representation of the reading material and reinforce how to perform correct clinical procedures.
   d. *Video Evaluation:* The video evaluation sheets assess the student's knowledge of key points in the clinical skills presented in the procedural videos presented on the Evolve site (http://evolve.elsevier.com/Bonewit).

I want to thank the staff at Elsevier for their assistance and support in preparing this Study Guide. I would also like to express my appreciation to the following individuals who provided encouragement and friendship throughout this endeavor: Daniel Baldwin, Marlene Donovan, Dawn Shingler, Deborah Murray, Rob Bonewit, Hollie Bonewit-Cron, and Tristen West.

Kathy Bonewit-West, BS, MEd

Message to the Student

This Study Guide has been designed to facilitate the attainment of competency in the clinical theory and procedures in your textbook. Each chapter of the manual has been organized into the ten components outlined below. By completing each component, it is hoped that your ability to assimilate the theory and perform the clinical skills will be greatly enhanced.

1. TEXTBOOK AND STUDY GUIDE ASSIGNMENT SHEETS
A. Each time your instructor makes an assignment from the textbook, Study Guide, or Evolve site, document the date due in the appropriate space on the Textbook or Study Guide Assignment Sheet.
B. Complete each assignment by the due date. Place a checkmark in the appropriate space on the Textbook or Study Guide Assignment Sheet after completing each assignment.
C. Grade the assignment according to the directions stipulated by your instructor.
D. Record your points earned in the appropriate space on the Textbook or Study Guide Assignment Sheet.

2. LABORATORY ASSIGNMENT SHEET
A. Your instructor will assign the procedures to be completed for each laboratory practice session. Check the assigned procedures in the appropriate space on the Laboratory Assignment Sheet.
B. Refer to the page numbers on the Laboratory Assignment Sheet for the Practice for Competency and Evaluation of Competency worksheets required for each procedure your instructor assigned.
C. Locate and tear out the worksheets required for each procedure to be performed, and bring them to your laboratory practice session.
D. Record the score you earned on the Evaluation of Competency Performance Evaluation Checklist in the appropriate space on the Laboratory Assignment Sheet. This will provide you with a record of your progress on clinical procedures.

3. PRETEST AND POSTTEST
A. Complete the Pretest before beginning a study of each chapter. Complete the Posttest after completing the study of the chapter. Place a checkmark in the appropriate space on the Study Guide Assignment Sheet after completing each test.
B. Check your work for accuracy against the textbook, and correct any errors.
C. Grade the tests according to the directions stipulated by your instructor.
D. Record the points you earned in the appropriate space on the Study Guide Assignment Sheet.
E. Review the Pretest and Posttest before taking your chapter test.

4. KEY TERM ASSESSMENT
A. Study the Terminology Review section located at the end of each chapter in the textbook.
B. Match the medical terms with the definitions and complete the word parts table. Place a checkmark in the appropriate space on the Study Guide Assignment Sheet after completing the exercise.
C. Check your work for accuracy against the textbook, and correct any errors.
D. Grade the exercise according to the directions stipulated by your instructor.
E. Record the points you earned in the appropriate space on the Study Guide Assignment Sheet.
F. Review the Key Term Assessment before taking your chapter test.

5. EVALUATION OF LEARNING QUESTIONS
A. Read the textbook chapter.
B. Complete the Evaluation of Learning questions. Place a checkmark in the appropriate space on the Study Guide Assignment Sheet after completing the questions.
C. Check your work for accuracy against the textbook, and correct any errors.
D. Grade the questions according to the directions stipulated by your instructor.
E. Record the points you earned in the appropriate space on the Textbook Assignment Sheet.
F. Review the Evaluation of Learning questions before taking your chapter test.

6. **CRITICAL THINKING ACTIVITIES**
    A. Review the information required to complete the Critical Thinking Activities.
    B. Obtain any additional materials or resources required.
    C. Complete each Critical Thinking Activity. Place a checkmark in the appropriate space on the Study Guide Assignment Sheet after completing each assigned activity.
    D. Grade each Critical Thinking Activity according to the directions stipulated by your instructor.
    E. Record the points you earned in the appropriate space on the Textbook Assignment Sheet.

7. **EVOLVE SITE ACTIVITIES**
    A. Complete each Evolve site activity listed on the Study Guide Assignment Sheet. Place a checkmark in the appropriate space on the Assignment Sheet after completing each assigned activity.
    B. Record the points you earned in the appropriate space on the Assignment Sheet.

8. **VIDEO EVALUATION**
    A. View the procedural videos assigned by your instructor (available on the Evolve site).
    B. Complete the video evaluation questions on the Evolve site, and place a checkmark in the appropriate space on the Study Guide Assignment Sheet.
    C. Check your work for accuracy, and correct any errors.
    D. Grade the questions according to the directions stipulated by your instructor.
    E. Record the points you earned in the appropriate space on the Study Guide Assignment Sheet.
    F. Review the Video Evaluation questions before being evaluated on each clinical skill by your instructor.

9. **PRACTICE FOR COMPETENCY**
    A. Your instructor will assign procedures to be completed for each laboratory practice session. For each procedure assigned, place a checkmark in the appropriate space on the Laboratory Assignment Sheet.
    B. Refer to the page numbers on the Laboratory Assignment Sheet for the Practice for Competency and Evaluation of Competency sheets required for each procedure your instructor assigned. Locate and tear out the sheets required for each procedure to be performed, and bring them to your laboratory practice session.
    C. Practice each assigned procedure the required number of times indicated on the Laboratory Assignment Sheet or as designated by your instructor. Use the following guidelines when practicing the procedure to attain competency over each procedure:
       1. Information indicated on the Practice for Competency sheet
          a. Record your practices in the chart provided.
       2. Procedure as presented in your textbook
       3. Video of the procedure (on the Evolve site)
          a. View each procedure several times to make sure you understand the correct technique and theory.
       4. Evaluation of Competency Performance Checklist
          a. Ensure that you can perform each procedure according to the criteria stipulated under conditions and standards.
       5. Peer evaluation
          a. If directed by your instructor, obtain a peer evaluation using the Evaluation of Competency Performance Evaluation Checklist.
    D. Bring the completed Practice for Competency sheet to your laboratory testing session, and present it to your instructor for his or her review before testing on the procedure.

10. **EVALUATION OF COMPETENCY PERFORMANCE CHECKLIST**
    A. Write your name and date in the space indicated on the Evaluation of Competency Performance Evaluation Checklist.
       1. Do not chart the procedure (in advance) on the Evaluation of Competency sheet. You do this after you have been tested on the procedure.
    B. For each procedure being evaluated, bring the following to your laboratory testing session, and present them to your instructor:
       1. Completed Practice for Competency sheet
       2. Evaluation of Competency Performance Checklist
       3. Outcome Assessment Record
    C. Demonstrate the proper procedure for performing the clinical skill for your instructor.
    D. Document results (if required) in the chart provided on the Evaluation of Competency Checklist.

E. Obtain your instructor's initials on your Outcome Assessment Record, indicating you have performed the procedure with competency.

F. Record the score you earned in the appropriate space on your Laboratory Assignment Sheet.

After you have completed each chapter in this Study Guide, place the perforated sheet into a three-ring notebook. This will provide an ongoing record of your academic progress. The notebook provides a classroom reference and a certification examination review resource.

I hope that this Study Guide will assist in your attainment of competency in clinical medical assisting procedures and will facilitate your transition from the classroom to the workplace.

Kathy Bonewit-West, BS, MEd

Outcome Assessment Record

This list of outcomes is used to maintain an ongoing record of classroom and practicum outcome assessment. Your instructor should initial each outcome when you have performed it with competency in the classroom. When you have performed the outcome with competency at your externship facility, it should be initialled by your practicum supervisor. Space is provided for three externship experiences in the event that you extern at more than one practicum site.

Name_____	Classroom Performance	Practicum	Practicum	Practicum
THE MEDICAL RECORD				
Complete or assist the patient in completing a health history form.				
Obtain and document a patient's symptoms.				
MEDICAL ASEPSIS AND THE OSHA STANDARD				
Perform handwashing.				
Apply an alcohol-based hand rub.				
Apply and remove clean disposable gloves.				
Demonstrate the proper use of a sharps container.				
Prepare regulated waste for pickup by a medical waste service.				
STERILIZATION AND DISINFECTION				
Sanitize instruments.				
Chemically disinfect contaminated articles.				
Wrap an instrument for autoclaving.				
Sterilize articles in the autoclave.				
VITAL SIGNS				
Measure oral body temperature.				
Measure axillary body temperature.				
Measure rectal body temperature.				
Measure aural body temperature.				

Name_____	Classroom Performance	Practicum	Practicum	Practicum
Measure temporal artery body temperature.				
Measure radial pulse and respiration.				
Measure apical pulse.				
Perform pulse oximetry.				
Measure blood pressure.				
THE PHYSICAL EXAMINATION				
Measure weight and height.				
Demonstrate proper body mechanics.				
Position and drape a patient.				
Transfer a patient from and to a wheelchair.				
Prepare the examining room.				
Prepare a patient for a physical examination.				
Assist the provider with a physical examination.				
EYE AND EAR PROCEDURES				
Assess distance visual acuity.				
Assess color vision.				
Perform an eye irrigation.				
Perform an eye instillation.				
Perform an ear irrigation.				
Perform an ear instillation.				
PHYSICAL AGENTS TO PROMOTE TISSUE HEALING				
Apply a heating pad.				
Apply a hot soak.				
Apply a hot compress.				
Apply an ice bag.				

Name_____	Classroom Performance	Practicum	Practicum	Practicum
Apply a cold compress.				
Apply a chemical cold and hot pack.				
Assist with the application and removal of a cast.				
Instruct a patient in proper cast care.				
Apply a splint.				
Apply a brace.				
Measure an individual for axillary crutches.				
Instruct an individual in mastering crutch gaits.				
Instruct an individual in the use of a cane.				
Instruct an individual in the use of a walker.				
THE GYNECOLOGIC EXAMINATION AND PRENATAL CARE				
Provide instructions for a breast self-examination.				
Assist with a gynecologic examination.				
Assist with a prenatal examination.				
THE PEDIATRIC EXAMINATION				
Carry an infant in the following positions: cradle and upright.				
Measure the weight and length of an infant.				
Measure the head circumference of an infant.				
Measure the chest circumference of an infant.				
Plot pediatric measurements on a growth chart.				
Apply a pediatric urine collector.				
Collect a specimen for a newborn screening test.				

Outcome Assessment Record

Name_____	Classroom Performance	Practicum	Practicum	Practicum
MINOR OFFICE SURGERY				
Apply and remove sterile gloves.				
Open a sterile package.				
Add an article to a sterile field from a peel-apart package.				
Pour a sterile solution into a container on a sterile field.				
Change a sterile dressing.				
Remove sutures.				
Remove staples.				
Apply and remove adhesive skin closures.				
Set up a tray for minor office surgery.				
Assist the provider with minor office surgery.				
Apply the following bandage turns: circular, spiral, spiral-reverse, figure-eight, and recurrent.				
Apply a tubular gauze bandage.				
ADMINISTRATION OF MEDICATION				
Prepare and administer oral medication.				
Prepare an injection from a vial.				
Prepare an injection from an ampule.				
Reconstitute a powdered drug.				
Administer a subcutaneous injection.				
Locate the following intramuscular injection sites: dorsogluteal, deltoid, vastus lateralis, and ventrogluteal.				
Administer an intramuscular injection.				
Administer an injection using the Z-track method.				
Administer an intradermal injection.				

Name_____	Classroom Performance	Practicum	Practicum	Practicum
Administer a tuberculin skin test and read the test results.				
CARDIOPULMONARY PROCEDURES				
Record an electrocardiogram.				
Instruct a patient in the guidelines for wearing a Holter monitor.				
Apply a Holter monitor.				
Perform a spirometry test.				
Measure a patient's peak flow rate.				
COLON PROCEDURES				
Instruct a patient for a fecal occult blood test.				
Develop a fecal occult blood test.				
Instruct a patient in the preparation for a sigmoidoscopy.				
Assist the provider with a sigmoidoscopy.				
Instruct a patient in the preparation for a colonoscopy.				
Provide instructions for a testicular self-examination.				
RADIOLOGY AND DIAGNOSTIC IMAGING				
Instruct a patient in the proper preparation required for each of the following x-ray examinations: mammogram, bone density scan, upper gastrointestinal (GI), lower GI, and intravenous pyelogram.				
Instruct a patient in the proper preparation required for each of the following: ultrasonography, computed tomography, magnetic resonance imaging, and nuclear medicine study.				
INTRODUCTION TO THE CLINICAL LABORATORY				
Operate an emergency eyewash station.				
Complete a laboratory request form.				

xv

Name_____	Classroom Performance	Practicum	Practicum	Practicum
Instruct the patient in advance preparation requirements for a laboratory test.				
Collect a specimen.				
Properly handle and store a specimen.				
Review a laboratory report.				
URINALYSIS				
Instruct a patient in clean-catch midstream urine specimen collection.				
Instruct a patient in 24-hour urine specimen collection.				
Assess the color and appearance of a urine specimen.				
Perform a CLIA-waived chemical assessment of a urine specimen.				
Prepare a urine specimen for microscopic analysis.				
Perform a rapid urine culture test.				
Perform a CLIA-waived urine pregnancy test.				
PHLEBOTOMY				
Perform a venipuncture using the vacuum tube method.				
Perform a venipuncture using the butterfly method.				
Separate serum from a blood specimen.				
Perform a capillary puncture.				
Reusable semiautomatic lancet device.				
HEMATOLOGY				
Perform a CLIA-waived hemoglobin determination.				
Perform a CLIA-waived hematocrit determination.				
Prepare a blood smear.				
Perform a CLIA-waived PT/INR test.				

Name_____	Classroom Performance	Practicum	Practicum	Practicum
BLOOD CHEMISTRY AND IMMUNOLOGY				
Perform a CLIA-waived blood glucose test.				
Perform a CLIA-waived blood chemistry test.				
Perform a CLIA-waived rapid mononucleosis test.				
MICROBIOLOGY				
Use a microscope.				
Collect a throat specimen.				
Obtain a specimen using a collection and transport system.				
Perform a CLIA-waived rapid strep test.				
Perform a CLIA-waived rapid influenza test.				
NUTRITION				
Instruct a patient according to patient's special dietary needs.				
EMERGENCY PREPAREDNESS AND PROTECTIVE PRACTICES				
Demonstrate proper use of a fire extinguisher.				
Participate in a mock exposure event.				
ADDITIONAL OUTCOMES (List)				

Outcome Assessment Record

Name_____	Classroom Performance	Practicum	Practicum	Practicum

Outcome Assessment Record

The Medical Record

CHAPTER ASSIGNMENTS

√ After Completing	Date Due	Study Guide Pages	STUDY GUIDE ASSIGNMENTS (CTA = Critical Thinking Activity)	Possible Points	Points You Earned
		5	Pretest	10	
		6	Key Term Assessment	11	
		6-12	Evaluation of Learning questions	60	
		13	**CTA A: Medical Abbreviations**	20	
		13	CTA B: Chief Complaint	6	
		14	CTA C: Crossword Puzzle	23	
			Evolve Site: Road to Recovery: Medical Abbreviations (Record points earned)		
		22-28	Taking Patient Symptoms: Supplemental Education for Chapter 1 (10 points for each problem)	60	
			Evolve Site: Apply Your Knowledge questions	10	
			Evolve Site: Video Evaluation	12	
		5	Posttest	10	
			ADDITIONAL ASSIGNMENTS		
			Total points		

√ When Assigned by Your Instructor	Study Guide Pages	Practices Required	LABORATORY ASSIGNMENTS (Procedure Number and Name)	Score*
	15	1	Practice for Competency Health History Form Textbook reference: pp. 8-10	
	15-18	5	Practice for Competency 1-1: Obtaining and Documenting Patient Symptoms Textbook reference: pp. 22-23	
	19-21		Evaluation of Competency 1-1: Obtaining and Recording Patient Symptoms	*
			ADDITIONAL ASSIGNMENTS	

Name: _____ Date: _____

True or False

_____ 1. The medical record serves as a legal document.

_____ 2. PHI includes health information in any form that contains patient-identifiable information.

_____ 3. A therapeutic service report documents the assessment and treatment designed to restore a patient's ability to function.

_____ 4. An example of a hospital document is a discharge summary report.

_____ 5. Diabetes mellitus is an example of a familial disease.

_____ 6. The medical assistant should make sure to document a procedure before performing it.

_____ 7. A symptom is any change in the body or its functioning that indicates the presence of disease.

_____ 8. A feeling of dizziness or light-headedness is known as vertigo.

_____ 9. Excessive perspiration is known as flatulence.

_____ 10. Pain is an example of an objective symptom.

📄❓ **POSTTEST**

True or False

_____ 1. The purpose of HIPAA is to provide patients with more control over the use and disclosure of their health information.

_____ 2. An example of a diagnostic procedure report is a urinalysis report.

_____ 3. A laboratory report is a report of the analysis or examination of body specimens.

_____ 4. The health history provides subjective data about a patient to assist the provider in arriving at a diagnosis.

_____ 5. The family history is a review of the health status of the patient's blood relatives.

_____ 6. The chief complaint is the symptom causing the patient the most trouble.

_____ 7. The social history includes information on the patient's lifestyle, such as health habits and living environment.

_____ 8. The patient's name must be included at the beginning of each entry documented in the patient's medical record.

_____ 9. A decrease in the amount of water in the body is known as edema.

_____ 10. Cyanosis is an example of an objective symptom.

Directions: Match each medical term (numbers) with its definition (letters).

_____ 1. Diagnosis

_____ 2. Diagnostic procedure

_____ 3. Documenting

_____ 4. Electronic medical record

_____ 5. Familial disease

_____ 6. Health history report

_____ 7. Medical record

_____ 8. Objective symptom

_____ 9. Patient-based patient record

_____ 10. Subjective symptom

_____ 11. Symptom

A. A collection of subjective data about a patient
B. A symptom felt by the patient but not observed by an examiner
C. The process of recording information about a patient in the medical record
D. Any change in the body or its functioning that indicates the presence of disease
E. A medical record that is stored on a computer
F. A written record of the important information regarding a patient
G. A symptom that can be observed by an examiner
H. The scientific method of determining and identifying a patient's condition
I. A condition that occurs in or affects blood relatives more frequently than would be expected by chance
J. A procedure performed to assist in the diagnosis, management, or treatment of a patient's condition
K. A medical record in paper form

EVALUATION OF LEARNING

Directions: Fill in each blank with the correct answer.

1. List three functions of the medical record.

_____

_____

_____

2. What is the meaning of the acronym HIPAA?

_____

3. What is the purpose of the HIPAA Privacy Rule?

_____

_____

4. Who must comply with HIPAA?

_____

5. What is a Notice of Privacy Practices?

_____

6. What is protected health information?

_____

_____

7. List examples of when HIPAA does not require written consent for the use or disclosure of protected health information in the following categories:

a. Treatment: _____

b. Payment: _____

c. Health care operations: _____

8. What must be done before the medical office can disclose protected health information (PHI) to a business associate?

_____

9. What are some examples of business associates to whom the medical office may disclose PHI?

_____

_____

10. How must medical office employees be informed of the privacy and security measures that must be followed with respect to PHI?

_____

11. List three examples of medical office administrative documents.

_____

_____

12. List five examples of medical office clinical documents.

_____

_____

13. What is a laboratory report, and what is its purpose?

_____

_____

14. What is a diagnostic procedure?

_____

_____

15. What information is included in a diagnostic procedure report?

_____

_____

16. List five examples of diagnostic procedure reports.

_____

_____

17. What information is documented in a therapeutic service report?

_____

_____

18. List three examples of therapeutic service reports.

_____

_____

19. What is the purpose of hospital documents?

_____

_____

20. Who is responsible for preparing hospital documents?

_____

21. List five examples of hospital documents.

_____

_____

22. What are consent forms?

_____

23. List two examples of consent documents.

_____

24. What types of forms are typically included in a paper-based patient record (PPR)?

_____

_____

25. What is an EMR?

_____

_____

26. What are the general functions performed by an EMR software program?

_____

_____

27. List and describe the advantages of the electronic medical record.

_____

_____

_____

_____

28. How are paper documents entered into a patient's electronic medical record?

_____

_____

29. What is the function of an optical character recognition (OCR) program?

_____

_____

30. What is a health history report?

_____

_____

31. List four functions of a health history report.

_____

_____

_____

32. What are three ways in which a health history can be entered into the EMR?

_____

_____

_____

33. State the purpose of the following seven sections of the health history:

   a. Identification data: _____

   b. Chief complaint: _____

   _____

   c. Present illness: _____

   _____

   d. Past history: _____

   _____

   e. Family history: _____

   _____

   f. Social history: _____

   _____

   g. Review of systems: _____

   _____

34. What is a chief complaint?

_____

35. List five guidelines that must be followed in documenting the chief complaint.

_____

_____

_____

36. What is the present illness, and how is this information usually obtained?

_____

_____

37. What is the past history, and how is it usually obtained?

_____

_____

38. List six examples of information included in the past medical history.

_____

_____

_____

_____

_____

39. List three examples of familial diseases.

_____

_____

_____

40. Explain the importance of the social history.

_____

_____

41. What specific areas are included in the social history?

_____

_____

42. What is the review of systems (ROS), and how is it usually obtained?

_____

_____

43. Explain the importance of good documentation.

_____

_____

44. What may result if the medical assistant documents information in the wrong patient's medical record?

_____

_____

45. Why is it important for the medical assistant to use the commonly accepted abbreviations, medical terms, and symbols when documenting in the medical record?

_____

_____

46. Why is it important to document immediately after performing a procedure?

_____

47. Why is it important to adhere to the following guidelines when documenting in the PPR?

a. Use black ink: _____

_____

b. Write in legible handwriting: _____

_____

c. Draw a single line through unneeded space: _____

_____

d. Never erase or obliterate an entry: _____

_____

48. What should be done if an error is made when documenting in a PPR?

_____

_____

49. What are progress notes?

_____

_____

50. What is the purpose of progress notes? _____

_____

51. What is a symptom? _____

_____

52. What is the difference between a subjective symptom and an objective symptom?

_____

_____

53. List three examples of subjective symptoms.

_____

_____

_____

54. List three examples of objective symptoms.

_____

_____

_____

55. In general, what information should be documented regarding a procedure performed on a patient?

_____

_____

56. What information should be documented regarding medication administered to a patient?

_____

_____

57. What information should be documented regarding a specimen collected from a patient?

_____

_____

58. Why is it important to document diagnostic procedures and laboratory tests ordered for a patient?

_____

_____

59. What is the importance of having a patient sign a form indicating he or she has read and understands instructions relayed to him or her?

_____

_____

60. Why is it important for the medical assistant to witness the patient's signature on an instruction sheet provided to the patient?

_____

_____

CRITICAL THINKING ACTIVITIES

A. Medical Abbreviations

Write a paragraph describing a visit to your doctor's office in the space provided using at least 20 abbreviations and symbols outlined in Table 1-1 of your textbook.

_____

_____

_____

_____

_____

_____

_____

_____

_____

_____

_____

_____

B. Chief Complaint

Indicate whether each of the following statements is an incorrect (I) or correct (C) example of documenting a chief complaint (CC). If the example is incorrect, explain which documentation guideline is not being followed.

_____ 1. CC: Low back pain _____

_____ 2. CC: Sore throat and fever for the past 2 days _____

_____ 3. CC: Dyspnea, paleness, and fatigue, similar to that associated with anemia, that have lasted for

2 weeks _____

_____ 4. CC: Poor health for the past several months _____

_____ 5. CC: Weakness and fatigue related to poor eating habits and lack of exercise

_____

_____ 6. CC: Heart palpitations occurring after drinking coffee in the morning before work

_____

_____

C. Crossword Puzzle: Symptoms

Directions: Complete the crossword puzzle using the terms provided.

Across

2 Stool is hard and dry
4 Blue skin from lack of O_2
5 Nosebleed
10 Skin eruption
11 Dizziness
14 No appetite
15 Yellow skin
18 Severe itching
19 Involuntary contractions of muscles
20 Gas
21 Head pain

Down

1 Fast pulse rate
2 Shivering
3 May be productive or nonproductive
5 Fluid retention
6 Ejection of stomach contents
7 Decreased H_2O levels in the body
8 Red face
9 Elevated temp
12 Bad all over
13 Loose, watery stools
16 Sensation of stomach discomfort
17 Feeling of distress or suffering

PRACTICE FOR COMPETENCY

Health History Form

Complete the health history form (pages 8 to 10) using yourself as the patient.

Procedure 1-1: Obtaining and Documenting Patient Symptoms

Practice obtaining patient symptoms, by completing Taking Patient Symptoms: Supplemental Education for Chapter 1 (pages 22 to 28 in this study guide).

PATIENT HEALTH HISTORY

A IDENTIFICATION DATA   Please print the following information.

Today's date _____

Name _____   ___ Male ___ Female

Address _____   ___ Married ___ Separated ___ Divorced ___ Widowed ___ Single

_____   Date of Birth _____

Telephone _____ _____
    Home number   Work number

B PAST HISTORY

Have you ever had the following: (Circle "no" or "yes"; leave blank if uncertain)

Measles_____ no yes	Heart Disease_____ no yes	Diabetes_____ no yes	Hemorrhoids_____ no yes
Mumps_____ no yes	Arthritis_____ no yes	Cancer_____ no yes	Asthma_____ no yes
Chickenpox_____ no yes	Sexually Transmitted no yes Disease	Polio_____ no yes	Allergies_____ no yes
Whooping Cough___ no yes	Anemia_____ no yes	Glaucoma_____ no yes	Eczema_____ no yes
Scarlet Fever_____ no yes	Bladder Infections___ no yes	Hernia_____ no yes	AIDS or HIV+_____ no yes
Diphtheria_____ no yes	Epilepsy_____ no yes	Blood or Plasma___ no yes Transfusions	Infectious Mono____ no yes
Pneumonia_____ no yes	Migraine Headaches__ no yes	Back Trouble____ no yes	Bronchitis_____ no yes
Rheumatic Fever___ no yes	Tuberculosis_____ no yes	High Blood_____ no yes Pressure	Mitral Valve Prolapse no yes
Stroke_____ no yes	Ulcer_____ no yes	Thyroid Disease___ no yes	Any other disease__ no yes Please list: _____
Hepatitis_____ no yes	Kidney Disease____ no yes	Bleeding Tendency_ no yes	_____

MAJOR HOSPITALIZATIONS: If you have ever been hospitalized for any major medical illness or operation, write in your most recent hospitalizations below.

Hospitalizations	Year	Operation or illness	Name of hospital	City and state
1st Hospitalization				
2nd Hospitalization				
3rd Hospitalization				
4th Hospitalization				

TESTS AND IMMUNIZATIONS: Mark an X next to those that you have had.

Tests: Immunizations:

☐ TB Test   ☐ Electrocardiogram   ☐ Influenza

☐ Rectal/Hemoccult   ☐ Chest X-ray   ☐ Hepatitis B

☐ Sigmoidoscopy   ☐ Mammogram   ☐ Tetanus

☐ Colonoscopy   ☐ Pap Test   ☐ MMR

                                             ☐ Polio

ALLERGIES: List all allergies (foods, drugs, environment). ☐ None

_____

_____

_____

_____

CURRENT MEDICATIONS: List the following that you are currently taking: Prescription medications, over-the-counter (OTC) medications, vitamin supplements, and herbal supplements.   ☐ None

Medication   Frequency

_____

_____

_____

ACCIDENTS/INJURIES: Describe all serious accidents, severe injuries, head injury, or fractures. Include the date each occurred. ☐ None

Accident/Injury: Date:

_____

_____

_____

_____

(Continued)

C | FAMILY HISTORY

For each member of your family, follow the purple or blue line across the page and check boxes for:
1. Their present state of health
2. Any illnesses they have had

	Good Health	Poor Health	Deceased	If deceased, write in age and cause of death.	Allergies or Asthma	Diabetes	Heart Disease	Stroke	Cancer	High Blood Pressure	Glaucoma	Arthritis	Ulcer	Kidney Disease	Mental Health Problems	Alcohol/Drug Abuse	Obesity	High Cholesterol	Thyroid Disease
Father:																			
Mother:																			
Brothers/Sisters:																			

D | SOCIAL HISTORY

EDUCATION _____ High school _____ College _____ Postgraduate

Occupation _____ Years _____

Previous occupations _____ Years _____

_____ Years _____

Have you ever been exposed to any of the following in your environment?

☐ Excess dust (coal, lime, rock)   ☐ Cleaning fluids/solvents   ☐ Radiation   ☐ Other toxic materials
☐ Sand   ☐ Hair spray   ☐ Insecticides
☐ Chemicals   ☐ Smoke or auto exhaust fumes   ☐ Paints

Please answer the follwing questions by placing an X in the box in front of the word Yes or No, except where you are asked for specific information. This information is obviously highly confidential and will be released to other health professionals or insurance carriers ONLY with your consent.

DIET:

Do you eat a good breakfast?	☐ Yes	☐ No
Do you snack between meals (soft drinks, chips, candy bars)?	☐ Yes	☐ No
Do you eat fresh fruits and vegetables each day?	☐ Yes	☐ No
Do you eat whole grain breads and cereals?	☐ Yes	☐ No
Is your diet high in fat content?	☐ Yes	☐ No
Is your diet high in cholesterol content?	☐ Yes	☐ No
Is your diet high in salt content?	☐ Yes	☐ No
Are you allergic to any foods?	☐ Yes	☐ No

How many glasses of water do you drink each day? _____

How would you describe your overall eating habits?
☐ Excellent
☐ Good
☐ Fair
☐ Poor

PERSONAL HISTORY:

Do you find it hard to make decisions?	☐ Yes	☐ No
Do you find it hard to concentrate or remember?	☐ Yes	☐ No
Do you feel depressed?	☐ Yes	☐ No
Do you have difficulty relaxing?	☐ Yes	☐ No
Do you have a tendency to worry a lot?	☐ Yes	☐ No
Have you gained or lost much weight recently?	☐ Yes	☐ No
Do you lose your temper often?	☐ Yes	☐ No
Are you disturbed by any work or family problems?	☐ Yes	☐ No
Are you having sexual difficulties?	☐ Yes	☐ No
Have you ever considered committing suicide?	☐ Yes	☐ No
Have you ever desired or sought psychiatric help?	☐ Yes	☐ No

EXERCISE:

Do you exercise on a regular basis?	☐ Yes	☐ No
Does your job require strenuous, sustained physical work?	☐ Yes	☐ No

SLEEP PATTERNS:

Do you seem to feel exhausted or fatigued most of the time?	☐ Yes	☐ No
Do you have difficulty either falling asleep or staying asleep?	☐ Yes	☐ No

USE OF TOBACCO/ALCOHOL/CAFFEINE/DRUGS:

How much do you smoke per day?   ☐ Cigarettes ___   Amt:
☐ Don't smoke   ☐ Cigars/pipes ___

Do you take two or more alcoholic drinks per day?	☐ Yes	☐ No
Do you drink six or more cups of coffee or tea per day?	☐ Yes	☐ No
Are you a regular user of sleeping pills, marijuana, tranquilizers, painkillers, etc.?	☐ Yes	☐ No
Have you ever used heroin, cocaine, LSD, PCP, etc.?	☐ Yes	☐ No

List any country outside the United States you have visited in the past six months. _____

When did you have your last physical examination? _____

Patient's Name _____

REVIEW OF SYSTEMS

HEAD AND NECK
_____ Frequent headaches
_____ Neck pain
_____ Neck lumps or swelling

EYES
_____ Wears glasses
_____ Blurry vision
_____ Eyesight worsening
_____ Sees double
_____ Sees halo
_____ Eye pain or itching
_____ Watering eyes
_____ Eye trouble

EARS
_____ Hearing difficulties
_____ Earaches
_____ Running ears
_____ Buzzing in ears
_____ Motion sickness

MOUTH
_____ Dental problems
_____ Swellings on gums or jaws
_____ Sore tongue
_____ Taste changes

NOSE AND THROAT
_____ Congested nose
_____ Running nose
_____ Sneezing spells
_____ Head colds
_____ Nosebleeds
_____ Sore throat
_____ Enlarged tonsils
_____ Hoarse voice

RESPIRATORY
_____ Wheezes or gasps
_____ Coughing spells
_____ Coughs up phlegm
_____ Coughed up blood
_____ Chest colds
_____ Excessive sweating,
        night sweats

CARDIOVASCULAR
_____ High blood pressure
_____ Racing heart
_____ Chest pains
_____ Dizzy spells
_____ Shortness of breath
_____ Shortness of breath at night
_____ More pillows to breathe
_____ Swollen feet or ankles
_____ Leg cramps
_____ Heart murmur

DIGESTIVE
_____ Heartburn
_____ Bloated stomach
_____ Belching
_____ Stomach pains
_____ Nausea
_____ Vomited blood
_____ Difficulty swallowing
_____ Constipation
_____ Loose bowels
_____ Black stools
_____ Gray stools
_____ Pain in rectum
_____ Rectal bleeding

URINARY
_____ Night frequency
_____ Day frequency
_____ Wets pants or bed
_____ Burning on urination
_____ Brown, black, or bloody urine
_____ Difficulty starting urine
_____ Urgency

MALE GENITAL
_____ Weak urine stream
_____ Prostate trouble
_____ Burning or discharge
_____ Lumps on testicles
_____ Painful testicles

FEMALE GENITAL
_/_/_ Last menstrual period
_/_/_ Last Pap test
_____ Postmenopausal or hysterectomy
_____ Noticed vaginal bleeding
_____ Abnormal LMP
_____ Heavy bleeding during periods
_____ Bleeding between periods
_____ Bleeding after intercourse
_____ Recent vaginal itching/discharge
_____ No monthly breast exam
_____ Lump or pain in breasts
_____ Complications with birth control

OBSTETRIC HISTORY
_____ Gravida
_____ Para
_____ Preterm
_____ Miscarriages
_____ Stillbirths
_____ Has had an abortion

MUSCULOSKELETAL
_____ Aching muscles
_____ Swollen joints
_____ Back or shoulder pains
_____ Painful feet
_____ Disability

SKIN
_____ Skin problems
_____ Itching or burning skin
_____ Bleeds easily
_____ Bruises easily

NEUROLOGICAL
_____ Faintness
_____ Numbness
_____ Convulsions
_____ Change in handwriting
_____ Trembles

PROGRESS NOTES

Date	

Notes

Procedure 1-1: Obtaining and Documenting Patient Symptoms

Name: _____   Date: _____

Evaluated by: _____   Score: _____

Performance Objective

Outcome:	Obtain and document patient symptoms.
Conditions:	Given the following: medical record of the patient to be interviewed and a pen with black ink.
Standards:	Time: 10 minutes. Student completed procedure in _____ minutes.
	Accuracy: Satisfactory score on the Performance Evaluation Checklist.

Performance Evaluation Checklist

Trial 1	Trial 2	Point Value	Performance Standards
		•	Assembled equipment.
		•	Made sure to obtain or access the correct patient record.
		•	Went to the waiting room and asked the patient to come back.
		•	Escorted the patient to a quiet room.
		•	In a calm and friendly manner, greeted the patient and introduced yourself.
		•	Identified the patient by full name and date of birth.
		•	Asked the patient to be seated.
		•	Seated yourself facing the patient at a distance of 3 to 4 feet.
		▷	Explained the purpose of this seating arrangement.
			Used good communication skills.
		•	Used the patient's name of choice.
		•	Demonstrated genuine interest and concern for the patient.
		•	Maintained appropriate eye contact.
		•	Used terminology the patient could understand.
		•	Listened carefully and attentively to the patient.
		•	Paid attention to the patient's nonverbal messages.
		•	Avoided judgmental comments.
		•	Avoided rushing the patient.
		•	Located the progress note sheet in the PPR or progress note template in the EMR.

Trial 1	Trial 2	Point Value	Performance Standards
		•	Documented the date, time, and CC abbreviation.
		•	Used an open-ended question to obtain the chief complaint.
		▷	Explained why an open-ended question should be used.
			Documented the chief complaint in the PPR:
		•	Limited the CC to one or two symptoms.
		•	Referred to a specific rather than a vague symptom.
		•	Documented concisely and briefly.
		•	Used the patient's own words as much as possible.
		•	Included the duration of the symptom.
		•	Avoided using names of diseases.
			Documented the chief complaint in the EMR by completing each field of the chief complaint template.
		•	Obtained additional information regarding the chief complaint.
		•	Thanked the patient and proceeded to the next step in the patient workup.
		•	Informed the patient approximately how long he or she will need to wait for the provider.
		•	If using a PPR, placed the medical record in the appropriate location for review by the provider.
			Demonstrated the following affective behavior(s) during this procedure:
		Ⓐ	Demonstrate (a) empathy (b) active listening (c) nonverbal communication
		Ⓐ	Demonstrated the principles of self-boundaries.
		★	Completed the procedure within 10 minutes.
			Totals

CHART

Date	

Evaluation of Student Performance

EVALUATION CRITERIA			COMMENTS
Symbol	**Category**	**Point Value**	
★	Critical Step	16 points	
•	Essential Step	6 points	
Ⓐ	Affective Competency	6 points	
▷	Theory Question	2 points	

Score calculation: 100 points

− _____ points missed

_____ Score

Satisfactory score: 85 or above

CAAHEP Competencies Achieved

Psychomotor (Skills)

☑ V. 1. Use feedback techniques to obtain patient information including a. reflection, b. restatement, and c. clarification.

☑ V. 3. Use medical terminology correctly and pronounced accurately to communicate information to providers and patients.

☑ V.11 Report relevant information concisely and accurately.

Affective (Behavior)

☑ V.1. Demonstrate (a) empathy (b) active listening (c) nonverbal communication

☑ V.2. Demonstrate the principles of self-boundaries.

ABHES Competencies Achieved

☑ 3. d. Define and use medical abbreviations when appropriate and acceptable.

☑ 4. a. Follow documentation guidelines.

☑ 7. a. Gather and process documents.

☑ 7. g. Display professionalism through written and verbal communication.

☑ 8. b. Obtain vital signs, obtain patient history, and formulate chief complaint.

Taking a patient's symptoms is a frequent and important responsibility of the medical assistant, who must have a thorough knowledge of symptoms and related terminology. A **symptom** is defined as any change in the body or its functioning that indicates the presence of disease. The medical assistant can observe **objective symptoms** presented by the patient, such as coughing, rash, and swelling. The medical assistant must rely on information relayed by the patient to obtain data on **subjective symptoms**. Examples of subjective symptoms include pain, pruritus, and vertigo.

This section is designed as supplemental education for Chapter 1 (The Medical Record) in your textbook. Completion of the exercises in this section can assist you in documenting a patient's symptoms effectively and thoroughly, which is essential to an accurate diagnosis by the provider.

Learning Objectives

After completing this chapter, you should be able to do the following:
1. Explain the purpose of analyzing a symptom.
2. State the seven basic types of information that must be obtained to analyze a symptom.
3. Analyze a symptom by using direct questions.

Analysis of a Symptom

Before a symptom can be analyzed, the **chief complaint** (CC) must first be identified. The chief complaint is the patient's reason for seeking care or the symptom causing the patient the most trouble. An open-ended question should be used to elicit the chief complaint from the patient, and it should be documented following the documentation guidelines presented in your textbook. The next step is to analyze the chief complaint in detail from the time of its onset. The purpose of this is to provide a complete description of the current status of the chief complaint.

Analyzing the chief complaint requires a combination of good listening and writing skills. The medical assistant must know what information should be documented for each symptom and the questions to ask the patient to obtain this information. A list of symptoms, explanation of the information required for each symptom, and examples of questions to ask the patient are provided.

Type of Information Required

The following information is needed for each symptom to provide a full description of the current status of the chief complaint:

1. Location of the symptom. This refers to the specific area of the body where the symptom is located. Locating the symptom is the first step in determining the cause of the patient's disease. The patient may refer to the location in general terms, such as the head, arm, stomach, or back. The medical assistant must be more specific than this and determine the exact location using descriptions, such as "occurs in the lower back" or "occurs under the sternum." Several questions can assist in accomplishing this.
   - Where exactly does it hurt?
   - Can you show me where it hurts?
   - Do you feel it anywhere else?

2. Quality of the symptom. The quality of the symptom includes a complete and concise description of the symptom. The medical assistant should use informative terms to describe the character of each symptom. For example, if the patient complains of pain, the character of the pain must be included. Several terms can be used to describe pain.
   - Burning
   - Aching
   - Sharp
   - Dull
   - Throbbing
   - Cramplike
   - Squeezing

   If the patient has vomited, the medical assistant should indicate the color, odor, and consistency of the vomitus. If the patient has a cough, the medical assistant should indicate whether it is productive or nonproductive and whether blood is present. Refer to the list of terms on pages 27 and 28 of this manual, which can assist in describing symptoms. Specific examples of questions that are helpful in determining the quality of the symptom are as follows:
   - Describe it (the symptom) to me as fully as possible.
   - What is it (the symptom) like?

3. Severity of the symptom. Severity refers to the quantitative aspect of the symptom. It includes the following:
   - Intensity of the symptom (e.g., mild, moderate, severe)
   - Number (e.g., of convulsions, of nosebleeds)
   - Volume (e.g., of vomitus, of blood, of mucus)
   - Size or extent (e.g., of the rash, edema, lumps, or masses)

   This information assists the provider in determining the extensiveness or seriousness of the illness. Questions to determine severity are often specific to that symptom. For example, if the patient has a productive cough, the medical assistant should determine how much phlegm is being coughed up (e.g., teaspoon, half of a cup). At first, this area may appear difficult, but as you practice taking symptoms, you will learn what questions to ask the patient, and it eventually will become automatic. The examples at the end of this section and the student practice problems provide guidance in developing skill in this area. Some examples of general questions that can be used to determine the severity of a symptom are as follows:
   - How bad is it (the symptom)?
   - Does it (the symptom) limit your normal activities?

4. Chronology and timing of the symptom. Chronology and timing include a sequential account of the symptom up to the time the patient came to the medical office for treatment. This information is important in determining the duration of the symptom and change in it since it first occurred. Chronology and timing include the following four areas:
   a. Date of onset: The date of onset of the symptom should be indicated, if possible, as a calendar date and clock time. The patient may need some time to recall this information. Examples of questions that help obtain this information are as follows:
      - When did you experience this (the symptom) for the first time?
      - Exactly when did this begin?
   b. Duration: The duration of the symptom refers to how long the symptom lasts after it occurs, for example: 10 minutes, 2 hours, continuously. Examples of questions to obtain this information are as follows:
      - How long does it last after occurring?
      - For what length of time do you experience this symptom?
   c. Frequency: The frequency of the symptom refers to how often the symptom occurs, such as twice daily or a single attack every 2 weeks. Examples of questions to obtain this information are as follows:
      - How often does it occur?
      - How often has the symptom recurred?
   d. Change over time: This area refers to any change in the symptom since it first occurred. A change in a symptom reflects the nature of the underlying disease, which assists the provider in making a diagnosis. Examples of questions to obtain this information are as follows:
      - Has the symptom changed since it first occurred?
      - Is it (the symptom) getting better, worse, or staying the same?

5. Manner of onset. The manner of onset refers to what the patient was doing when the symptom first occurred and exactly what was experienced by the patient when the symptom began. These data help provide information on the pathologic process responsible for the symptom. For example, the patient may have been lifting a heavy object before experiencing low back pain. This information helps the provider in making an accurate diagnosis. Examples of questions that are helpful in determining the manner of onset are as follows:
   - What exactly did you experience when it (the symptom) first occurred?
   - What was the first thing you noticed?
   - Did it (the symptom) come on suddenly or gradually?
   - What were you doing when it (the symptom) began?
   - Where were you when this happened?
   - How were you feeling before it (the symptom) began?

6. Modifying factors. Symptoms are often influenced by activities or physiological processes such as physical exercise, change in weather, bodily functions (e.g., bowel movements, eating, coughing), pregnancy, emotional states, and fatigue. Some activities may aggravate the symptom, while others may alleviate it. These influences may help to determine what is causing the problem. For example, pain that becomes worse after the patient eats but is relieved after taking an antacid assists the provider in focusing on gastrointestinal disorders. Questions to assist in determining modifying factors are as follows:
   - Does anything make it (the symptom) better?
   - Does anything make it worse?
   - What have you done to make it better?
   - What did you do to help it?
   - Are you taking any medication for it? Did it help?

7. Associated symptoms. There is usually more than one symptom associated with a disease process. Determining these additional symptoms gives the provider a complete picture of the illness. Examples of questions that help to identify the presence of additional symptoms are as follows:
   - Are you having any other symptoms?
   - What other problems have you noticed since you became ill?

Examples

The following examples illustrate how to analyze a symptom. The chief complaint is listed first, followed by questions to ask the patient from the seven basic categories of information.

> *Example: Chief complaint: Headaches that began 2 months ago.*

1. Using your finger, point to the location of the headache.
2. Describe the pain. Is it sharp, dull, throbbing?
3. Are you able to carry on normal activities when you have a headache?
4. Is it sometimes more severe than usual?
5. When exactly did your headaches begin?
6. How long does your headache last when it occurs?
7. How often do you get a headache?
8. Since your headaches began, have they gotten better or worse, or have they stayed the same?
9. What were you doing the first time you experienced a headache?
10. What was your health status before your headaches began?
11. Do you get a headache before, during, or after a particular activity, such as reading or watching TV?
12. Does anything make your headache better?
13. Are you taking any medication for your headache? Does it help?
14. Have you had any other problems since your headaches began, such as nausea, vomiting, dizziness, or problems with vision?

> *Example: Chief complaint: The patient has been coughing for the past 3 days.*

1. Does it hurt when you cough? Where? Show me with one of your fingers.
2. What is the cough like?
3. Can you cough for me?
4. Do you bring up any phlegm when you cough? What color is it? Is blood present?
5. Describe the pain. Is it sharp, dull, squeezing?
6. Do you become exhausted when you cough?
7. How much phlegm do you bring up? A teaspoon? Half a cup?
8. How much blood is present in the phlegm?
9. When did your cough first begin?
10. Does it seem like an attack? How long does the attack last?
11. How often do you get a coughing attack?
12. Does your cough seem to be getting better or worse?
13. What was the first thing you noticed when you became ill?
14. How were you feeling before your symptoms began?
15. Is there anything that makes your cough better?
16. Is there anything that makes your cough worse?
17. Do you cough more at night or during the day?
18. Are you taking any medication for it? Does it help?
19. Are you having any other problems?

Practice Problems

In the space provided, indicate examples of direct questions to ask the patient to obtain the necessary information for the symptoms presented in the chief complaint.

Problem 1

Chief complaint: Earache and fever for the past 2 days.

Questions:

_____

_____

_____

_____

_____

_____

_____

_____

_____

_____

Problem 2

Chief complaint: Rash with itching that began 3 days ago.

Questions:

_____

_____

_____

_____

_____

_____

_____

_____

_____

_____

Problem 3

> *Chief complaint: Pain during urination that began yesterday.*

Questions:

_____

_____

_____

_____

_____

_____

_____

_____

_____

Problem 4

> *Chief complaint: Low back pain for the past 3 months.*

Questions:

_____

_____

_____

_____

_____

_____

_____

_____

_____

Problem 5

> *Chief complaint: Sore throat and fever for the past 24 hours.*

Questions:

_____

_____

_____

_____

_____

_____

_____

_____

Problem 6

> *Chief complaint: Chest pain that occurred this morning.*

Questions:

_____

_____

_____

_____

_____

_____

_____

_____

_____

Terms for Describing Symptoms

Pain

Burning, aching, sharp, dull, throbbing, cramping, squeezing

Radiating, transient, constant

Localized, superficial, deep

Respirations

Rapid, irregular, shallow, deep, labored, gasping, noisy, wheezing

Apnea, dyspnea, orthopnea

Discomfort, pain, cyanosis, cough

Cough

Nonproductive, productive

Persistent, dry, hacking, barking, spasmodic

Phlegm: color, consistency, presence or absence of blood

Exhausting or painful

Cardiovascular system

Pain, palpitations

Sharp, radiating

Dyspnea, orthopnea

Cyanosis

Gastrointestinal system

Abdomen: flaccid, rigid, distended

Appetite: anorexia, intolerance to foods

Heartburn, pain after eating, belching, nausea, vomiting, flatulence, change in bowel habits, constipation, diarrhea, black stools

Urine or Stool

 Abnormality: color, odor, consistency, frequency

 Contents: sediment, mucus, blood

 Elimination: urgency, nocturia, pain, burning

Skin

 Rash: pruritus, red, swelling, distribution

 Lesions: color, character, distribution

 Pallor: flushing, jaundice, warm, dry, cold, clammy

 Ecchymosis, petechiae, cyanosis, edema

 Pruritus, sweating, change in color, bruises easily

Ears

 Pain, loss of hearing, tinnitus, vertigo

 Discharge, infection

Eyes

 Itching, burning, blurry vision, seeing double, photophobia

 Discharge, watering, infection

CHAPTER ASSIGNMENTS

√ After Completing	Date Due	Study Guide Pages	STUDY GUIDE ASSIGNMENTS (CTA = Critical Thinking Activity)	Possible Points	Points You Earned
		33	Pretest	10	
		34-35	Key Term Assessment		
		34	A. Definitions	24	
		35	B. Word Parts (Add 1 point for each key term)	15	
		35-41	Evaluation of Learning questions	55	
		42	CTA A: Infection Process Cycle	5	
		42-43	CTA B: Handwashing	8	
		43	CTA C: Personal Protective Equipment: Gloves	8	
		43-44	CTA D: Personal Protective Equipment	30	
		44-45	CTA E: OSHA Standard	10	
		46	CTA F: Discarding Medical Waste	20	
			Evolve Site: Discard It! (Record points earned)		
		47	CTA G: Crossword Puzzle	25	
			Evolve Site: Quiz Show (Record points earned)		
			Evolve Site: Apply Your Knowledge questions (Record points earned)	10	
			Evolve Site: Video Evaluation	56	
		33	Posttest	10	
			ADDITIONAL ASSIGNMENTS		
			Total points		

√ When Assigned by Your Instructor	Study Guide Pages	Practices Required	LABORATORY ASSIGNMENTS (Procedure Number and Name)	Score*
	49	5	**Practice for Competency** 2-1: Handwashing Textbook reference: pp. 30-32	
	51-52		**Evaluation of Competency** 2-1: Handwashing	*
	49	4	**Practice for Competency** 2-2: Applying an Alcohol-Based Hand Rub Textbook reference: pp. 33	
	53-54		**Evaluation of Competency** 2-2: Applying an Alcohol-Based Hand Rub	*
	49	5	**Practice for Competency** 2-3: Application and Removal of Clean Disposable Gloves Textbook reference: pp. 34-35	
	55-56		**Evaluation of Competency** 2-3: Application and Removal of Clean Disposable Gloves	*
	57-58	3	**Evaluation of Competency** 2-A: Proper Use of a Sharps Container	*
	59-60	3	**Evaluation of Competency** 2-B: Disposal of Hazardous Material	*
			ADDITIONAL ASSIGNMENTS	

Notes

Name: _____   Date: _____

?≣ **PRETEST**

True or False

_____ 1. A microorganism is a tiny living plant or animal that cannot be seen with the naked eye.

_____ 2. A disease-producing microorganism is known as a nonpathogen.

_____ 3. Microorganisms grow best in an acidic environment.

_____ 4. Coughing and sneezing help to force pathogens from the body.

_____ 5. An alcohol-based hand rub should be used to sanitize hands that are visibly soiled.

_____ 6. OSHA stands for Occupational Safety and Health Administration.

_____ 7. A biohazard warning label must be fluorescent orange or an orange-red color.

_____ 8. Prescription eyeglasses are acceptable eye protection when handling blood.

_____ 9. Hepatitis B is an infection of the liver caused by a virus.

_____ 10. AIDS cannot be transmitted through casual contact.

?≣ **POSTTEST**

True or False

_____ 1. Bacteria and viruses are examples of microorganisms.

_____ 2. An anaerobe can exist only in the presence of oxygen.

_____ 3. The optimum growth temperature is the temperature at which a microorganism grows the best.

_____ 4. Medical asepsis refers to practices that inhibit the growth and hinder the transmission of pathogenic microorganisms.

_____ 5. Resident flora are picked up in the course of daily activities and are usually pathogenic.

_____ 6. The purpose of the OSHA Standard is to prevent exposure of employees to bloodborne pathogens.

_____ 7. OSHA requires the Exposure Control Plan to be updated annually.

_____ 8. An engineering control includes all measures and devices that isolate or remove the bloodborne pathogens hazard from the workplace.

_____ 9. A reagent strip that has been used to test urine is an example of regulated medical waste.

_____ 10. Patients with chronic hepatitis B face an increased risk of developing pancreatitis.

Chapter **2** **Medical Asepsis and the OSHA Standard**

A. Definitions

Directions: Match each key term with its definition.

_____ 1. Aerobe

_____ 2. Anaerobe

_____ 3. Antiseptic

_____ 4. Bloodborne pathogens

_____ 5. Cilia

_____ 6. Contaminated

_____ 7. Exposure incident

_____ 8. Hand hygiene

_____ 9. Infection

_____ 10. Medical asepsis

_____ 11. Microorganism

_____ 12. Nonintact skin

_____ 13. Nonpathogen

_____ 14. Occupational exposure

_____ 15. Opportunistic infection

_____ 16. Optimal growth temperature

_____ 17. Pathogen

_____ 18. Parenteral

_____ 19. pH

_____ 20. Postexposure prophylaxis

_____ 21. Regulated medical waste

_____ 22. Reservoir host

_____ 23. Sharps

_____ 24. Transient flora

A. A disease-producing microorganism

B. Microorganisms that reside on the superficial skin layers and are picked up in the course of daily activities

C. A microorganism that needs oxygen to live and grow

D. Reasonably anticipated skin, eye, mucous membrane, or parenteral contact with bloodborne pathogens or other potentially infectious materials that may result from the performance of an employee's duties

E. Practices that are employed to inhibit the growth and hinder the transmission of pathogenic microorganisms

F. The piercing of the skin barrier or mucous membranes, such as through needlesticks, human bites, cuts, and abrasions

G. Skin that has a break in the surface

H. The temperature at which an organism grows best

I. The degree to which a solution is acidic or basic

J. A specific eye, mouth, other mucous membrane, nonintact skin, or parenteral contact with blood or other potentially infectious materials that results from an employee's duties

K. Pathogenic microorganisms capable of causing disease that are present in human blood

L. The condition in which the body, or part of it, is invaded by a pathogen

M. Any waste containing infectious material that may pose a threat to health and safety

N. Slender, hairlike processes that constantly beat toward the outside to remove microorganisms from the body

O. A microorganism that does not normally produce disease

P. A microscopic plant or animal

Q. A microorganism that grows best in the absence of oxygen

R. The presence or reasonably anticipated presence of blood or OPIM on an item or surface

S. The organism that becomes infected by a pathogen and also serves as a source of transfer of pathogens to others

T. An infection resulting from a defective immune system that cannot defend the body from pathogens normally found in the environment

U. An agent that inhibits the growth of or kills microorganisms

V. The process of cleaning or sanitizing the hands

W. Treatment administered to an individual after exposure to an infectious disease to prevent the disease

X. Objects that can penetrate the skin such as needles and lancets

B. Word Parts

Directions: Indicate the meaning of each word part in the space provided. List as many medical terms as possible that incorporate the word part in the space provided.

Word Part	Meaning of Word Part	Medical Terms That Incorporate Word Part
1. aer/o		
2. an-		
3. anti-		
4. -septic		
5. a-		
6. micro-		
7. non-		
8. path/o		
9. -gen		
10. para-		
11. enter/o		
12. -al		
13. post-		
14. pro-		
15. -phylaxis		

EVALUATION OF LEARNING

Directions: Fill in each blank with the correct answer.

1. List four types of microorganisms.

_____

_____

2. Define medical asepsis.

_____

_____

3. What type of microorganism may remain on an object that is considered medically aseptic?

_____

4. List the six growth requirements needed by microorganisms to survive.

_____

_____

_____

5. What is the name given to the organism that uses organic or living substances for food?

_____

6. Why do most microorganisms prefer a neutral pH?

_____

_____

7. List three examples of how a microorganism can be transmitted from one person to another.

_____

_____

_____

_____

_____

_____

8. List five examples of how microorganisms can enter the body.

_____

_____

_____

9. List four examples of factors that would make a host more susceptible to the entrance of a pathogen.

_____

_____

_____

_____

10. List five protective devices of the body that prevent the entrance of microorganisms.

_____

_____

_____

11. What is the difference between resident flora and transient flora?

_____

_____

_____

12. List three examples of when handwashing should be performed in the medical office.

_____

_____

_____

13. How does antiseptic handwashing sanitize the hands?

_____

_____

14. List five examples of when an alcohol-based hand rub may be used to sanitize the hands.

_____

_____

_____

15. What are the advantages and disadvantages of alcohol-based hand rubs?

Advantages:

_____

Disadvantages:

_____

16. List six medical aseptic practices the medical assistant should follow in the medical office.

_____

_____

_____

_____

_____

_____

17. What is a disadvantage of latex gloves?

_____

_____

_____

18. What are the symptoms of a mild and severe latex hypersensitivity reaction?

a. Mild latex glove allergy: _____

_____

b. Severe latex glove allergy: _____

_____

19. What guidelines should be followed when working with gloves?

_____

_____

_____

_____

37

20. List examples of non-latex gloves.

_____

_____

_____

_____

21. What does the acronym OSHA stand for, and what is the purpose of OSHA?

_____

_____

22. What is the purpose of the OSHA Occupational Exposure to Bloodborne Pathogens Standard?

_____

_____

23. Who must follow the OSHA Bloodborne Pathogens Standard? List examples.

_____

_____

_____

24. What is occupational exposure?

_____

_____

25. What are sharps? List examples of sharps.

_____

_____

26. List five examples of other potentially infectious materials (OPIMs).

_____

_____

_____

_____

27. List examples of nonintact skin.

_____

_____

28. What is an exposure incident? List examples of exposure incidents.

_____

_____

_____

29. What is the purpose of the exposure control plan (ECP)? How often must it be updated?

_____

_____

30. List three examples of items to which a biohazard warning label must be attached.

_____

_____

31. What is the purpose of a sharps injury log? What types of offices must maintain this log?

_____

_____

32. Define an engineering control, and list three examples of engineering controls.

_____

_____

_____

33. What is a safer medical device?

_____

_____

34. What is a work practice control?

_____

35. List examples of work practice controls required by the OSHA Standard.

_____

_____

_____

36. What should you do if you splash blood in your eyes?

_____

37. What is personal protective equipment (PPE)? List examples of PPE.

_____

_____

_____

Chapter **2** **Medical Asepsis and the OSHA Standard**

38. List six guidelines that must be followed when using PPE.

_____

_____

_____

_____

_____

_____

39. List examples of housekeeping procedures required by the OSHA Standard.

_____

_____

_____

_____

40. List four guidelines that must be followed with respect to biohazard sharps containers.

_____

_____

_____

_____

_____

41. Who must be offered the hepatitis B vaccination?

_____

42. When does an employer *not* have to offer the hepatitis B vaccine to medical office personnel?

_____

_____

43. What must be done if a medical office employee declines the hepatitis B vaccination?

_____

44. What is regulated medical waste? What are examples of regulated medical waste?

_____

_____

_____

45. Explain how to prepare regulated medical waste for pickup by a medical waste service.

_____

_____

_____

46. How should regulated medical waste be stored while waiting for pickup by the medical waste service? Explain why.

_____

_____

_____

47. What information is included on a regulated medical waste tracking form?

_____

_____

_____

48. What is the most likely means of contracting hepatitis B in the health care setting?

_____

_____

49. What side effects may occur after the administration of a hepatitis B vaccine?

_____

_____

50. What postexposure prophylaxis (PEP) is recommended for an unvaccinated individual who has been exposed to hepatitis B?

_____

_____

_____

51. What may eventually occur in a patient with chronic hepatitis C?

_____

52. What is the difference between HIV and AIDS?

_____

_____

53. How is HIV transmitted? How is it not transmitted?

_____

_____

_____

54. What is an opportunistic infection?

_____

55. What are the characteristics of AIDS?

_____

_____

Chapter **2** **Medical Asepsis and the OSHA Standard**

A. Infection Process Cycle

Carefully review the infection process cycle and the requirements for growth needed by microorganisms. Create an environment in a medical office that would function to interrupt the infection process cycle and discourage the growth of pathogens.

_____

_____

_____

_____

B. Handwashing

Using the principles outlined in the handwashing procedure, explain what may happen under the following circumstances:

1. The medical assistant's uniform touches the sink during the handwashing procedure.

_____

_____

_____

2. The hands are not held lower than the elbows during the handwashing procedure.

_____

_____

_____

3. Friction is not used to wash the hands.

_____

_____

_____

4. Water is splashed on the medical assistant's uniform during the handwashing procedure.

_____

_____

_____

5. The medical assistant continually uses water that is too cold to wash hands.

_____

_____

_____

6. The medical assistant turns off the running water with his or her bare hands.

_____

_____

_____

7. The medical assistant does not clean his or her fingernails daily.

_____

_____

_____

8. The medical assistant's skin becomes chapped.

_____

_____

_____

C. Personal Protective Equipment: Gloves

In which of the following situations does OSHA require the use of clean disposable gloves? Indicate your answer by placing a check mark in the space provided.

_____ 1. Performing a urinalysis on a urine specimen that contains blood.

_____ 2. Sanitizing operating scissors for sterilization.

_____ 3. Performing a finger puncture.

_____ 4. Performing a vision screening test on a school-aged child.

_____ 5. Cleaning up a blood spill on a laboratory worktable.

_____ 6. Drawing blood from an elderly patient.

_____ 7. Measuring the weight of a college student.

_____ 8. Testing a blood specimen for glucose.

D. Personal Protective Equipment

Create a collage of items or articles that can and cannot be used as PPE following these guidelines:

1. Using items cut from a magazine, colored pencils, or markers, create a collage of items that are designated as PPE by OSHA.

2. On the reverse side of the sheet, create a collage of items or articles that are not permitted to be used as PPE.

3. In the classroom, choose a partner and trade sheets. For each PPE item, provide examples of the procedures or tasks that may require its use. For each item that is not PPE, explain why it should not be used as PPE.

Examples of PPE:

_____

_____

_____

_____

Not examples of PPE:

_____

_____

_____

_____

E. OSHA Standard

The following situations may occur in the medical office. For each situation, indicate an appropriate action to take that complies with the OSHA Bloodborne Pathogens Standard.

1. **Situation:** You just gave an injection to a patient, and after withdrawing the needle, you notice that there is no sharps container in the room.
   Action:

   _____

   _____

   _____

2. **Situation:** You are getting ready to apply gloves and notice that you have a cut on your finger.
   Action:

   _____

   _____

   _____

3. **Situation:** You accidentally get some blood on your bare hands while removing your gloves.
   Action:

   _____

   _____

   _____

4. **Situation:** A part-time clinical medical assistant was just hired. She is not immunized against hepatitis B.
   Action:

   _____

   _____

   _____

5. **Situation:** A clinical medical assistant who has worked at the office for 5 years changes her mind and decides she wants the hepatitis B vaccine.
   Action:

   _____

   _____

   _____

6. **Situation:** You are wearing a protective laboratory coat over your scrubs. While performing a laboratory test, some blood splashes onto your lab coat, but it does not penetrate through to your scrubs.
   Action:

   _____

   _____

   _____

7. **Situation:** You go into an examining room and notice that the biohazard sharps container in that room is completely full.
   Action:

   _____

   _____

   _____

8. **Situation:** You have collected three tubes of blood from a patient using glass tubes. You accidentally drop one of the blood tubes, and it breaks.
   Action:

   _____

   _____

   _____

9. **Situation:** You are wearing a protective lab coat over your scrubs, and you are getting ready to leave for the day.
   Action:

   _____

   _____

   _____

10. **Situation:** You remove your gloves after giving an injection to a patient and accidentally discard them into the biohazard sharps container.
    Action:

    _____

    _____

    _____

Chapter **2** **Medical Asepsis and the OSHA Standard**

F. Discarding Medical Waste

Indicate where each of the following (used) items should be discarded using these acronyms:

RWC: regular waste container
BSC: biohazard sharps container
BB: biohazard bag waste container

_____ 1. Urine testing strip

_____ 2. Lancet

_____ 3. Gloves with blood on them

_____ 4. Blood tube

_____ 5. Tongue depressor

_____ 6. Razor blade

_____ 7. Capillary pipet

_____ 8. Dressing saturated with blood

_____ 9. Patient drape

_____ 10. An empty urine container

_____ 11. Sutures caked with blood

_____ 12. Thermometer probe cover

_____ 13. Patient gown

_____ 14. Disposable diaper

_____ 15. Dressing saturated with a purulent discharge

_____ 16. Clean disposable gloves

_____ 17. Disposable vaginal speculum

_____ 18. An outdated vaccine

_____ 19. Syringe and needle

_____ 20. Examining table paper

G. Crossword Puzzle: Medical Asepsis and the OSHA Standard

Directions: Complete the crossword puzzle using the clues provided.

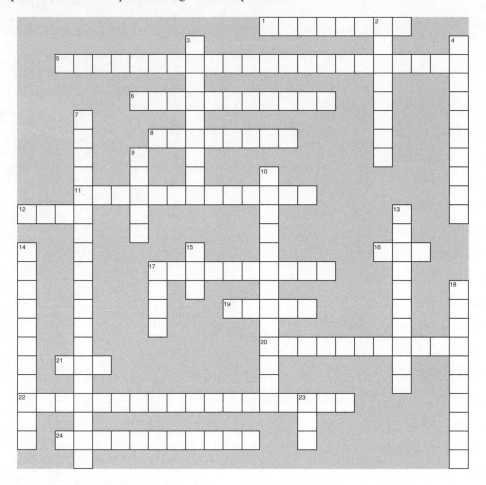

Across

1 Grows best without oxygen
5 Infection resulting from a defective immune system
6 HBV serious complication
8 Microorganism that causes disease
11 Normally live on the skin
12 Vaginal secretions (example)
16 Protector of public health
17 Can live dry for 1 week
19 Traps microorganisms
20 Low resistance
21 After exposure: may prevent disease
22 Isolates or removes bloodborne pathogens hazard
24 Eats "live stuff"

Down

2 Example of a microorganism
3 Body invasion by a pathogen
4 Found in antimicrobial soap
7 Way to prevent a needlestick injury
9 HIV screening test
10 Broken skin
13 No. 1 chronic viral disease in the United States
14 No. 1 aseptic practice
15 Scrubs are not this
17 Hepatitis B passive immunizing agent
18 Piercing of the skin barrier
23 Discard in a biohazard container

Chapter **2** Medical Asepsis and the OSHA Standard

Notes

PRACTICE FOR COMPETENCY

Procedure 2-1: Handwashing

Perform the handwashing procedure. List five medically aseptic steps that must be followed during this procedure.

1. _____

_____

2. _____

_____

3. _____

_____

4. _____

_____

5. _____

_____

Procedure 2-2: Applying an Alcohol-Based Hand Rub

Apply an alcohol-based hand rub. Practice applying a gel and a foam hand rub. List the brand names of the hand rubs you applied, and list the ingredients contained in them.

_____

_____

Procedure 2-3: Application and Removal of Clean Disposable Gloves

Apply and remove clean disposable gloves. What size gloves fits you best?

_____

_____

Procedure 2-A: Proper Use of a Sharps Container

Demonstrate the proper use of a sharps container by discarding contaminated sharps into the sharps container. In the space provided, indicate the items you discarded into the sharps container.

_____

_____

Procedure 2-B: Disposal of Hazardous Material

Handle and prepare regulated medical waste for pickup by a medical waste service.

_____

_____

Chapter **2** **Medical Asepsis and the OSHA Standard**

ℯ Procedure 2-1: Handwashing

Name: _____ Date: _____

Evaluated by: _____ Score: _____

Performance Objective

Outcome:	Perform handwashing.
Conditions:	Using a sink.
	Given liquid soap and paper towels.
Standards:	Time: 5 minutes. Student completed procedure in _____ minutes.
	Accuracy: Satisfactory score on the Performance Evaluation Checklist.

Performance Evaluation Checklist

Trial 1	Trial 2	Point Value	Performance Standards
		•	Removed watch or pushed it up on the forearm.
		•	Removed rings.
		▷	Stated the reason for removing rings.
		•	Stood at sink with clothing away from edge of sink.
		•	Turned on faucets with paper towel.
		▷	Explained the reason for turning on faucets with paper towel.
		•	Adjusted the water to a warm temperature.
		•	Discarded towel into trash can.
		•	Wet hands and forearms with water.
		•	Held hands lower than elbows at all times.
		▷	Explained why the hands should be held lower than elbows.
		•	Did not touch the inside of sink with hands.
		•	Applied soap to hands.
		•	Washed palms and backs of hands with 10 circular motions and friction.
		▷	Explained why circular motions and friction are needed to wash hands.
		•	Washed fingers with 10 circular motions.
		•	Washed fingers while interlaced using friction and circular motions.
		•	Rinsed well (keeping hands lower than elbows).
		•	Washed wrists and forearms using friction and circular motions.
		•	Cleaned fingernails using manicure stick.
		•	Rinsed arms and hands.

Trial 1	Trial 2	Point Value	Performance Standards
		•	Repeated handwashing procedure (if necessary).
		•	Dried hands gently and thoroughly.
		▷	Stated the reason for drying hands gently and thoroughly.
		•	Turned off faucets using paper towel.
		•	Did not touch sink area with bare hands.
		▷	Explained the reason for not touching sink area with bare hands.
			Demonstrated the following affective behavior(s) during this procedure:
		Ⓐ	Recognized the implications for failure to comply with Centers for Disease Control (CDC) regulations in health care settings.
		★	Completed the procedure within 5 minutes.
			Totals

Evaluation of Student Performance

EVALUATION CRITERIA			COMMENTS
Symbol	**Category**	**Point Value**	
★	Critical Step	16 points	
•	Essential Step	6 points	
Ⓐ	Affective Competency	6 points	
▷	Theory Question	2 points	

Score calculation: 100 points
− _____ points missed
_____ Score

Satisfactory score: 85 or above

CAAHEP Competencies Achieved

Psychomotor (Skills)
☑ III. 3. Perform handwashing.

Affective (Behavior)
☑ III. 1. Recognize the implications for failure to comply with Centers for Disease Control (CDC) regulations in health care settings.

ABHES Competencies Achieved

☑ 4. f. Comply with federal, state, and local health laws and regulations as they relate to health care settings.
☑ 9. a. Practice standard precautions and perform disinfection/sterilization techniques.

Procedure 2-2: Applying an Alcohol-Based Hand Rub

Name: _____ Date: _____

Evaluated by: _____ Score: _____

Performance Objective

Outcome:	Apply an alcohol-based hand rub.
Conditions:	Given an alcohol-based hand rub.
Standards:	Time: 2 minutes. Student completed procedure in _____ minutes.
	Accuracy: Satisfactory score on the Performance Evaluation Checklist.

Performance Evaluation Checklist

Trial 1	Trial 2	Point Value	Performance Standards
		•	Inspected the hands to make sure they are not visibly soiled.
		▷	Stated the procedure to follow if the hands are visibly soiled.
		•	Removed watch or pushed it up on the forearm.
		•	Removed rings.
			Applied the alcohol-based hand rub to the palm of one hand as follows:
		•	*Gel or lotion:* Applied an amount of gel or lotion approximately equal to the size of a dime.
		•	*Foam:* Applied an amount of foam approximately equal to the size of a walnut.
		▷	Explained why it is important not to use more than the recommended amount of hand rub.
		•	Thoroughly spread the hand rub over the surface of both hands up to $^1/_2$ inch above the wrist.
		•	Spread the hand rub around and under the fingernails.
		▷	Explained why it is important to cover the entire surface of the hands.
		•	Rubbed the hands together until they were dry.
		•	Did not touch anything until the hands were dry.
			Demonstrated the following affective behavior(s) during this procedure:
		Ⓐ	Recognized the implications for failure to comply with Centers for Disease Control (CDC) regulations in health care settings.
		★	Completed the procedure within 2 minutes.
			Totals

53

Evaluation of Student Performance

EVALUATION CRITERIA			COMMENTS
Symbol	**Category**	**Point Value**	
★	Critical Step	16 points	
•	Essential Step	6 points	
Ⓐ	Affective Competency	6 points	
▷	Theory Question	2 points	

Score calculation: 100 points
− _____ points missed
_____ Score
Satisfactory score: 85 or above

CAAHEP Competencies Achieved

Psychomotor (Skills)
☑ III. 3. Perform handwashing.

Affective (Behavior)
☑ III. 1. Recognize the implications for failure to comply with Centers for Disease Control (CDC) regulations in health care settings.

ABHES Competencies Achieved

☑ 4. f. Comply with federal, state, and local health laws and regulations as they relate to health care settings.
☑ 8. a. Practice standard precautions and perform disinfection/sterilization techniques.

ℯ Procedure 2-3: Application and Removal of Clean Disposable Gloves

Name: _____   Date: _____

Evaluated by: _____   Score: _____

Performance Objective

Outcome:	Apply and remove clean disposable gloves.
Conditions:	Given the appropriate-sized clean disposable gloves.
Standards:	Time: 5 minutes. Student completed procedure in _____ minutes.
	Accuracy: Satisfactory score on the Performance Evaluation Checklist.

Performance Evaluation Checklist

Trial 1	Trial 2	Point Value	Performance Standards
			Application of Clean Gloves
		•	Removed all rings.
		▷	Stated why rings should be removed.
		•	Sanitized the hands.
		•	Chose the appropriate-sized gloves.
		▷	Explained what can happen if the gloves are too small or too large.
		•	Applied the gloves.
		•	Adjusted the gloves so that they fit comfortably.
		•	Inspected the gloves for tears.
		▷	Stated the procedure to follow if a glove is torn.
			Removal of Clean Gloves
		•	Grasped the outside of the left glove 1 to 2 inches from the top with the gloved right hand.
		•	Slowly pulled left glove off the hand.
		•	Pulled the left glove free, and scrunched it into a ball with the gloved right hand.
		•	Placed the index and middle fingers of the left hand on the inside of the right glove.
		•	Did not allow the clean hand to touch outside of the glove.
		•	Pulled the glove off the right hand, enclosing the balled-up left glove.
		•	Discarded both gloves in an appropriate waste container.
		▷	Stated when gloves should be discarded in a biohazardous waste container.
		•	Sanitized the hands.
		▷	Stated why the hands should be sanitized after removing gloves.

55

Trial 1	Trial 2	Point Value	Performance Standards
			Demonstrated the following affective behavior(s) during this procedure:
		Ⓐ	Recognized the implications for failure to comply with Centers for Disease Control (CDC) regulations in health care settings.
		★	Completed the procedure in 5 minutes.
			Totals

Evaluation of Student Performance

EVALUATION CRITERIA			COMMENTS
Symbol	**Category**	**Point Value**	
★	Critical Step	16 points	
•	Essential Step	6 points	
Ⓐ	Affective Competency	6 points	
▷	Theory Question	2 points	

Score calculation: 100 points
−_____ points missed
_____ Score
Satisfactory score: 85 or above

CAAHEP Competencies Achieved

Psychomotor (Skills)
☑ III. 2. Select appropriate barrier/personal protective equipment (PPE).

Affective (Behavior)
☑ III. 1. Recognize the implications for failure to comply with Centers for Disease Control (CDC) regulations in health care settings.

ABHES Competencies Achieved

☑ 4. f. Comply with federal, state, and local health laws and regulations as they relate to health care settings.
☑ 8. a. Practice standard precautions and perform disinfection/sterilization techniques.

Procedure 2-A: Proper Use of a Sharps Container

Name: _____   Date: _____

Evaluated by: _____   Score: _____

Performance Objective

Outcome:	Demonstrate the proper use of a sharps container.
Conditions:	Given the following: Sharps container and a contaminated sharp.
Standards:	Time: 3 minutes. Student completed procedure in _____ minutes.
	Accuracy: Satisfactory score on the Performance Evaluation Checklist.

Performance Evaluation Checklist

Trial 1	Trial 2	Point Value	Performance Standards
		•	Ensured that the sharps container met the following OSHA Standards: a. Was closable b. Was puncture resistant c. Was leakproof d. Was labeled with a biohazard warning label e. Was color-coded in red
		•	Located the sharps container as close as possible to the area of use.
		▷	Stated why the sharps container should be located close to the area of use.
		•	Made sure the sharps container was maintained in an upright position.
		•	Immediately after use, placed the contaminated sharp in the sharps container.
		•	Dropped the contaminated sharp into the container without touching the sides of the container.
		•	Stated examples of items that must be discarded in a sharps container.
		•	Did not reach into the sharps container with the hands.
		•	Replaced the sharps container on a regular basis and did not allow it to overfill.
		▷	Stated when a sharps container should be replaced.
			Demonstrated the following affective behavior(s) during this procedure:
		Ⓐ	Recognized the implications for failure to comply with CDC and OSHA regulations in a health care setting.
		★	Completed the procedure within 5 minutes.
			Totals

Evaluation of Student Performance

EVALUATION CRITERIA			COMMENTS
Symbol	**Category**	**Point Value**	
★	Critical Step	16 points	
•	Essential Step	6 points	
Ⓐ	Affective Competency	6 points	
▷	Theory Question	2 points	

Score calculation: 100 points
−   _____   points missed
_____   Score
Satisfactory score: 85 or above

CAAHEP Competencies Achieved

Psychomotor (Skills)
☑ III. 1. Participate in bloodborne pathogen training.
☑ III.10. Demonstrate proper disposal of biohazardous material
   a. Sharps
   b. Regulated waste
☑ X11. 2. Demonstrate proper use of:
   d. Eyewash equipment
   e. Fire extinguishers
   f. Sharps disposal containers

Affective (Behavior)
☑ III. 1. Recognize the implications for failure to comply with Centers for Disease Control (CDC) regulations in health care settings.

ABHES Competencies Achieved

☑ 4. f. Comply with federal, state, and local health laws and regulations as they relate to health care settings.
☑ 8. a. Practice standard precautions and perform disinfection/sterilization techniques.
☑ 9. c. Dispose of biohazardous materials.

Procedure 2-B: Disposal of Hazardous Material

Name: _____ Date: _____

Evaluated by: _____ Score: _____

Performance Objective

Outcome:	Handle and prepare regulated waste for pickup by a medical waste service.
Conditions:	Given the following: disposable gloves, biohazard sharps container, biohazards bags, cardboard box with biohazard labels, packing tape, tracking record.
Standards:	Time: 5 minutes. Student completed procedure in _____ minutes.
	Accuracy: Satisfactory score on the Performance Evaluation Checklist.

Performance Evaluation Checklist

Trial 1	Trial 2	Point Value	Performance Standards
			Handling regulated waste
		•	Sanitized hands and applied gloves.
		•	Closed and locked the lid of the full sharps container before removing it from the examining room.
		▷	Stated the reason for closing the lid of the sharps container before removing it from the examining room.
		•	Did not open, empty, or clean the sharps container.
		•	If the sharps container was leaking, placed it in a second container that is closable, leakproof, and appropriately labeled.
		•	Securely closed the full biohazard bag before removing it from an examining room.
		•	If required by the medical office policy, double-bag by placing the primary bag inside a second biohazard bag.
		•	Transported the biohazard containers to a secure area away from the general public.
			Preparing regulated waste for pickup by a medical waste service
		•	Placed sharps containers and biohazard bags into a cardboard box provided by the medical waste service.
		•	Removed gloves and sanitized the hands.
		•	Securely sealed the box with packing tape.
		•	Made sure that a biohazard warning label appeared on two opposite sides of the box.
		•	Stored the biohazard box in a labeled locked room inside the facility or in a labeled locked collection container outside the facility.
		▷	Stated why biohazard boxes awaiting pickup must be stored in a locked storage area.
		•	Completed a tracking record, if required by your state.

Trial 1	Trial 2	Point Value	Performance Standards
		▷	Stated what information is included on a tracking record.
			Demonstrated the following affective behavior(s) during this procedure:
		Ⓐ	Recognized the implications for failure to comply with CDC and OSHA regulations in a health care setting.
		★	Completed the procedure within 5 minutes.
			Totals

Evaluation of Student Performance

EVALUATION CRITERIA			COMMENTS
Symbol	**Category**	**Point Value**	
★	Critical Step	16 points	
•	Essential Step	6 points	
Ⓐ	Affective Competency	6 points	
▷	Theory Question	2 points	

Score calculation: 100 points

− _____ points missed

_____ Score

Satisfactory score: 85 or above

CAAHEP Competencies Achieved

Psychomotor (Skills)

☑ III. 1. Participate in bloodborne pathogen training.

☑ III.10. Demonstrate proper disposal of biohazardous material
c. Sharps
d. Regulated waste

Affective (Behavior)

☑ III. 1. Recognize the implications for failure to comply with Centers for Disease Control (CDC) regulations in health care settings.

ABHES Competencies Achieved

☑ 4. f. Comply with federal, state, and local health laws and regulations as they relate to health care settings.

☑ 8. a. Practice standard precautions and perform disinfection/sterilization techniques.

☑ 9. c. Dispose of biohazardous materials.

3 Sterilization and Disinfection

CHAPTER ASSIGNMENTS

√ After Completing	Date Due	Study Guide Pages	STUDY GUIDE ASSIGNMENTS (CTA = Critical Thinking Activity)	Possible Points	Points You Earned
		65	Pretest	10	
		66	Term Key Term Assessment	14	
		66-72	Evaluation of Learning questions	56	
		72-73	CTA A: Safety Data Sheet	16	
		73-75	CTA B: Obtaining a Safety Data Sheet	18	
		75-76	CTA C: Sanitization	8	
		76	CTA D: Storage of a Chemical Disinfectant	4	
		77	CTA E: Sterilization	10	
			Evolve Site: Chapter 3 What Happens Now? (Record points earned)		
			Evolve Site: Chapter 3 Quiz Show (Record points earned)		
			Evolve Site: Apply Your Knowledge questions (Record points earned)	10	
			Evolve Site: Video Evaluation	36	
		62	Posttest	10	
			ADDITIONAL ASSIGNMENTS		
			Total points		

√ When Assigned by Your Instructor	Study Guide Pages	Practices Required	LABORATORY ASSIGNMENTS (Procedure Number and Name)	Score*
	79	3	**Practice for Competency** 3-1: Sanitization of Instruments Textbook reference: pp. 62-65	
	81-83		**Evaluation of Competency** 3-1: Sanitization of Instruments	
	79		**Practice for Competency** 3-2: Chemical Disinfection of Articles Textbook reference: pp. 68-70	
	85-86		**Evaluation of Competency** 3-2: Chemical Disinfection of Articles	*
	79	Paper: 3 Muslin: 3	**Practice for Competency** 3-3: Wrapping Instruments Using Paper or Muslin Textbook reference: pp. 75-76	
	87-88		**Evaluation of Competency** 3-3: Wrapping Instruments Using Paper or Muslin	*
	79	3	**Practice for Competency** 3-4: Wrapping Instruments Using a Pouch Textbook reference: p. 77	
	89-90		**Evaluation of Competency** 3-4: Wrapping Instruments Using a Pouch	*
	79	3	**Practice for Competency** 3-5: Sterilizing Articles in the Autoclave Textbook reference: pp. 81-84	
	91-93		**Evaluation of Competency** 3-5: Sterilizing Articles in the Autoclave	*
			ADDITIONAL ASSIGNMENTS	

Notes

Name: _____ Date: _____

True or False

_____ 1. A bacterial spore consists of a hard, thick-walled capsule that can resist adverse conditions.

_____ 2. The purpose of sanitization is to remove all microorganisms and spores from a contaminated article.

_____ 3. According to OSHA, gloves do not need to be worn during the sanitization process.

_____ 4. Glutaraldehyde (Cidex) is a high-level disinfectant.

_____ 5. High-level disinfection kills all microorganisms but not spores.

_____ 6. Sterilization is the process of destroying all forms of microbial life except for bacterial spores.

_____ 7. Autoclave tape indicates whether an autoclaved item is sterile.

_____ 8. The wrapper used to autoclave articles should prevent contaminants from getting in during handling and storage.

_____ 9. Tap water should be used in the autoclave.

_____ 10. The inside of the autoclave should be wiped every day with a damp cloth.

? POSTTEST

True or False

_____ 1. The agent used to destroy microorganisms on an article depends on the size of the article.

_____ 2. The purpose of the Hazard Communication Standard is to make sure that employees do not use hazardous chemicals in the workplace.

_____ 3. The Hazard Communication Standard requires that the label of a hazardous chemical include GHS hazard pictograms.

_____ 4. Stethoscopes must be decontaminated using a high-level disinfectant.

_____ 5. The most common temperature and pressure for autoclaving is 212°F at 15 lb of pressure per square inch.

_____ 6. A sterilization strip should be positioned in the center of a wrapped pack.

_____ 7. The best means of determining the effectiveness of the sterilization process are biologic indicators.

_____ 8. The proper time for sterilizing an article in the autoclave depends on what is being autoclaved.

_____ 9. A pack that has been in the storage cupboard for 4 weeks should be resterilized.

_____ 10. Ethylene oxide gas is used by medical manufacturers to sterilize disposable items.

Directions: Match each key term with its definition.

F 1. Autoclave
E 2. Critical item
G 3. Detergent
J 4. Disinfectant
N 5. Hazardous chemical
A 6. Incubate
I 7. Load
C 8. Noncritical item
K 9. Safety Data Sheet
L 10. Sanitization
H 11. Semicritical item
D 12. Spore
M 13. Sterilization
B 14. Thermolabile

A. To provide proper conditions for growth and development
B. Easily affected or changed by heat
C. An item that comes in contact with intact skin but not mucous membranes
D. A hard, thick-walled capsule formed by some bacteria that contains only the essential parts of the protoplasm of the bacterial cell
E. An item that comes in contact with sterile tissue or the vascular system
F. An apparatus for the sterilization of materials, using steam under pressure
G. An agent that cleanses by emulsifying dirt and oil
H. An item that comes in contact with nonintact skin or intact mucous membranes
I. The articles that are being sterilized
J. An agent used to destroy pathogenic microorganisms but not their spores (usually applied to inanimate objects)
K. A sheet that provides information regarding a chemical and its hazards, and measures to take to avoid injury and illness when handling the chemical
L. A process to remove organic matter from an article and to lower the number of microorganisms to a safe level as determined by public health requirements
M. The process of destroying all forms of microbial life, including bacterial spores
N. Any chemical that is classified as a health or physical hazard

EVALUATION OF LEARNING

Directions: Fill in each blank with the correct answer.

1. How does one determine what type of physical or chemical agent to use to destroy microorganisms on an article?

Inventory of Hazardous Chemical

Employer is responsible for developing and maintaining a list of hazardous chemicals that are used and stored in the workplace. The office staff has an obligation to follow these guidelines.

2. List two diseases that are caused by bacteria that produce spores.

_____

_____

3. What are the characteristics of bacterial spores?

_____

_____

4. What is the purpose of the Hazard Communication Standard?

_____

_____

5. What is the difference between a health hazard and a physical hazard?

_____

_____

6. What is the purpose of the Globally Harmonized System of Classification and Labeling of Chemicals (GHS)?

_____

_____

_____

7. List four examples of hazardous chemicals that may be used in the medical office.

_____

_____

8. What information must be included on a hazardous chemical label?

_____

_____

_____

9. What is the purpose of a GHS signal word?

_____

_____

10. What is the meaning of the following GHS signal words?

a. Danger: _____

b. Warning: _____

11. What is the difference between a GHS hazard statement and a GHS precautionary statement?

_____

_____

_____

12. What is a GHS hazard pictogram, and what is its purpose?

_____

_____

13. List and briefly describe the information that must be included on a Safety Data Sheet.

1. Identification - product name, brand name, address and phone #, emergency #
2. Hazards Identification - hazard classification of the chemical, signal word
3. Composition/Information on Ingredients - list of ingredients
4. First aid Measures - exposed the hazardous chemical - different route
5. fire fighting measures - fighting fire caused by the chemical - suitable extinguishing agents
6. Accidental Release measures - personal protective measures
7. Handling and Storage - handling and safe storage
8. exposure controls/Personal Protection - personal Protective measures PEL +
9. Physical and Chemical Properties
10. Stability and Reactivity
11. Toxicological

14. What is the purpose of sanitizing an article?

_____

_____

15. What is the advantage of using the ultrasound method to clean instruments?

_____

_____

16. Why should gloves be worn during the sanitization procedure?

Protects the MA from bloodborne pathogens and other potentially infectious materials.
Heavy duty gloves should be worn when working with sharp instruments and chemicals

17. Why should instruments be handled carefully?

_____

18. Why should a chemical not be used past its expiration date?

_____

19. Why must a cleaning agent with a neutral pH be used to sanitize instruments?

_____

_____

20. What type of brush should be used to clean the following parts of an instrument?

   a. Surface of an instrument: _____

   b. Grooves, crevices, or serrations: _____

21. How should each of the following be checked for defects and proper working condition?

   a. Blades of an instrument: _____

   b. Tips of an instrument: _____

   c. Instrument with a box lock: _____

   d. Cutting edge of a sharp instrument: _____

   e. Scissors: _____

22. What is the purpose of lubricating an instrument?

_____

_____

23. What is the definition of high-level disinfection?

_____

_____

24. List one example of an item that requires high-level disinfection. List one example of a high-level disinfectant.

_____

_____

25. List two examples of items that can be disinfected through intermediate-level disinfection. List one example of an intermediate-level disinfectant.

_____

_____

26. List two examples of items that are disinfected by low-level disinfection.

_____

27. What disinfectant does OSHA recommend for the decontamination of blood spills?

10% bleach 90% wipe up leaving solution for 20 mins - then wipe up remain solution.

28. Why is it important to remove all organic matter from an article before it is disinfected?

incomplete sterilization or disinfection - organic material for an article acts as a barrier preventing chemical agent reaching the surface.
to kill microorganisms.

29. Explain the difference between the shelf life and use life of a chemical disinfectant.

_____

_____

_____

30. What is the purpose of sterilization?

_____

31. What is a critical item? List examples of critical items.

_____

_____

32. What is the purpose of the pressure used in the autoclaving process?

_____

_____

33. Why is it important that all air be removed from the autoclave during the sterilization process?

_____

_____

34. What temperature and pressure are the most commonly used to sterilize materials with the autoclave?

15 pounds of pressure per a square inch (psi) at a temperature of 250°F

_____

Chapter **3** **Sterilization and Disinfection**

35. What information does the Centers for Disease Control and Prevention (CDC) recommend be documented in an autoclave log regarding each cycle?

① Date and time of each the cycle   ⑤ Initials of the operator
② Description of the Load   ⑥ results of Sterilization indicator
③ exposure temperature,   Some Autoclaves recorders that autoprint
④ results of the sterilization indicator

36. What is the purpose of a sterilization indicator?

to determine the effectiveness of the Sterilization - proper temperature
If the Sterization Indicator does not change colors there may be a problem with the Autoclave.

37. What should be done if a sterilization indicator does not change properly?

_____

_____

38. How should sterilization indicators be stored?

_____

39. What are the advantages and disadvantages of autoclave tape?

_____

_____

40. How should a sterilization strip be placed in a wrapped pack?

_____

41. How often should a biologic indicator be used to monitor an autoclave?

_____

42. What is the purpose of wrapping articles to be autoclaved?

to avoid recontamination

_____

43. List two properties of a good wrapper for use in autoclaving.

_____

_____

44. List three examples of wrapping materials used for the autoclave and identify an advantage of each type.

_____

_____

_____

45. Why shouldn't tap water be used to fill the water reservoir of an autoclave?

_____

_____

46. How should the following be positioned in the autoclave?

    a. Small packs: _____

    b. Large packs: _____

    c. Jars and glassware: _____

    d. Sterilization pouches: _____

47. Why is more time needed to autoclave a large minor office surgery pack?

_____

_____

48. What determines the amount of time required to sterilize articles in the autoclave?

_____

49. Why must a sterilized load be allowed to dry before it is removed from the autoclave?

_____

_____

50. What is event-related sterility?

_____

_____

51. How should sterilized packs be stored?

_____

_____

52. Describe the care an autoclave should receive on a daily basis.

1. Wipe the outside of the autoclave

2. Wipe the interior of the autoclave and trays with damp cloth

3. Clean the rubber gasket on the autoclave. Make sure the gasket is intact

4. Inspect the gasket for damage that could prevent good seal

53. Why is a longer exposure period needed to ensure sterilization when using the dry-heat oven?

_____

_____

54. What effect does moist heat have on instruments with sharp cutting edges?

_____

55. How does the medical manufacturing industry use ethylene oxide gas sterilization?

_____

_____

_____

56. What guidelines must be followed when using cold sterilization?

_____

_____

_____

_____

CRITICAL THINKING ACTIVITIES

A. Safety Data Sheet

Refer to the Safety Data Sheet (SDS) in the textbook (see Fig. 3-4), and answer the following questions.

1. What is the brand name of this chemical?

_____

2. What is the recommended use of glutaraldehyde?

_____

3. What is the GHS hazard classification of glutaraldehyde?

_____

_____

_____

4. What is the signal word of glutaraldehyde?

_____

5. What GHS hazard statements are associated with glutaraldehyde?

_____

_____

_____

6. What are the first aid measures for glutaraldehyde for each of the following?

a. Skin contact: _____

_____

b. Eye contact: _____

_____

_____

c. Inhalation: _____

_____

_____

d. Ingestion: _____

_____

7. What should be done if glutaraldehyde is spilled?

_____

_____

_____

8. How should glutaraldehyde be stored?

_____

9. What type of personal protective equipment should be used with glutaraldehyde?

_____

10. Describe the appearance and odor of glutaraldehyde.

_____

11. What conditions should be avoided with glutaraldehyde?

_____

12. What symptoms can occur from overexposure to glutaraldehyde for each of the following?

    a. Inhalation: _____

    b. Skin contact: _____

    c. Eye contact: _____

    d. Ingestion: _____

13. What medical conditions are aggravated by exposure to glutaraldehyde?

_____

14. Does glutaraldehyde cause cancer?

_____

15. What is the disposal method for glutaraldehyde?

_____

_____

_____

16. When was the SDS last revised?

_____

_____

B. Obtaining a Safety Data Sheet

Obtain an SDS for one of the following hazardous chemicals, and answer the questions.

    To locate an SDS on the Internet, enter the name of the chemical into a search engine with the abbreviation "SDS." (Example: Cidex SDS)

- Cidex
- MetriCide
- Cidex OPA

73

- CaviCide
- MadaCide
- SaniZide
- Wavicide
- Biozide
- Sporox II
- Vesphene
- Envirocide
- Clorox bleach

1. What is the product name of this hazardous chemical?

   Cidex

2. What is the brand or trade name of this chemical?

   Cidex® OPH Solution

3. Who manufactures this chemical?

   Advance Sterilization Products

4. What number would you call if an emergency occurred with this chemical?

   _(703) 527-3887_

5. What is the recommended use of this chemical?

   High Level disinfectant

6. What is the GHS hazard classification of this chemical?

   Acute toxicity Oral GHS Category 3
   Skin irritation GHS Category 1
   Acute aquatic toxicity GHS Category 1

7. What is the signal word for this chemical?

   _____

8. What GHS hazard statements are associated with this chemical?

   _____

   _____

9. Sketch the GHS hazard pictograms associated with this chemical below:

10. What are the GHS precautionary statements associated with this chemical?

_____

_____

_____

11. What are the first aid measures for this chemical?

_____

_____

_____

12. What should be done if this chemical is spilled?

_____

13. What are the precautions for safe handling of this chemical?

_____

_____

14. How should this chemical be stored?

_____

15. What type of personal protective equipment should be used with this chemical?

_____

_____

16. What are the acute health hazards associated with this chemical?

_____

_____

_____

17. What medical conditions are aggravated by exposure to this chemical?

_____

_____

18. What is the disposal method for this chemical?

_____

_____

C. Sanitization

For each of the following situations involving sanitization, write C if the technique is correct and I if the technique is incorrect. If the situation is correct, state the principle underlying the technique. If the situation is incorrect, explain what might happen if the technique were performed in the incorrect manner.

_____I_____ 1. A contaminated surgical instrument is left in the examination room.

_____

_____

___I___ 2. The medical assistant does not wear gloves when sanitizing surgical instruments.

The gloves protects the medical Assistant from blood borne and other potentially infectious materials

___I___ 3. The medical assistant piles instruments while preparing them for sanitization.

This could risk the integrity of the instruments causing damage.

___I___ 4. The medical assistant forgets to read the Safety Data Sheet before decontaminating some surgical instruments in Cidex.

The Medical Assistant should thoroughly rinse the instruments and read the SDS on the disinfectant - check the expiration date

___I___ 5. The medical assistant uses laundry detergent to sanitize surgical instruments.

No No! rinse the surgical instruments - check the list of hazardous for the appropiate Chemical

___I___ 6. Dried blood is not completely cleansed from hemostatic forceps before they are sterilized in the autoclave.

creates a barrier to the surface of the forceps - So the surface of the instrument is not being cleaned.

___I___ 7. The medical assistant checks all instruments for proper working condition before sterilizing them.

after sterilization of the instruments - cleaning, rinsing and drying

___I___ 8. The medical assistant lubricates hemostatic forceps with a steam-penetrable lubricant before sterilizing them.

lubricate after the finial rinse

D. Storage of a Chemical Disinfectant

You have just received a 0.5-gallon container of Cidex Plus. You look at the label on the container and notice the following:

- Expiration date: 8/7/20
- Use life: 28 days
- Reuse life: 28 days

Based on this information, answer the following questions.

1. If the Cidex Plus is left unopened on the shelf, when would it expire and need to be discarded?

2. You open and activate the Cidex Plus on 9/1/18. What date should you write on the container?

3. You next fill a disinfectant container with the Cidex Plus and disinfect some articles in it. On what date would the Cidex Plus be unusable and need to be disposed?

4. On what date would you need to discard the rest of the container of Cidex Plus if it is not used?

E. Sterilization

For each of the following situations involving sterilization of articles in the autoclave, write C if the technique is correct, and I if the technique is incorrect. If the situation is correct, state the principle underlying the technique. If the situation is incorrect, explain what might happen if the technique were performed in the incorrect manner.

_C_ 1. The medical assistant opens a hemostat before placing it in a sterilization pouch.

_____

_____

_I_ 2. Tap water is used to fill the water reservoir of the autoclave.

distilled water needs to be used - to reduce calcium build up.

_I_ 3. When loading the autoclave, the medical assistant places glass jars in an upright position.

0919 Glass Jars should be placed on their sides in the autoclave with their lids removed. If they are placed upright air may get trapped in them, and they would not be

_I_ 4. The medical assistant places four sterilization pouches on top of one another in the autoclave.

Sterilization pouches should be positioned on their sides to maximize steam circulation and to and to facilitate the drying process

_C_ 5. The medical assistant places small packs to be sterilized approximately 1 to 3 inches apart in the autoclave.

Placing the articles too close together retards the flow of steam.

_____ 6. Spore strips are placed in the autoclave where steam will penetrate them most easily.

_____

_____

_____ 7. The medical assistant begins timing the load in the autoclave after the proper temperature of 250°F has been reached.

_____

_____

_I_ 8. The medical assistant removes the load from the autoclave while it is still wet.

_____

_____

_C_ 9. The medical assistant notices a tear in one of the wrappers while removing articles from the autoclave. He or she rewraps and resterilizes the article.

_____

_____

_I_ 10. The medical assistant notices that a sterilized wrapped article stored on the storage shelf has opened up. He or she retapes the pack and places it back on the storage shelf.

_____

_____

Chapter **3** **Sterilization and Disinfection**

Procedure 3-1: Sanitization of Instruments

Sanitize instruments. In the space provided, indicate the following:

A. Name of the disinfectant _____

B. Name of the instrument cleaner _____

C. Names of instruments sanitized _____

_____

Procedure 3-2: Chemical Disinfection of Articles

Chemically disinfect contaminated articles. In the space provided, indicate the following:

A. Name of the disinfectant

_____

B. Names of articles disinfected

_____

_____

Procedure 3-3: Wrapping Instruments Using Paper or Muslin, and Procedure 3-4: Wrapping Instruments Using a Pouch

Wrap articles for autoclaving. In the space provided, list the information you indicated on the label of each pack that includes the contents of the pack, the date, and your initials.

   Information indicated on the label of the wrapped article:

_____

_____

_____

_____

_____

_____

_____

Procedure 3-5: Sterilizing Articles in the Autoclave

Sterilize articles in the autoclave. In the space provided, indicate the articles you sterilized.

_____

_____

_____

_____

Procedure 3-1: Sanitization of Instruments

Name: _____   Date: _____

Evaluated by: _____   Score: _____

Performance Objective

Outcome:	Sanitize instruments.
Conditions:	Given the following: disposable gloves, utility gloves, contaminated instruments, chemical disinfectant and SDS, disinfectant container, cleaning solution and SDS, basin, nylon brush, wire brush, paper towels, cloth towel, and instrument lubricant.
Standards:	Time: 10 minutes. Student completed procedure in _____ minutes.
	Accuracy: Satisfactory score on the Performance Evaluation Checklist.

Performance Evaluation Checklist

Trial 1	Trial 2	Point Value	Performance Standards
		•	Reviewed the SDS for hazardous chemicals being used.
		•	Applied gloves.
		•	Transported the contaminated instruments to the cleaning area.
		•	Applied heavy duty utility gloves over the disposable gloves.
		▷	Stated the purpose of the utility gloves.
		•	Separated sharp instruments and delicate instruments from other instruments.
		▷	Explained why instruments should be separated.
		•	Immediately rinsed the instruments thoroughly under warm running water.
		▷	Stated why the instruments should be rinsed immediately.
			Decontamination of the Instruments
		•	Checked the expiration date of the chemical disinfectant.
		▷	Explained why an expired disinfectant should not be used.
		•	Observed all personal safety precautions listed on the label.
		•	Followed label directions for proper mixing and use of the disinfectant.
		•	Labeled the disinfecting container with the name of the disinfectant and the reuse expiration date.
		•	Poured the disinfectant into the labeled container.
		•	Completely submerged the articles in the disinfectant.
		•	Covered the disinfectant container.
		▷	Stated the reason for covering the container.

Trial 1	Trial 2	Point Value	Performance Standards
		•	Disinfected the articles for 10 minutes.
		▷	Explained the reason for decontaminating the instruments.
			Cleaning the Instruments: Manual Method
		•	Checked the expiration date of the cleaning agent.
		•	Observed all personal safety precautions.
		•	Followed label directions for proper use and mixing of the cleaning agent.
		•	Removed articles from disinfectant and placed them in the cleaning solution.
		•	Cleaned the surface of the instruments with a nylon brush.
		•	Cleaned grooves, crevices, or serrations with a wire brush.
		•	Removed stains using commercial stain remover.
		•	Scrubbed the instruments until they were visibly clean.
		▷	Explained why all organic matter must be removed.
			Cleaning the Instruments: Ultrasound Method
		•	Prepared the cleaning solution in the ultrasonic cleaner.
		•	Observed all personal safety precautions listed on label.
		•	Removed the articles from the disinfectant.
		•	Separated instruments of dissimilar metals.
		•	Properly placed the instruments in the ultrasonic cleaner.
		•	Positioned hinged instruments in an open position.
		▷	Stated why hinged instruments must be in an open position.
		•	Ensured that sharp instruments did not touch other instruments.
		•	Checked to make sure all instruments were fully submerged.
		•	Placed the lid on the ultrasonic cleaner.
		•	Turned on the ultrasonic cleaner.
		•	Cleaned the instruments for the length of time recommended by the manufacturer.
		•	Removed the instruments from the machine.
		•	Rinsed each instrument thoroughly with warm water for 20 to 30 seconds.
		▷	Explained why instruments should be rinsed thoroughly.
		•	Dried each instrument with a paper towel.
			Completion of the Procedure
		•	Placed instrument on a towel for additional drying.

Trial 1	Trial 2	Point Value	Performance Standards
		▷	Stated the reason for drying the instruments.
		•	Checked each instrument for defects and proper working condition.
		•	Lubricated hinged instruments in an open position.
		•	Opened and closed the instrument to distribute the lubricant.
		•	Placed the lubricated instrument on a towel to drain.
		▷	Stated the reason for lubricating instruments.
		•	Disposed of the cleaning solution according to the manufacturer's instructions.
		•	Removed both sets of gloves.
		•	Sanitized hands.
		•	Wrapped the instruments.
		•	Sterilized the instruments in the autoclave.
		★	Completed the procedure within 10 minutes.
			Totals

Evaluation of Student Performance

EVALUATION CRITERIA			COMMENTS
Symbol	**Category**	**Point Value**	
★	Critical Step	16 points	
•	Essential Step	6 points	
Ⓐ	Affective Competency	6 points	
▷	Theory Question	2 points	

Score calculation: 100 points
− _____ points missed
_____ Score

Satisfactory score: 85 or above

CAAHEP Competency Achieved

Psychomotor (Skills)
☑ III. 4. Prepare items for autoclaving.

ABHES Competency Achieved

☑ 8. a. Practice standard precautions and perform disinfection/sterilization techniques.

Notes

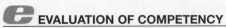 **EVALUATION OF COMPETENCY**

Procedure 3-2: Chemical Disinfection of Articles

Name: _____ Date: _____

Evaluated by: _____ Score: _____

Performance Objective

Outcome:	Chemically disinfect articles.
Conditions:	Given the following: disposable gloves, utility gloves, contaminated articles, chemical disinfectant and SDS, disinfectant container, and paper towels.
Standards:	Time: 10 minutes. Student completed procedure in _____ minutes.
	Accuracy: Satisfactory score on the Performance Evaluation Checklist.

Performance Evaluation Checklist

Trial 1	Trial 2	Point Value	Performance Standards
		•	Applied gloves and sanitized the articles.
		•	Reviewed the SDS for the chemical disinfectant.
		▷	Described what information is included on an SDS.
		•	Checked the expiration date of the disinfectant.
		▷	Explained why an expired disinfectant should not be used.
		•	Observed all personal safety precautions listed on the container label.
		•	Followed the directions on the label for proper use and reuse of the disinfectant.
		•	Completely immersed articles in the chemical disinfectant.
		•	Covered disinfectant container.
		▷	Stated the reason for covering the container.
		•	Disinfected articles for the proper length of time as indicated on the label of the container.
		•	Rinsed the articles thoroughly.
		▷	Stated the reason for rinsing the articles.
		•	Dried the articles.
		•	Properly disposed of the disinfectant.
		▷	Stated the purpose of proper disposal of the disinfectant.
		•	Removed gloves.
		•	Sanitized hands.
		•	Properly stored the articles.
		★	Completed the procedure within 10 minutes.
			Totals

Evaluation of Student Performance

EVALUATION CRITERIA			COMMENTS
Symbol	Category	Point Value	
★	Critical Step	16 points	
•	Essential Step	6 points	
▷	Theory Question	2 points	

Score calculation: 100 points
− _____ points missed
_____ Score

Satisfactory score: 85 or above

CAAHEP Competencies Achieved

Psychomotor (Skills)

☑ XII. 1. Comply with safety signs, symbols, and labels.

ABHES Competencies Achieved

☑ 8. a. Practice standard precautions and perform disinfection/sterilization techniques.

Procedure 3-3: Wrapping Instruments Using Paper or Muslin

Name: _____ Date: _____

Evaluated by: _____ Score: _____

Performance Objective

Outcome:	Wrap an instrument for autoclaving.
Conditions:	Given the following: sanitized instrument, wrapping material, sterilization indicator strip, autoclave tape, and a permanent marker.
Standards:	Time: 5 minutes. Student completed procedure in _____ minutes.
	Accuracy: Satisfactory score on the Performance Evaluation Checklist.

Performance Evaluation Checklist

Trial 1	Trial 2	Point Value	Performance Standards
		•	Sanitized hands.
		•	Assembled equipment.
		•	Selected the appropriate-sized wrapping material.
		•	Checked the expiration date on the sterilization indicator box.
		▷	Stated why outdated strips should not be used.
		•	Placed wrapping material on clean, flat surface.
		•	Turned the wrap in a diagonal position.
		•	Placed instrument in the center of wrapping material.
		•	Placed instruments with movable joints in an open position.
		▷	Stated why instruments with movable joints must be placed in an open position.
		•	Placed a sterilization indicator in the center of the pack.
		•	Folded wrapping material up from the bottom and doubled back a small corner.
		•	Folded over one edge of wrapping material and doubled back the corner.
		•	Folded over the other edge of wrapping material and doubled back the corner.
		•	Folded the pack up from the bottom and secured with autoclave tape.
		•	Ensured that the pack was firm enough for handling, but loose enough to permit proper circulation of steam.
		▷	Stated why instruments are wrapped for autoclaving.
		•	Labeled and dated the pack. Included initials.
		▷	Stated the purpose of dating the pack.
		★	Completed the procedure within 5 minutes.
			Totals

Evaluation of Student Performance

EVALUATION CRITERIA			COMMENTS
Symbol	**Category**	**Point Value**	
★	Critical Step	16 points	
•	Essential Step	6 points	
Ⓐ	Affective Competency	6 points	
▷	Theory Question	2 points	

Score calculation: 100 points
− _____ points missed
_____ Score

Satisfactory score: 85 or above

CAAHEP Competency Achieved

Psychomotor (Skills)

☑ III. 4. Prepare items for autoclaving.

ABHES Competency Achieved

☑ 8. a. Practice standard precautions and perform disinfection/sterilization techniques.

Procedure 3-4: Wrapping Instruments Using a Pouch

Name: _____ Date: _____

Evaluated by: _____ Score: _____

Performance Objective

Outcome:	Wrap an instrument for autoclaving.
Conditions:	Given the following: sanitized instrument, sterilization pouch, and a permanent marker.
Standards:	Time: 5 minutes. Student completed procedure in _____ minutes.
	Accuracy: Satisfactory score on the Performance Evaluation Checklist.

Performance Evaluation Checklist

Trial 1	Trial 2	Point Value	Performance Standards
		•	Sanitized hands.
		•	Assembled equipment.
		•	Selected the appropriate-sized pouch.
		•	Placed the pouch on a clean, flat surface.
		•	Labeled and dated the pack. Included initials.
		•	Inserted the instrument into the open end of the pouch.
		•	Sealed the pouch.
		•	Sterilized the pack in the autoclave.
		▷	Stated how long the pack is sterile once it has been autoclaved.
		★	Completed the procedure within 5 minutes.
			Totals

Evaluation of Student Performance

EVALUATION CRITERIA			COMMENTS
Symbol	**Category**	**Point Value**	
★	Critical Step	16 points	
•	Essential Step	6 points	
Ⓐ	Affective Competency	6 points	
▷	Theory Question	2 points	

Score calculation: 100 points
       − _____ points missed
       _____ Score

Satisfactory score: 85 or above

89

CAAHEP Competency Achieved

Psychomotor (Skills)

☑ III. 4. Prepare items for autoclaving.

ABHES Competency Achieved

☑ 8. a. Practice standard precautions and perform disinfection/sterilization techniques.

Procedure 3-5: Sterilizing Articles in the Autoclave

Name: _____ Date: _____

Evaluated by: _____ Score: _____

Performance Objective

Outcome:	Sterilize articles in the autoclave.
Conditions:	Using an autoclave.
Standards:	Time: 10 minutes. Student completed procedure in _____ minutes.
	Accuracy: Satisfactory score on the Performance Evaluation Checklist.

Performance Evaluation Checklist

Trial 1	Trial 2	Point Value	Performance Standards
		•	Assembled equipment.
		•	Checked the water level in the autoclave.
		•	Properly loaded the autoclave.
		▷	Stated how far apart to place small packs and large packs.
		▷	Explained two ways for positioning pouches in the autoclave.
			Manual Operation of the Autoclave
		•	Determined the sterilizing time for the types of articles being autoclaved.
		•	Turned on the autoclave.
		•	Filled the chamber with water.
		•	Closed and latched the door.
		•	Set the timing control.
		▷	Stated when the timer should be set.
		•	Vented the chamber of steam.
		•	Dried the load.
		▷	Stated the reason for drying the load.
			Automatic Operation of the Autoclave
		•	Closed and latched the door.
		•	Turned on the autoclave.
		•	Determined the sterilization program.
		•	Pressed the appropriate program button.

Trial 1	Trial 2	Point Value	Performance Standards
		•	Pressed the start button.
		▷	Stated the purpose of each control or indicator on the autoclave.
			Completion of the Procedure
		•	Turned off the autoclave.
		•	Removed the load with heat-resistant gloves.
		▷	Stated the reason for using heat-resistant gloves.
		•	Inspected the packs as they were removed for damage.
		▷	Explained what should be done if a pack is torn.
		•	Checked the sterilization indicators on the outside of the packs.
		•	Documented information in the autoclave log.
		•	Stored the articles in a clean dust-proof area.
		•	Placed the most recently sterilized packs behind previously sterilized packs.
		•	Maintained appropriate daily care of the autoclave.
		▷	Described the care the autoclave should receive each day.
			Demonstrated the following affective behavior(s) during this procedure:
		Ⓐ	Recognized the implications for failure to comply with Centers for Disease Control (CDC) regulations in health care settings.
		★	Completed the procedure within 10 minutes.
			Totals

Evaluation of Student Performance

EVALUATION CRITERIA			COMMENTS
Symbol	**Category**	**Point Value**	
★	Critical Step	16 points	
•	Essential Step	6 points	
Ⓐ	Affective Competency	6 points	
▷	Theory Question	2 points	

Score calculation: 100 points

− _____ points missed

_____ Score

Satisfactory score: 85 or above

Chapter **3** **Sterilization and Disinfection**

CAAHEP Competencies Achieved

Psychomotor (Skills)

☑ III. 5. Perform sterilization procedures.

☑ VI. 8. Perform routine maintenance of administrative or clinical equipment.

Affective (Behavior)

☑ III. 1. Recognize the implications for failure to comply with Centers for Disease Control (CDC) regulations in health care settings.

ABHES Competency Achieved

☑ 4. f. Comply with federal, state, and local health laws and regulations as they relate to health care settings.

☑ 8. a. Practice standard precautions and perform disinfection/sterilization techniques.

4 Vital Signs

√ After Completing	Date Due	Study Guide Pages	STUDY GUIDE ASSIGNMENTS (CTA = Critical Thinking Activity)	Possible Points	Points You Earned
		99	📋 Pretest	10	
		100-102	🔑 Key Term Assessment		
		100-101	A. Definitions	55	
		102	B. Word Parts (Add 1 point for each key term)	30	
		103-112	📖 Evaluation of Learning questions	93	
		112-113	CTA A: Measurement of Body Temperature	17	
		114	CTA B: Alterations in Body Temperature	5	
		114	CTA C: Pulse Sites	6	
		114-115	CTA D: Pulse and Respiratory Rates	3	
		115-116	CTA E: Pulse Oximetry	11	
		116-117	CTA F: Blood Pressure Measurement	10	
		117-118	CTA G: Proper BP Cuff Selection	12	
		118	CTA H: Reading Blood Pressure Values	24	
			🅔 Evolve Site: Under Pressure (Record points earned)		
		118-119	CTA I: Interpreting Blood Pressure Readings	10	
		119	CTA J: Hypertension	20	
		121	CTA K: Crossword Puzzle	30	
			🅔 Evolve Site: Road to Recovery Game: Vital Signs Terminology (Record points earned)		
			🅔 Evolve Site: Apply Your Knowledge questions (Record points earned)	11	

√ After Completing	Date Due	Study Guide Pages	STUDY GUIDE ASSIGNMENTS (CTA = Critical Thinking Activity)	Possible Points	Points You Earned
			e Evolve Site: Video Evaluation	86	
		99	Posttest	10	
			ADDITIONAL ASSIGNMENTS		
			Total points		

√ When Assigned by Your Instructor	Study Guide Pages	Practices Required	LABORATORY ASSIGNMENTS	Score*
	123	5	**Practice for Competency** 4-1: Measuring Oral Body Temperature—Electronic Thermometer Textbook reference: pp. 97-99	
	125-127		**Evaluation of Competency** 4-1: Measuring Oral Body Temperature—Electronic Thermometer	*
	123	3	**Practice for Competency** 4-2: Measuring Axillary Body Temperature—Electronic Thermometer Textbook reference: pp. 99-100	
	129-130		**Evaluation of Competency** 4-2: Measuring Axillary Body Temperature—Electronic Thermometer	*
	123	3	**Practice for Competency** 4-3: Measuring Rectal Body Temperature—Electronic Thermometer Textbook reference: pp. 100-102	
	131-133		**Evaluation of Competency** 4-3: Measuring Rectal Body Temperature—Electronic Thermometer	*
	123	5	**Practice for Competency** 4-4: Measuring Aural Body Temperature—Tympanic Membrane Thermometer Textbook reference: pp. 102-104	
	135-137		**Evaluation of Competency** 4-4: Measuring Aural Body Temperature—Tympanic Membrane Thermometer	*
	123	5	**Practice for Competency** 4-5: Measuring Temporal Body Temperature Textbook reference: pp. 104-106	
	139-141		**Evaluation of Competency** 4-5: Measuring Temporal Body Temperature	*
	124	10	**Practice for Competency** 4-6: Measuring Pulse and Respiration Textbook reference: pp. 117-118	
	143-145		**Evaluation of Competency** 4-6: Measuring Pulse and Respiration	*
	124	5	**Practice for Competency** 4-7: Measuring Apical Pulse Textbook reference: pp. 119-120	
	147-148		**Evaluation of Competency** 4-7: Measuring Apical Pulse	*

√ When Assigned by Your Instructor	Study Guide Pages	Practices Required	LABORATORY ASSIGNMENTS	Score*
	124	5	**Practice for Competency** 4-8: Performing Pulse Oximetry Textbook reference: pp. 120-122	
	149-151		**Evaluation of Competency** 4-8: Performing Pulse Oximetry	*
	124	10	**Practice for Competency** 4-9: Measuring Blood Pressure Textbook reference: pp. 133-136	
	153-155		**Evaluation of Competency** 4-9: Measuring Blood Pressure	*
			ADDITIONAL ASSIGNMENTS	

Name: _____   Date: _____

True or False

_____ 1. The heat-regulating center of the body is the medulla.

_____ 2. A vague sense of body discomfort, weakness, and fatigue that often marks the onset of a disease is known as the blahs.

_____ 3. If an axillary temperature of 100° F was taken orally, it would register as 101° F.

_____ 4. If the lens of a tympanic membrane thermometer is dirty, the reading may be falsely low.

_____ 5. Chemical thermometers should be stored in the freezer.

_____ 6. The femoral pulse site can be used to assess circulation to the foot.

_____ 7. The term used to describe an irregularity in the heart's rhythm is dysrhythmia.

_____ 8. Pulse oximetry provides the provider with information on the amount of oxygen being delivered to the tissues.

_____ 9. Blood pressure measures the contraction and relaxation of the heart.

_____ 10. When taking blood pressure, the stethoscope is placed over the brachial artery

?≡ **POSTTEST**

True or False

_____ 1. A temperature of 100° F is classified as a low-grade fever.

_____ 2. The rectal site should not be used to take the temperature of a newborn.

_____ 3. A tympanic membrane thermometer should not be used to measure temperature on a child younger than 6 years of age.

_____ 4. A temporal artery temperature reading is the same as an oral reading.

_____ 5. Excessive pressure should not be applied when measuring a pulse because it could obstruct the pulse.

_____ 6. A child has a faster pulse rate than an adult.

_____ 7. The normal respiratory rate of an adult ranges between 10 and 18 respirations per minute.

_____ 8. The term used to describe a bluish discoloration of the skin due to a lack of oxygen is hypoxia.

_____ 9. The oxygen saturation level of a healthy individual falls between 85% and 90%.

_____ 10. When measuring blood pressure, the patient's arm should be positioned above the level of the heart.

A. Definitions

Temperature

Directions: Match each key term with its definition.

_____ 1. Afebrile

_____ 2. Antipyretic

_____ 3. Axilla

_____ 4. Celsius scale

_____ 5. Conduction

_____ 6. Convection

_____ 7. Crisis

_____ 8. Disinfectant

_____ 9. Fahrenheit scale

_____ 10. Febrile

_____ 11. Fever

_____ 12. Frenulum linguae

_____ 13. Hyperpyrexia

_____ 14. Hypothermia

_____ 15. Malaise

_____ 16. Radiation

A. An extremely high fever

B. An agent used to destroy disease-producing microorganisms but not necessarily their spores (usually applied to inanimate objects)

C. A body temperature that is below normal

D. The armpit

E. The transfer of energy, such as heat, through air currents

F. A body temperature that is above normal (pyrexia)

G. An agent that reduces fever

H. A temperature scale on which the freezing point of water is 32° and the boiling point of water is 212°

I. The transfer of energy, such as heat, in the form of waves

J. A temperature scale on which the freezing point of water is 0° and the boiling point is 100°

K. The midline fold that connects the undersurface of the tongue with the floor of the mouth

L. Pertaining to fever

M. The transfer of energy from one object to another by direct contact

N. A sudden falling of an elevated body temperature to normal

O. Without fever; the body temperature is normal

P. A vague sense of body discomfort, weakness, and fatigue often marking the onset of a disease and continuing through the course of the illness

Pulse

Directions: Match each key term with its definition.

_____ 1. Antecubital space

_____ 2. Aorta

_____ 3. Bounding pulse

_____ 4. Bradycardia

_____ 5. Dysrhythmia

_____ 6. Intercostal

_____ 7. Pulse rhythm

_____ 8. Pulse volume

_____ 9. Tachycardia

_____ 10. Thready pulse

A. Between the ribs

B. A pulse with an increased volume that feels very strong and full

C. The strength of the heartbeat

D. The space located at the front of the elbow

E. An abnormally fast heart rate (more than 100 beats per minute)

F. The major trunk of the arterial system of the body

G. The time interval between heartbeats

H. A pulse with a decreased volume that feels weak and thin

I. An irregular rhythm

J. An abnormally slow heart rate (less than 60 beats per minute)

Respiration and Pulse Oximetry

Directions: Match each key term with its definition.

_____ 1. Alveolus

___D___ 2. Apnea

_____ 3. Bradypnea

_____ 4. Cyanosis

_____ 5. Dyspnea

_____ 6. Eupnea

_____ 7. Exhalation

_____ 8. Hyperpnea

_____ 9. Hyperventilation

_____ 10. Hypopnea

_____ 11. Hypoxemia

_____ 12. Hypoxia

_____ 13. Inhalation

_____ 14. Orthopnea

_____ 15. Pulse oximeter

_____ 16. Pulse oximetry

_____ 17. SaO_2

___L___ 18. SpO_2

___S___ 19. Tachypnea

A. The act of breathing out
B. A reduction in the oxygen supply to the tissues of the body
C. A decrease in the oxygen saturation of the blood; may lead to hypoxia
D. The temporary cessation of breathing
E. An abnormal increase in the respiratory rate of more than 20 respirations per minute
F. A computerized device consisting of a probe and monitor used to measure the oxygen saturation of arterial blood
G. An abnormal decrease in the rate and depth of respiration
H. A thin-walled air sac of the lungs in which the exchange of oxygen and carbon dioxide takes place
I. The use of a pulse oximeter to measure the oxygen saturation of arterial blood
J. The act of breathing in
K. A bluish discoloration of the skin and mucous membranes first observed in the nail beds and lips
L. Abbreviation for the percentage of hemoglobin that is saturated with oxygen in arterial blood
M. The condition in which breathing is easier when an individual is in a standing or sitting position
N. Shortness of breath or difficulty in breathing
O. Abbreviation for the percentage of hemoglobin that is saturated with oxygen in arterial blood as measured by a pulse oximeter
P. Normal respiration
Q. An abnormally fast and deep type of breathing usually associated with acute anxiety conditions
R. An abnormal decrease in the respiratory rate of less than 10 respirations per minute
S. An abnormal increase in the rate and depth of respiration

Blood Pressure

Directions: Match each key term with its definition.

_____ 1. Diastole

_____ 2. Diastolic pressure

_____ 3. Hypertension

_____ 4. Hypotension

_____ 5. Meniscus

_____ 6. Pulse pressure

_____ 7. Sphygmomanometer

_____ 8. Stethoscope

_____ 9. Systole

_____ 10. Systolic pressure

A. The curved surface on a column of liquid in a tube
B. High blood pressure
C. The point of maximum pressure on the arterial walls
D. The phase in the cardiac cycle in which the heart relaxes between contractions
E. An instrument for measuring arterial blood pressure
F. The point of lesser pressure on the arterial walls
G. Low blood pressure
H. The phase in the cardiac cycle in which the ventricles contract, sending blood out of the heart and into the aorta and pulmonary aorta
I. An instrument for amplifying and hearing sounds produced by the body
J. The difference between the systolic and diastolic pressures

B. Word Parts

Directions: Indicate the meaning of each word part in the space provided. List as many medical terms as possible that incorporate the word part in the space provided.

Word Part	Meaning of Word Part	Medical Terms That Incorporate Word Part
1. anti-		
2. pyr/o		
3. -ic		
4. -pnea		
5. brady-		
6. cardi/o		
7. -ia		
8. a-		
9. cyan/o		
10. -osis		
11. dys-		
12. eu-		
13. ex-		
14. hyper-		
15. hypo-		
16. -tension		
17. therm/o		
18. ox/i		
19. in-		
20. inter-		
21. cost/o		
22. -al		
23. -mal		
24. -meter		
25. orth/o		
26. -metry		
27. sphygm/o		
28. steth/o		
29. -scope		
30. tachy-		

Temperature

Directions: Fill in each blank with the correct answer.

1. Define a vital sign.

   _____

   _____

2. What are the four vital signs?

   _____

   _____

   _____

3. What general guidelines should be followed when measuring vital signs?

   _____

   _____

   _____

   _____

4. List four ways in which heat is produced in the body.

   _____

   _____

   _____

   _____

5. List four ways in which heat is lost from the body.

   _____

   _____

   _____

   _____

6. What is the normal body temperature range? What is the average body temperature?

   _____

7. What is a fever?

   _____

   _____

8. How do diurnal variations affect body temperature?

_____

_____

9. How do emotional states affect body temperature?

_____

10. How does vigorous physical exercise affect body temperature?

_____

11. What symptoms occur with a fever?

_____

_____

12. Describe the following fever patterns:

   a. Continuous fever

   _____

   _____

   b. Intermittent fever

   _____

   _____

   c. Remittent fever

   _____

   _____

13. What is the subsiding stage of a fever?

_____

14. What five sites are used for taking body temperature?

_____

15. List three instances in which the axillary site for taking body temperature would be preferred over the oral site.

_____

_____

_____

16. Why does the rectal method for taking body temperature provide a very accurate temperature measurement?

_____

_____

_____

17. When can the rectal method be used to take body temperature?

_____

18. When can the aural method be used to take body temperature?

_____

_____

19. How does a temperature taken through the rectal and axillary methods compare (in terms of degrees) with a temperature taken through the oral method?

_____

_____

20. List and describe the four types of thermometers available for taking body temperature.

_____

_____

_____

21. Describe the advantages of a tympanic membrane thermometer.

_____

_____

22. Explain how a tympanic membrane thermometer measures body temperature.

_____

_____

_____

23. Explain how to clean the lens of a tympanic membrane thermometer.

_____

_____

_____

24. What is the purpose of placing a probe cover on a tympanic membrane thermometer?

_____

_____

25. List three reasons why the temporal artery is a good site to measure body temperature.

_____

_____

26. How does the temperature obtained through the temporal site compare with oral, rectal, and axillary body temperatures?

_____

_____

_____

27. List four factors that can result in an inaccurate temporal artery temperature reading.

_____

_____

28. Where should a chemical thermometer be stored? Explain why.

_____

_____

Pulse

Directions: Fill in each blank with the correct answer.

1. What causes the pulse to occur?

_____

_____

_____

2. What is the unit of measurement for pulse rate?

_____

3. How does physical activity affect the pulse rate?

_____

4. What is the most common site for taking the pulse?

_____

5. List two reasons for taking the pulse at the apical pulse site.

_____

_____

6. Where is the apex of the heart located?

_____

_____

7. When is the brachial artery used as a pulse site?

_____

8. When is the carotid artery used as a pulse site?

_____

9. When is the femoral artery used as a pulse site?

_____

10. What two pulse sites can be used to assess circulation to the foot?

_____

11. List two reasons for measuring the pulse rate.

_____

_____

12. State the normal range for a pulse rate for an adult.

_____

13. What is the normal pulse range for the following age groups:

    a. Infant: _____

    b. Toddler: _____

    c. Preschooler: _____

    d. School-age: _____

    e. Adult after age 60: _____

14. What is the normal pulse range for a well-trained athlete?

_____

15. What may cause tachycardia?

_____

16. How is an apical-radial pulse taken?

_____

17. What is a pulse deficit?

_____

18. If the rhythm and volume of a patient's pulse are normal, the medical assistant documents the information as

_____

Respiration

Directions: Fill in each blank with the correct answer.

1. What is the purpose of respiration?

_____

_____

2. What is the purpose of inhalation?

_____

_____

3. What is the purpose of exhalation?

_____

_____

4. What is included in one complete respiration?

_____

_____

5. The exchange of oxygen and carbon dioxide between the body cells and blood is known as

_____

6. What is the name of the control center for involuntary respiration?

_____

7. Why must respiration be measured without the patient's awareness?

_____

8. What is the normal respiratory rate (range) for a normal adult?

_____

9. What is the ratio of respirations to pulse beats?

_____

10. List two factors that can increase the respiratory rate.

_____

_____

11. Describe a normal rhythm for respiration.

_____

_____

12. What can cause hyperventilation?

_____

13. What type of patient may experience hypopnea?

_____

14. Where is cyanosis first observed?

_____

_____

15. What can cause cyanosis?

_____

16. What are two conditions in which dyspnea may occur?

_____

_____

17. Describe the character of normal breath sounds.

_____

_____

18. Describe the characteristics of the following abnormal breath sounds:

a. Crackles:

_____

_____

b. Rhonchi:

_____

_____

c. Wheezes:

_____

_____

Pulse Oximetry

Directions: Fill in each blank with the correct answer.

1. What is the purpose of pulse oximetry?

_____

_____

2. What is the function of hemoglobin?

_____

3. What is the oxygen saturation level of a healthy individual?

_____

4. What can occur if the oxygen saturation level falls between 85% and 90%?

_____

_____

5. List three patient conditions that can cause a decreased SpO_2 value.

_____

_____

_____

6. When can pulse oximetry be used for the short-term continuous monitoring of a patient?

_____

_____

_____

7. What is the purpose of the pulse oximeter power-on self-test (POST)?

_____

_____

8. What type of site must be used for applying a pulse oximeter probe?

_____

_____

9. How can dark fingernail polish cause a falsely low SpO_2 reading?

_____

_____

10. How can patient movement cause an inaccurate SpO_2 reading?

_____

_____

11. What types of patients may make it difficult to properly align the oximeter probe?

_____

_____

12. List three conditions that can cause poor peripheral blood flow.

_____

_____

13. Why must a reusable oximeter probe be free of all dirt and grime before it is used?

_____

_____

Blood Pressure
Directions: Fill in each blank with the correct answer.

1. What does blood pressure measure?

_____

_____

2. Why is the diastolic pressure lower than the systolic pressure?

_____

_____

_____

3. What is considered normal blood pressure for an adult?

_____

4. State the blood pressure range for each of the following:

   a. Prehypertension: _____

   b. Hypertension, stage 1: _____

   c. Hypertension, stage 2: _____

110

5. Why should blood pressure readings always be interpreted using the patient's baseline blood pressure?

_____

_____

6. How does age affect blood pressure?

_____

7. How do diurnal variations affect blood pressure?

_____

_____

8. What are the two types of stethoscope chest pieces and the use of each?

_____

_____

_____

_____

9. What are the parts of a sphygmomanometer?

_____

_____

10. How often should an aneroid sphygmomanometer be recalibrated?

_____

11. When would each of the following cuffs be used to measure blood pressure?

    a. Child: _____

    b. Adult: _____

    c. Thigh: _____

12. Explain how to determine the proper cuff size for a patient.

_____

_____

13. What may occur if blood pressure is taken using a cuff that is too small or too large?

_____

_____

14. How should the blood pressure be measured if the patient's arm circumference is greater than 50 cm (20 inches)?

_____

_____

_____

15. List the five phases included in the Korotkoff sounds, and describe what type of sound is heard during each phase.

_____

_____

_____

_____

_____

16. List five advantages of an automated blood pressure monitor.

_____

_____

_____

_____

_____

CRITICAL THINKING ACTIVITIES

A. Measurement of Body Temperature

For each of the following situations involving the measurement of body temperature, write C if the technique is correct and I if the technique is incorrect. If the situation is correct, state the principle underlying the technique. If the situation is incorrect, explain what might happen if the technique were performed in the incorrect manner.

Electronic Thermometer

_____ 1. The medical assistant takes a patient's oral temperature immediately after the patient has consumed a cup of coffee.

_____

_____

_____ 2. The medical assistant instructs the patient not to talk while his or her oral temperature is being measured.

_____

_____

_____ 3. The medical assistant forgets to lubricate the rectal probe before taking a patient's rectal temperature.

_____

_____

_____ 4. An axillary temperature reading is documented as follows: 102.2° F.

_____

_____

_____ 5. The medical assistant discards a used rectal probe in a regular waste container.

_____

_____

_____ 6. The medical assistant's bare fingers accidentally touch a used oral probe cover while discarding it.

_____

_____

Tympanic Membrane Thermometer

_____ 1. A thermometer with a dirty probe lens is used to take the patient's temperature.

_____ 2. The ear canal is straightened before taking a patient's aural temperature.

_____ 3. The medical assistant does not seal the opening of the ear canal with the probe when taking aural temperature.

_____ 4. The probe is positioned toward the opposite temple when taking aural temperature.

_____ 5. The medical assistant waits 30 seconds before taking the patient's temperature in the same ear.

Temporal Artery Thermometer

_____ 1. The medical assistant checks to make sure the probe lens is clean and intact before using a temporal artery thermometer.

_____ 2. The medical assistant brushes hair away from the patient's forehead before measuring the patient's temperature.

_____ 3. The medical assistant slides the temporal artery probe across the patient's forehead while continually depressing the scan button.

_____ 4. The medical assistant quickly scans the patient's forehead during temporal artery temperature measurement.

_____ 5. After scanning the forehead, the medical assistant documents the patient's temporal artery temperature reading.

_____ 6. The medical assistant cleans the temporal artery thermometer by immersing it in warm, sudsy water.

B. Alterations in Body Temperature

Label the following diagram with the terms that describe the body temperature alteration.

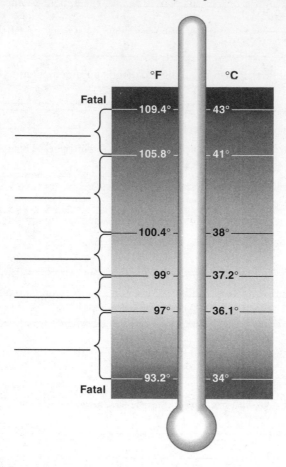

C. Pulse Sites

Locate the pulse at the following sites, and document the pulse rates below:

1. Brachial pulse _____

2. Temporal pulse _____

3. Carotid pulse _____

4. Femoral pulse _____

5. Popliteal pulse _____

6. Dorsalis pedis pulse _____

D. Pulse and Respiratory Rates

Take the pulse and respiration of a person before and after vigorous exercise, and document the results.

1. Before vigorous exercise

_____

_____

2. After vigorous exercise

_____

_____

3. Compare the results, and explain how exercise affects the pulse and respiratory rates.

_____

_____

E. Pulse Oximetry

Your provider asks you to measure the oxygen saturation level of the patients listed. For each situation, answer the following questions:

    a. What would you do in each situation to prevent an inaccurate pulse oximetry reading?

    b. What occurs with each of these situations and how does it affect the SpO_2 reading?

1. Kelly Collins, a patient with chronic bronchitis, is wearing navy blue nail polish.

_____

_____

2. Melvin Hosey has Parkinson's disease and is having difficulty controlling tremors in his hands.

_____

_____

3. Scott Kimes, a patient with emphysema, frequently experiences periods of prolonged coughing.

_____

_____

4. Nicole Lowe has returned to the office for a recheck of her viral pneumonia. You are getting ready to measure her oxygen saturation and notice that bright sunlight is coming through the window where she is seated and shining on her hand.

_____

_____

5. Rebecca Bensie, a patient on oxygen therapy, is morbidly obese, and you are having trouble properly aligning the oximeter probe on her finger.

_____

_____

6. Doug Habbershaw, a patient with peripheral vascular disease, has come to the office for a health checkup.

_____

_____

7. Emily Lacey has come to the office because she has been experiencing dyspnea. Her hands are very cold, and it is interfering with the pulse oximetry procedure.

_____

_____

8. Susan Boone, a patient with asthma, is wearing artificial fingernails.

_____

_____

9. Frank Stewart, a patient with congestive heart failure, is at the office to have a mole removed from his back. There are bright overhead lights in the room, and they cannot be turned off because the provider needs to have good lighting to perform the surgery.

_____

_____

10. Wanda Weaver is having a sebaceous cyst removed from her chest and has been sedated for the procedure. You have applied an automatic blood pressure cuff to her right arm. The provider asks you to apply an oximeter probe to Wanda's left finger to continuously monitor her oxygen saturation level during the procedure.

_____

_____

11. Which control, indicator, or display is involved when the following occurs?

a. The oximeter is searching for a pulse.

_____

b. The oximeter cannot find a pulse.

_____

c. The oximeter is portraying the strength of the pulse.

_____

d. The pulse is audibly broadcasted by a beeping sound.

_____

e. The oximeter displays the oxygen saturation level.

_____

f. The oximeter displays the pulse rate.

_____

g. The battery is low.

_____

h. You turn the oximeter off.

_____

F. Blood Pressure Measurement

Using the principles outlined in your textbook, explain what happens under the following circumstances:

1. The blood pressure is taken on a patient who has just undergone vigorous physical exercise.

_____

2. The blood pressure is taken on a patient with tight sleeves.

_____

_____

116

3. The blood pressure is taken on an apprehensive patient.

_____

_____

4. An adult cuff is used to measure blood pressure on a young child.

_____

_____

5. The blood pressure is taken over clothing.

_____

_____

6. The arm is below heart level during blood pressure measurement.

_____

_____

7. The patient's legs are crossed during blood pressure measurement.

_____

_____

8. The rubber bladder is not centered over the brachial artery.

_____

_____

9. The cuff is placed $1/2$ inch above the bend in the elbows.

_____

_____

10. The manometer is viewed from a distance of 4 feet.

_____

_____

G. Proper BP Cuff Selection
Measurements of the arm circumference (in centimeters) are given for various patients. Using Table 4.9 on page 126 of your textbook, indicate what size of blood pressure cuff (child, small adult, adult, large adult, or adult thigh) should be used with each of these patients.

1. 47 cm: _____

2. 20 cm: _____

3. 32 cm: _____

4. 16 cm: _____

5. 38 cm: _____

6. 27 cm: _____

7. 52 cm: _____

8. 24 cm: _____

Measure the arm circumference of four classmates with a centimeter tape measure, and document the values below. Next to each value, indicate what size blood pressure cuff should be used with each of these individuals.

1. _____

2. _____

3. _____

4. _____

H. Reading Blood Pressure Values

Read and document the following blood pressure measurements in the space provided.

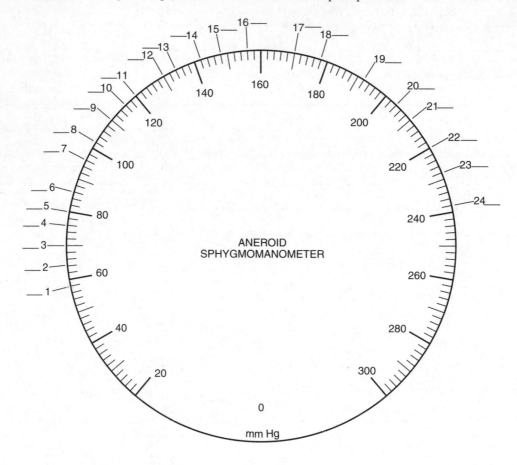

ANEROID
SPHYGMOMANOMETER

mm Hg

I. Interpreting Blood Pressure Readings

Classify each of the following blood pressure readings into its appropriate category. The readings are based on the average of two or more properly measured and seated blood pressure readings taken at each of two or more visits.

Normal
Prehypertension
Hypertension: Stage 1
Hypertension: Stage 2

1. 90/66: _____

2. 126/76: _____

3. 146/88: _____

4. 120/88: _____

5. 120/80: _____

118

6. 158/102: _____

7. 134/82: _____

8. 180/106: _____

9. 104/60: _____

10. 148/94: _____

J. Hypertension

Create a profile of an individual who is at risk for hypertension following these guidelines:

1. Using a blank piece of paper and colored pencils, crayons, or markers, draw a figure of an individual exhibiting risk factors for hypertension. Be as creative as possible.

2. Do not use any text in your drawing other than to label items you have drawn in your picture (e.g., cigarettes). A picture is worth a thousand words!

3. Include at least six risk factors for hypertension in your drawing. The Hypertension Patient Teaching Box in your textbook (page 125) can be used as a reference source.

4. In the classroom, choose a partner and trade drawings. Identify the risk factors for hypertension in your partner's drawing. Discuss with your partner what this person could do to lower his or her chances of developing hypertension.

K. Crossword Puzzle: Vital Signs

Directions: Complete the crossword puzzle using the clues provided.

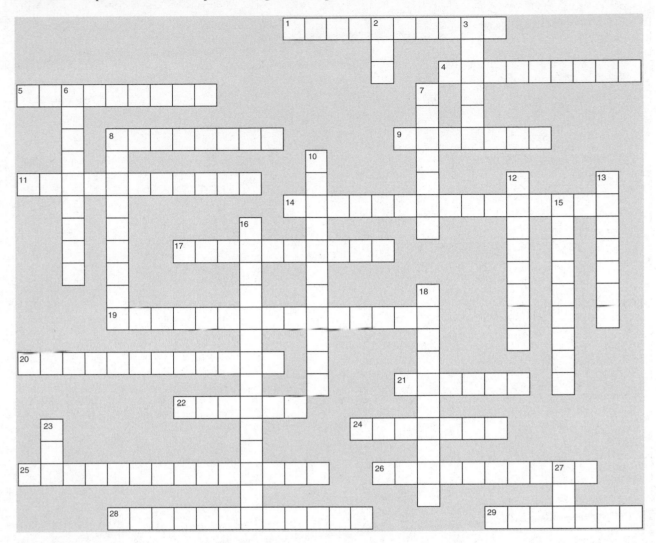

Across

1 Diaphragm or bell
4 Angled stethoscope earpieces
5 BP sounds
8 Has an S-shape
9 European temp measurement
11 Fever reducer
14 Fever increases this by 7% (for each °F)
17 U.S. temp measurement
19 Lowers pulse rate over time
20 Above 140/90
21 High BP might cause this
22 2400 mg or less per day
24 Asthma breath sounds
25 Center BP cuff over this
26 Risk factor for high BP
28 Cools body
29 Cracked earpieces can cause this

Down

2 Pulse range for exercising
3 Body temperature increaser
6 Fever that occurs with the flu
7 Invented the stethoscope
8 COPD example
10 Profuse perspiration
12 Do this after aerobic exercise
13 Leading cause of COPD
15 Fever causer
16 Drug to help COPD
18 BP position for patient's arm
23 220 minus your age
27 Good cholesterol

Notes

Measuring Body Temperature

Measure body temperature with each of the following types of thermometers, and document the results in the chart provided.

Procedures 4-1, 4-2, and 4-3: Electronic Thermometer (Oral, Axillary, and Rectal)
Procedure 4-4: Tympanic Membrane Thermometer (Aural)
Procedure 4-5: Temporal Artery Thermometer

CHART	
Date	

Measuring Pulse, Respiration, and Oxygen Saturation

Procedure 4-6: Pulse and Respiration

Measure the radial pulse and respiration. Describe the rhythm and volume of the pulse. Describe the rhythm and depth of the respirations. Document the results in the chart provided.

Procedure 4-7: Apical Pulse

Measure apical pulse. Describe the rhythm and volume of the pulse. Document the results in the chart provided.

Procedure 4-8: Pulse Oximetry

Measure the oxygen saturation level and document the results in the chart provided.

Measuring Blood Pressure

Procedure 4-9: Blood Pressure

Measure blood pressure. Document the results in the chart provided.

CHART	
Date	

Procedure 4-1: Measuring Oral Body Temperature—Electronic Thermometer

Name: _____ Date: _____

Evaluated by: _____ Score: _____

Performance Objective

Outcome:	Measure oral body temperature.
Conditions:	Given the following: electronic thermometer and oral probe, probe cover, and a waste container.
Standards:	Time: 5 minutes. Student completed procedure in _____ minutes.
	Accuracy: Satisfactory score on the Performance Evaluation Checklist.

Performance Evaluation Checklist

Trial 1	Trial 2	Point Value	Performance Standards
		•	Sanitized hands.
		•	Assembled equipment.
		•	Removed thermometer from its storage base.
		•	Attached oral probe to thermometer unit.
		•	Inserted probe into the thermometer.
		•	Greeted the patient and introduced yourself.
		•	Identified the patient and explained the procedure.
		•	Asked the patient whether he or she has ingested hot or cold beverages.
		▷	Explained what to do if the patient has recently ingested a hot or cold beverage.
		•	Removed probe from the thermometer.
		▷	Explained what occurs when probe is removed from the thermometer.
		•	Attached probe cover to probe.
		▷	Stated the purpose of the probe cover.
		•	Correctly inserted the probe in patient's mouth.
		•	Instructed the patient to keep the mouth closed.
		▷	Explained why the mouth should be kept closed.
		•	Held probe in place until an audible tone was heard.
		•	Noted patient's temperature reading on display screen.
		•	Removed probe from patient's mouth.
		•	Discarded probe cover in a regular waste container.
		•	Did not allow fingers to come in contact with cover.

Trial 1	Trial 2	Point Value	Performance Standards
		•	Returned probe to the thermometer unit.
		▷	Stated what occurs when probe is returned to the thermometer.
		•	Returned the thermometer unit to its storage base.
		•	Sanitized hands.
		•	Documented the results correctly.
		★	The temperature recording was identical to the reading on the display screen.
		▷	Stated the normal body temperature range for an adult (97° F to 99° F).
			Demonstrated the following affective behavior(s) during this procedure:
		Ⓐ	Incorporated critical thinking skills when performing patient assessment.
		★	Completed the procedure within 5 minutes.
			Totals

CHART

Date	

Evaluation of Student Performance

EVALUATION CRITERIA			COMMENTS
Symbol	**Category**	**Point Value**	
★	Critical Step	16 points	
•	Essential Step	6 points	
Ⓐ	Affective Competency	6 points	
▷	Theory Question	2 points	

Score calculation: 100 points
        −_____ points missed
        _____ Score
Satisfactory score: 85 or above

CAAHEP Competencies Achieved

Psychomotor (Skills)

☑ I. 1. b. Measure and record temperature.

Affective (Behavior)

☑ I. 1. Incorporate critical thinking skills when performing patient assessment.

ABHES Competency Achieved

☑ 8. b. Obtain vital signs, obtain patient history, and formulate chief complaint.

Notes

EVALUATION OF COMPETENCY

e Procedure 4-2: Measuring Axillary Body Temperature—Electronic Thermometer

Name: _____ Date: _____

Evaluated by: _____ Score: _____

Performance Objective

Outcome:	Measure axillary body temperature.
Conditions:	Given the following: electronic thermometer and oral probe, probe cover, and a waste container.
Standards:	Time: 5 minutes. Student completed procedure in _____ minutes.
	Accuracy: Satisfactory score on the Performance Evaluation Checklist.

Performance Evaluation Checklist

Trial 1	Trial 2	Point Value	Performance Standards
		•	Sanitized hands.
		•	Assembled equipment.
		•	Removed thermometer from its storage base.
		•	Attached oral probe to thermometer unit.
		•	Inserted probe into the thermometer.
		•	Greeted the patient and introduced yourself.
		•	Identified the patient and explained the procedure.
		•	Removed clothing from patient's shoulder and arm.
		•	Made sure that the axilla was dry.
		•	Removed probe from the thermometer.
		•	Attached probe cover to probe.
		•	Placed probe in the center of the patient's axilla.
		•	Ensured that the arm was held close to the body.
		▷	Explained why the arm must be held close to the body.
		•	Held probe in place until an audible tone was heard.
		•	Removed probe from patient's axilla.
		•	Noted patient's temperature reading on display screen.
		•	Discarded probe cover in a regular waste container.
		•	Did not allow fingers to come in contact with cover.
		•	Returned probe to the thermometer unit.
		•	Returned the thermometer unit to its storage base.

Trial 1	Trial 2	Point Value	Performance Standards
		•	Sanitized hands.
		•	Documented the results correctly.
		★	Temperature recording was identical to the reading on the display screen.
			Demonstrated the following affective behavior(s) during this procedure:
		Ⓐ	Incorporated critical thinking skills when performing patient assessment.
		★	Completed the procedure within 5 minutes.
			Totals

CHART

Date	

Evaluation of Student Performance

EVALUATION CRITERIA			COMMENTS
Symbol	**Category**	**Point Value**	
★	Critical Step	16 points	
•	Essential Step	6 points	
Ⓐ	Affective Competency	6 points	
▷	Theory Question	2 points	

Score calculation: 100 points
− _____ points missed
_____ Score

Satisfactory score: 85 or above

CAAHEP Competencies Achieved

Psychomotor (Skills)
☑ I. 1. b. Measure and record temperature.

Affective (Behavior)
☑ I. 1. Incorporate critical thinking skills when performing patient assessment.

ABHES Competency Achieved

☑ 8. b. Obtain vital signs, obtain patient history, and formulate chief complaint.

Procedure 4-3: Measuring Rectal Body Temperature—Electronic Thermometer

Name: _____ Date: _____

Evaluated by: _____ Score: _____

Performance Objective

Outcome:	Measure rectal body temperature.
Conditions:	Given the following: electronic thermometer, rectal probe, probe cover, lubricant, disposable gloves, tissues, and a waste container.
Standards:	Time: 5 minutes. Student completed procedure in _____ minutes.
	Accuracy: Satisfactory score on the Performance Evaluation Checklist.

Performance Evaluation Checklist

Trial 1	Trial 2	Point Value	Performance Standards
		•	Sanitized hands.
		•	Assembled equipment.
		•	Removed thermometer from its storage base.
		•	Attached rectal probe to thermometer unit.
		•	Inserted probe into the thermometer.
		•	Greeted the patient and introduced yourself.
		•	Identified the patient and explained the procedure.
		•	Applied gloves.
		▷	Stated the reason for applying gloves.
		•	Positioned and draped the patient.
		▷	Explained how to position an adult and an infant.
		•	Removed probe from the thermometer.
		•	Attached probe cover to probe.
		•	Applied lubricant up to a level of 1 inch.
		▷	Stated the purpose of the lubricant.
		•	Instructed patient to lie still.
		•	Separated the buttocks and properly inserted the thermometer.
		▷	Stated how far the thermometer should be inserted for adults, children, and infants.
		•	Held probe in place until an audible tone was heard.
		•	Removed the probe in the same direction as it was inserted.
		•	Noted patient's temperature reading on display screen.

131

Trial 1	Trial 2	Point Value	Performance Standards
		•	Discarded probe cover in a regular waste container.
		▷	Explained why the cover can be discarded in a regular waste container.
		•	Returned probe to the thermometer unit.
		•	Returned the thermometer unit to its storage base.
		•	Wiped the anal area with tissues.
		•	Removed gloves and sanitized hands.
		•	Documented the results correctly.
		★	The temperature recording was identical to the reading on the display screen.
			Demonstrated the following affective behavior(s) during this procedure:
		Ⓐ	Incorporated critical thinking skills when performing patient assessment.
		★	Completed the procedure within 5 minutes.
			Totals

CHART

Date	

Evaluation of Student Performance

EVALUATION CRITERIA			COMMENTS
Symbol	**Category**	**Point Value**	
★	Critical Step	16 points	
•	Essential Step	6 points	
Ⓐ	Affective Competency	6 points	
▷	Theory Question	2 points	

Score calculation: 100 points
−_____ points missed
_____ Score

Satisfactory score: 85 or above

CAAHEP Competencies Achieved

Psychomotor (Skills)

☑ I. 1. b. Measure and record temperature.

Affective (Behavior)

☑ I. 1. Incorporate critical thinking skills when performing patient assessment.

ABHES Competency Achieved

☑ 8. b. Obtain vital signs, obtain patient history, and formulate chief complaint.

Notes

Procedure 4-4: Measuring Aural Body Temperature—Tympanic Membrane Thermometer

Name: _____ Date: _____

Evaluated by: _____ Score: _____

Performance Objective

Outcome:	Measure aural body temperature.
Conditions:	Given the following: tympanic membrane thermometer, probe cover, and a waste container.
Standards:	Time: 5 minutes. Student completed procedure in _____ minutes.
	Accuracy: Satisfactory score on the Performance Evaluation Checklist.

Performance Evaluation Checklist

Trial 1	Trial 2	Point Value	Performance Standards
		•	Sanitized hands.
		•	Assembled equipment.
		•	Greeted the patient and introduced yourself.
		•	Identified the patient and explained the procedure.
		•	Removed thermometer from its storage base.
		•	Checked to make sure the probe lens was clean and intact.
		▷	Stated what might occur if the lens was dirty.
		•	Attached a cover on the probe.
		▷	Explained the purpose of the probe cover.
		•	Observed the screen to determine if the thermometer is ready to use.
		•	Held the thermometer in the dominant hand.
		•	Straightened the patient's ear canal with the nondominant hand.
		▷	Explained the purpose of straightening the ear canal.
		•	Inserted the probe into the patient's ear canal and sealed the opening without causing the patient discomfort.
		•	Pointed the tip of the probe toward the opposite temple.
		▷	Stated the reason for pointing the probe toward the opposite temple.
		•	Asked the patient to remain still.
		•	Depressed the activation button for 1 full second or until an audible tone is heard.
		•	Removed the thermometer from the ear canal and noted the patient's temperature on the display screen.
		▷	Stated what should be done if the temperature seems too low.

135

Trial 1	Trial 2	Point Value	Performance Standards
		•	Disposed of the probe cover in a waste container.
		•	Replaced the thermometer in its storage base.
		▷	Explained the reason for storing the thermometer in its base.
		•	Sanitized hands.
		•	Documented the results correctly.
		★	The temperature recording was identical to the reading on the display screen.
			Demonstrated the following affective behavior(s) during this procedure:
		Ⓐ	Incorporated critical thinking skills when performing patient assessment.
		★	Completed the procedure within 5 minutes.
			Totals

CHART	
Date	

Evaluation of Student Performance

EVALUATION CRITERIA			COMMENTS
Symbol	**Category**	**Point Value**	
★	Critical Step	16 points	
•	Essential Step	6 points	
Ⓐ	Affective Competency	6 points	
▷	Theory Question	2 points	

Score calculation: 100 points
− _____ points missed
_____ Score

Satisfactory score: 85 or above

CAAHEP Competencies Achieved

Psychomotor (Skills)

☑ I. 1. b. Measure and record temperature.

Affective (Behavior)

☑ I. 1. Incorporate critical thinking skills when performing patient assessment.

ABHES Competency Achieved

☑ 8. b. Obtain vital signs, obtain patient history, and formulate chief complaint.

Notes

Procedure 4-5: Measuring Temporal Body Temperature

Name: _____ Date: _____

Evaluated by: _____ Score: _____

Performance Objective

Outcome:	Measure temporal body temperature.
Conditions:	Given the following: temporal artery thermometer, disposable probe cover, antiseptic wipe, and a waste container.
Standards:	Time: 5 minutes. Student completed procedure in _____ minutes.
	Accuracy: Satisfactory score on the Performance Evaluation Checklist.

Performance Evaluation Checklist

Trial 1	Trial 2	Point Value	Performance Standards
		•	Sanitized the hands and assembled equipment.
		•	Greeted the patient and introduced yourself.
		•	Identified the patient and explained the procedure.
		•	Checked to make sure the probe lens is clean and intact.
		▷	Stated why the lens should be clean.
		•	Placed a disposable cover onto the probe or cleaned the probe with an antiseptic wipe and allowed it to dry.
		•	Selected an appropriate site (right or left side of the forehead).
		•	Brushed away any hair that is covering the scanning sites.
		▷	Explained why hair must be brushed away.
		•	Held the thermometer in the dominant hand with the thumb on the scan button.
		•	Gently positioned the probe of the thermometer on the center of the patient's forehead midway between the eyebrow and hairline.
		•	Depressed the scan button and kept it depressed for the entire measurement.
		▷	Stated why the scan button must be continually depressed.
		•	Slowly and gently slid the probe straight across the forehead midway between the eyebrow and the upper hairline.
		•	Continued until the hairline was reached, making sure to keep the probe flush against the forehead.
		•	Keeping the button depressed, lifted the probe from the forehead and placed it behind the earlobe for 1 to 2 seconds.
		▷	Stated why the probe is placed behind the earlobe.
		•	Released the scan button and noted the temperature on the display screen.

139

Trial 1	Trial 2	Point Value	Performance Standards
		•	Disposed of the probe cover in a regular waste container.
		•	Wiped the probe with an antiseptic wipe and allowed it to dry.
		•	Sanitized hands.
		•	Documented the results correctly.
		★	The temperature recording was identical to the reading on the display screen.
		•	Stored the thermometer in a clean, dry area.
			Demonstrated the following affective behavior(s) during this procedure:
		Ⓐ	Incorporated critical thinking skills when performing patient assessment.
		★	Completed the procedure within 5 minutes.
			Totals

CHART	
Date	

Evaluation of Student Performance

EVALUATION CRITERIA			COMMENTS
Symbol	**Category**	**Point Value**	
★	Critical Step	16 points	
•	Essential Step	6 points	
Ⓐ	Affective Competency	6 points	
▷	Theory Question	2 points	

Score calculation: 100 points
−_____ points missed
_____ Score

Satisfactory score: 85 or above

CAAHEP Competencies Achieved
Psychomotor (Skills) ☑ I. 1. b. Measure and record temperature. *Affective (Behavior)* ☑ I. 1. Incorporate critical thinking skills when performing patient assessment.

ABHES Competencies Achieved
☑ 8. b. Obtain vital signs, obtain patient history, and formulate chief complaint.

Notes

Procedure 4-6: Measuring Pulse and Respiration

Name: _____   Date: _____

Evaluated by: _____   Score: _____

Performance Objective

Outcome:	Measure radial pulse and respiration.
Conditions:	Using a watch with a second hand.
Standards:	Time: 5 minutes. Student completed procedure in _____ minutes.
	Accuracy: Satisfactory score on the Performance Evaluation Checklist.

Performance Evaluation Checklist

Trial 1	Trial 2	Point Value	Performance Standards
		•	Sanitized hands.
		•	Greeted the patient and introduced yourself.
		•	Identified the patient and explained the procedure.
		•	Observed patient for any signs that might affect the pulse rate or respiratory rate.
		▷	Stated two factors that would increase the pulse rate.
		•	Positioned the patient in a comfortable seated position.
		•	Placed three middle fingertips over the radial pulse site.
		▷	Explained why the pulse should not be taken with the thumb.
		•	Applied moderate, gentle pressure until the pulse was felt.
		▷	Stated what will occur if too much pressure is applied over the radial artery.
		•	Counted the pulse for 30 seconds and made a mental note of the number.
		•	Determined the rhythm and volume of the pulse.
		▷	Stated when the pulse should be measured for a full minute.
		•	Continued to hold the fingers on the patient's wrist.
		▷	Explained why respirations should be taken without the patient's awareness.
		•	Observed the rise and fall of patient's chest.
		•	Counted the number of respirations for 30 seconds and made a mental note of the number.
		▷	Stated what makes up one respiration.
		•	Determined the rhythm and depth of the respirations.
		•	Observed the patient's color.
		•	Sanitized hands.

Trial 1	Trial 2	Point Value	Performance Standards
		•	Multiplied the pulse and respiration values by 2.
		•	Documented the results correctly.
		★	The pulse rate was within ±2 beats of the evaluator's reading.
		★	The respiratory rate was within 1 respiration of the evaluator's measurement.
		▷	Stated the normal adult range for the pulse rate (60 to 100 beats/min).
		▷	Stated the normal adult range for the respiratory rate (12 to 20 respirations/minute).
			Demonstrated the following affective behavior(s) during this procedure:
		Ⓐ	Incorporated critical thinking skills when performing patient assessment.
		★	Completed the procedure within 5 minutes.
			Totals

CHART

Date	

Evaluation of Student Performance

EVALUATION CRITERIA			COMMENTS
Symbol	**Category**	**Point Value**	
★	Critical Step	16 points	
•	Essential Step	6 points	
Ⓐ	Affective Competency	6 points	
▷	Theory Question	2 points	

Score calculation: 100 points
          − _____ points missed
          _____ Score

Satisfactory score: 85 or above

CAAHEP Competencies Achieved

Psychomotor (Skills)

☑ I. 1. c. Measure and record pulse.

☑ I. 1. d. Measure and record respirations.

Affective (Behavior)

☑ I. 1. Incorporate critical thinking skills when performing patient assessment.

ABHES Competency Achieved

☑ 8. b. Obtain vital signs, obtain patient history, and formulate chief complaint.

Notes

Procedure 4-7: Measuring Apical Pulse

Name: _____   Date: _____

Evaluated by: _____   Score: _____

Performance Objective

Outcome:	Measure apical pulse.
Conditions:	Given the following: stethoscope and antiseptic wipe.
	Using a watch with a second hand.
Standards:	Time: 5 minutes. Student completed procedure in _____ minutes.
	Accuracy: Satisfactory score on the Performance Evaluation Checklist.

Performance Evaluation Checklist

Trial 1	Trial 2	Point Value	Performance Standards
		•	Sanitized hands.
		•	Greeted the patient and introduced yourself.
		•	Identified the patient and explained the procedure.
		•	Observed the patient for any signs that might affect the pulse rate.
		•	Assembled equipment.
		•	Rotated the chest piece to the bell position.
		•	Cleaned earpieces and chest piece with antiseptic wipe.
		▷	Stated the reason for cleaning stethoscope with an antiseptic.
		•	Asked the patient to unbutton or remove his or her shirt.
		•	Positioned patient in a sitting or lying position.
		•	Warmed chest piece of the stethoscope.
		▷	Explained the reason for warming chest piece.
		•	Inserted earpieces of stethoscope in a forward position in the ears.
		▷	Explained why the earpieces must be directed forward.
		•	Placed the chest piece over the apex of the heart.
		▷	Described the location of the apex of the heart.
		•	Counted the number of heartbeats for 30 seconds and multiplied by 2.
		★	The reading was within ±2 beats of the evaluator's reading.
		•	Sanitized hands.
		•	Documented the results correctly.

Trial 1	Trial 2	Point Value	Performance Standards
		•	Cleaned earpieces and chest piece with an antiseptic wipe.
			Demonstrated the following affective behavior(s) during this procedure:
		Ⓐ	Incorporated critical thinking skills when performing patient assessment.
		★	Completed the procedure within 5 minutes.
			Totals

CHART

Date	

Evaluation of Student Performance

EVALUATION CRITERIA			COMMENTS
Symbol	**Category**	**Point Value**	
★	Critical Step	16 points	
•	Essential Step	6 points	
Ⓐ	Affective Competency	6 points	
▷	Theory Question	2 points	

Score calculation: 100 points
− _____ points missed
_____ Score

Satisfactory score: 85 or above

CAAHEP Competencies Achieved

Psychomotor (Skills)
☑ I. 1. c. Measure and record pulse.

Affective (Behavior)
☑ I. 1. Incorporate critical thinking skills when performing patient assessment.

ABHES Competency Achieved

☑ 8. b. Obtain vital signs, obtain patient history, and formulate chief complaint.

Procedure 4-8: Performing Pulse Oximetry

Name: _____ Date: _____

Evaluated by: _____ Score: _____

Performance Objective

Outcome:	Perform pulse oximetry.
Conditions:	Given the following: handheld pulse oximeter, reusable finger probe, and an antiseptic wipe.
Standards:	Time: 5 minutes. Student completed procedure in _____ minutes.
	Accuracy: Satisfactory score on the Performance Evaluation Checklist.

Performance Evaluation Checklist

Trial 1	Trial 2	Point Value	Performance Standards
		•	Sanitized hands and assembled equipment.
		•	Ensured the probe opened and closed smoothly and that the windows were clean.
		•	Disinfected the probe windows and platforms and allowed them to dry.
		▷	Stated the purpose of disinfecting the probe windows.
		•	If necessary, connected the probe to the cable.
		•	Connected the cable to the monitor.
		•	Did not lift or carry the monitor by the cable.
		•	Greeted the patient and introduced yourself.
		•	Identified the patient and explained the procedure.
		•	Seated the patient in a chair with the lower arm supported and the palm facing down.
		▷	Explained why the arm should be supported.
		•	Selected an appropriate finger to apply the probe.
		•	Observed the patient's finger to make sure it is free of dark fingernail polish or an artificial nail.
		•	Checked to make sure the patient's fingertip is clean.
		•	Checked to make sure the patient's finger is not cold.
		▷	Explained what to do if the patient's finger is cold.
		•	Made sure that ambient light will not interfere with the measurement.
		▷	Explained why ambient light should be avoided.
		•	Positioned the probe securely on the fingertip with the fleshy tip of the finger covering the window.
		•	Allowed the cable to lie across the back of the hand and parallel to the arm of the patient.

149

Trial 1	Trial 2	Point Value	Performance Standards
		•	Instructed the patient to remain still and to breathe normally.
		▷	Stated why the patient must remain still.
		•	Turned on the pulse oximeter.
		•	Waited while the oximeter went through its power-on self-test (POST).
		▷	Explained the purpose of the POST.
		•	Allowed several seconds for the oximeter to detect the pulse and calculate the oxygen saturation.
		•	Ensured that the pulse strength indicator fluctuates with each pulsation and that the pulse signal is strong.
		▷	Stated what should be done if the oximeter is unable to locate a pulse.
		•	Left the probe in place until the oximeter displayed a reading.
		•	Noted the oxygen saturation value and pulse rate.
		★	The reading was identical to the evaluator's reading.
		▷	Stated the normal oxygen saturation level of a healthy adult (95% to 99%).
		▷	Stated what should be done if the oxygen saturation is less than 95%.
		•	Removed the probe from the patient's finger and turned off the oximeter.
		•	Sanitized hands.
		•	Documented the results correctly.
		•	Disconnected the cable from the monitor.
		•	Disinfected the probe with an antiseptic wipe.
		•	Properly stored the monitor in a clean, dry area.
			Demonstrated the following affective behavior(s) during this procedure:
		Ⓐ	Incorporated critical thinking skills when performing patient assessment.
		★	Completed the procedure within 5 minutes.
			Totals

CHART

Date	

Evaluation of Student Performance

EVALUATION CRITERIA			COMMENTS
Symbol	**Category**	**Point Value**	
★	Critical Step	16 points	
•	Essential Step	6 points	
Ⓐ	Affective Competency	6 points	
▷	Theory Question	2 points	

Score calculation: 100 points
    − _____ points missed
    _____ Score
Satisfactory score: 85 or above

CAAHEP Competencies Achieved

Psychomotor (Skills)
☑ I. 1. i. Measure and record pulse oximetry.

Affective (Behavior)
☑ I. 1. Incorporate critical thinking skills when performing patient assessment.

ABHES Competency Achieved

☑ 8. b. Obtain vital signs, obtain patient history, and formulate chief complaint.

Notes

Procedure 4-9: Measuring Blood Pressure

Name: _____   Date: _____

Evaluated by: _____   Score: _____

Performance Objective

Outcome:	Measure blood pressure.
Conditions:	Given the following: stethoscope, sphygmomanometer, and an antiseptic wipe.
Standards:	Time: 5 minutes. Student completed procedure in _____ minutes.
	Accuracy: Satisfactory score on the Performance Evaluation Checklist.

Performance Evaluation Checklist

Trial 1	Trial 2	Point Value	Performance Standards
		•	Sanitized hands.
		•	Assembled equipment.
		•	Rotated the chest piece to the diaphragm position.
		•	Cleaned earpieces and chest piece of stethoscope with an antiseptic wipe.
		•	Greeted the patient and introduced yourself.
		•	Identified the patient and explained the procedure.
		•	Observed patient for any signs that might influence the blood pressure reading.
		▷	Stated signs that would influence the blood pressure reading.
		•	Determined how high to pump the cuff (palpated systolic pressure or checked the patient's medical record).
		•	Positioned patient in a sitting position with the legs uncrossed.
		•	Made sure that the patient's arm was uncovered.
		▷	Explained why blood pressure should not be taken over clothing.
		•	Positioned patient's arm at heart level with the palm facing up.
		•	Selected the proper cuff size.
		▷	Explained how to determine the proper cuff size.
		▷	Made sure the cuff was completely deflated and there was no residual air in the cuff.
		•	Located the brachial pulse with the fingertips.
		▷	Stated the location of the brachial pulse.
		•	Centered bladder over the brachial pulse site.
		▷	Explained why the bladder should be centered over the brachial pulse site.

Trial 1	Trial 2	Point Value	Performance Standards
		•	Placed cuff on patient's arm 1 to 2 inches above bend in elbow.
		•	Wrapped cuff smoothly and snugly around patient's arm and secured it.
		•	Positioned self and/or manometer for direct viewing and at a distance of no more than 3 feet.
		•	Instructed the patient not to talk.
		•	Inserted earpieces of stethoscope in a forward position in the ears.
		•	Located the brachial pulse again.
		•	Placed diaphragm of the stethoscope over the brachial pulse site to make a tight seal.
		▷	Explained why there should be good contact of the chest piece with the skin.
		•	Made sure chest piece was not touching cuff.
		▷	Explained why the chest piece should not touch the cuff.
		•	Closed valve on bulb by turning thumbscrew to the right.
		•	Rapidly pumped air into cuff up to a level approximately 30 mm Hg above the palpated or previously measured systolic pressure.
		•	Did not overinflate the cuff.
		▷	Explained why the cuff should not be overinflated.
		•	Released pressure at a moderate, steady rate by turning thumbscrew to the left.
		•	Heard and noted the first clear tapping sound (systolic pressure).
		•	Continued to deflate the cuff for another 10 mm Hg.
		•	Heard and noted the point on the scale at which the sounds ceased (diastolic pressure).
		•	Quickly and completely deflated cuff to zero and removed earpieces from ears.
		▷	Stated how long to wait before taking the blood pressure again on the same arm.
		•	Carefully removed cuff from patient's arm.
		•	Sanitized hands.
		•	Documented the results correctly.
		★	The reading was within ±2 mm Hg of the evaluator's reading.
		▷	Stated the normal blood pressure for an adult (less than 120/80 mm Hg).
		•	Cleaned earpieces and chest piece with an antiseptic wipe.
			Demonstrated the following affective behavior(s) during this procedure:
		Ⓐ	Incorporated critical thinking skills when performing patient assessment.
		★	Completed the procedure within 5 minutes.
			Totals

CHART

Date	

Evaluation of Student Performance

EVALUATION CRITERIA			COMMENTS
Symbol	**Category**	**Point Value**	
★	Critical Step	16 points	
•	Essential Step	6 points	
Ⓐ	Affective Competency	6 points	
▷	Theory Question	2 points	

Score calculation: 100 points

－ _____ points missed

_____ Score

Satisfactory score: 85 or above

CAAHEP Competencies Achieved

Psychomotor (Skills)

☑ I. 1. a. Measure and record blood pressure.

Affective (Behavior)

☑ I. 1. Incorporate critical thinking skills when performing patient assessment.

ABHES Competency Achieved

☑ 8. b. Obtain vital signs, obtain patient history, and formulate chief complaint.

5 The Physical Examination

CHAPTER ASSIGNMENTS

√ After Completing	Date Due	Study Guide Pages	STUDY GUIDE ASSIGNMENTS (CTA = Critical Thinking Activity)	Possible Points	Points You Earned
		161	📰 Pretest	10	
		162	🔑 Term Key Term Assessment		
		162	A. Definitions	17	
		162	B. Word Parts	9	
			(Add 1 point for each key term)		
		163-166	📋 Evaluation of Learning questions	31	
		166-167	CTA A. Preparation of the Examining Room	10	
		167	CTA B: Reading Weight Measurements	15	
			_e_ Evolve Site: By the Pound (Record points earned)		
		168	CTA C: Reading Height Measurements	11	
			_e_ Evolve Site: Feet and Inches (Record points earned)		
		169	CTA D: Calculating BMI	12	
		169-170	CTA E: Patient Positions	10	
			_e_ Evolve Site: Let's Get Physical (Record points earned)		
		170	CTA F: Examination Techniques	10	
		171	CTA G: Crossword Puzzle	25	
			_e_ Evolve Site: Apply Your Knowledge questions	10	
			_e_ Evolve Site: Video Evaluation	54	
		161	📰 Posttest	10	

√ After Completing	Date Due	Study Guide Pages	STUDY GUIDE ASSIGNMENTS (CTA = Critical Thinking Activity)	Possible Points	Points You Earned
			ADDITIONAL ASSIGNMENTS		
			Total points		

√ When Assigned by Your Instructor	Study Guide Pages	Practices Required	LABORATORY ASSIGNMENTS (Procedure Number and Name)	Score*
	173	5	**Practice for Competency** 5-1: Measuring Weight and Height Textbook reference: pp. 151-153	
	175-177		**Evaluation of Competency** 5-1: Measuring Weight and Height	*
	173		**Practice for Competency** 5-A: Body Mechanics Textbook reference: pp. 153-156	
	179-181		**Evaluation of Competency** 5-A: Body Mechanics	*
	173	3	**Practice for Competency** 5-2: Sitting Position Textbook reference: p. 157	
	183-184		**Evaluation of Competency** 5-2: Sitting Position	*
	173	3	**Practice for Competency** 5-3: Supine Position Textbook reference: p. 158	
	185-186		**Evaluation of Competency** 5-3: Supine Position	*
	173	3	**Practice for Competency** 5-4: Prone Position Textbook reference: p. 159	
	187-188		**Evaluation of Competency** 5-4: Prone Position	*
	173	3	**Practice for Competency** 5-5: Dorsal Recumbent Position Textbook reference: p. 160	
	189-190		**Evaluation of Competency** 5-5: Dorsal Recumbent Position	*
	173	3	**Practice for Competency** 5-6: Lithotomy Position Textbook reference: pp. 161-162	
	191-193		**Evaluation of Competency** 5-6: Lithotomy Position	*
	173	3	**Practice for Competency** 5-7: Sims Position Textbook reference: pp. 162-163	

Chapter **5** **The Physical Examination**

√ When Assigned by Your Instructor	Study Guide Pages	Practices Required	LABORATORY ASSIGNMENTS (Procedure Number and Name)	Score*
	195-196		**Evaluation of Competency** 5-7: Sims Position	*
	173	3	**Practice for Competency** 5-8: Knee-Chest Position Textbook reference: pp. 163-164	
	197-199		**Evaluation of Competency** 5-8: Knee-Chest Position	*
	173	3	**Practice for Competency** 5-9: Fowler Position Textbook reference: pp. 164-165	
	201-202		**Evaluation of Competency** 5-9: Fowler Position	*
	173	3	**Practice for Competency** 5-10: Wheelchair Transfer Textbook reference: pp. 166-169	
	203-206		**Evaluation of Competency** 5-10: Wheelchair Transfer	*
	173	3	**Practice for Competency** 5-11: Assisting with the Physical Examination Textbook reference: pp. 174-177	
	207-210		**Evaluation of Competency** 5-11: Assisting with the Physical Examination	*
			ADDITIONAL ASSIGNMENTS	

PRETEST

True or False

_____ 1. A complete patient examination consists of a physical examination and laboratory tests.

_____ 2. Arthritis is an example of a chronic illness.

_____ 3. An otoscope is used to examine the eyes.

_____ 4. A patient should be identified by name and date of birth.

_____ 5. The reason for weighing a prenatal patient is to determine the baby's due date.

_____ 6. The height of an adult is measured during every office visit.

_____ 7. The lithotomy position is used to examine the vagina.

_____ 8. Inspection involves the observation of the patient for any signs of disease.

_____ 9. Measuring blood pressure is an example of auscultation.

_____ 10. The supine position is used to examine the back.

POSTTEST

True or False

_____ 1. The prognosis is what is wrong with the patient.

_____ 2. A risk factor means that a patient will develop a certain disease.

_____ 3. Electrocardiography is an example of a therapeutic procedure.

_____ 4. The function of a speculum is to open a body orifice for viewing.

_____ 5. The process of measuring the patient is called mensuration.

_____ 6. A reason for weighing a child is to determine drug dosage.

_____ 7. The purpose of draping a patient is to make it easier for the provider to examine the patient.

_____ 8. Sims position is used for flexible sigmoidoscopy.

_____ 9. Measuring pulse is an example of percussion.

_____ 10. BMI is the acronym for body mass index.

A. Definitions

Directions: Match each key term with its definition.

_____D_____ 1. Audiometer

_____J_____ 2. Auscultation

_____P_____ 3. Bariatrics

_____Q_____ 4. Body mechanics

_____B_____ 5. Clinical diagnosis

_____F_____ 6. Diagnosis

_____K_____ 7. Differential diagnosis

_____H_____ 8. Inspection

_____E_____ 9. Mensuration

_____A_____ 10. Ophthalmoscope

_____L_____ 11. Otoscope

_____M_____ 12. Palpation

_____G_____ 13. Percussion

_____N_____ 14. Percussion hammer

_____O_____ 15. Prognosis

_____C_____ 16. Speculum

_____I_____ 17. Symptom

A. An instrument for examining the interior of the eye

B. A tentative diagnosis obtained through the evaluation of the health history and the physical examination, without the benefit of laboratory or diagnostic tests

C. An instrument for opening a body orifice or cavity for viewing

D. An instrument used to measure hearing

E. The process of measuring a patient

F. The scientific method for determining and identifying a patient's condition

G. The process of tapping the body to detect signs of disease

H. The process of observing a patient to detect any signs of disease

I. Any change in the body or its functioning that indicates that a disease might be present

J. The process of listening to the sounds produced within the body to detect signs of disease

K. A determination of which of two or more diseases with similar symptoms is producing the patient's symptoms

L. An instrument for examining the external ear canal and tympanic membrane

M. The process of feeling with the hands to detect signs of disease

N. An instrument with a rubber head, used for testing reflexes

O. The probable course and outcome of a patient's condition and the patient's prospects for recovery

P. The branch of medicine that deals with the treatment and control of obesity and diseases associated with obesity

Q. Use of the correct muscles to maintain proper balance, posture, and body alignment to accomplish a task safely and efficiently

B. Word Parts

Directions: Indicate the meaning of each word part in the space provided. List as many medical terms as possible that incorporate the word part in the space provided.

Word Part	Meaning of Word Part	Medical Terms That Incorporate Word Part
1. audi/o		
2. -meter		
3. bar/o		
4. -iatrics		
5. dia-		
6. -gnosis		
7. ophthalm/o		
8. -scope		
9. ot/o		

Directions: Fill in each blank with the correct answer.

1. What are the three parts of a complete patient examination?

   _____

   _____

2. List two functions of the physical examination.

   _____

   _____

3. What is the purpose of establishing a final diagnosis?

   _____

   _____

4. Why is there a space for indicating the clinical diagnosis on the laboratory request form?

   _____

   _____

5. What is a risk factor?

   _____

   _____

6. What is an acute illness? List two examples of acute illnesses.

   _____

   _____

7. What is a chronic illness? List two examples of chronic illnesses.

   _____

   _____

8. What is the difference between a therapeutic procedure and a diagnostic procedure?

   _____

   _____

   _____

9. How should a patient be identified?

   _____

   _____

163

10. Why is it important to properly identify the patient?

_____

_____

11. How can patient apprehension be reduced during a physical examination?

_____

_____

12. Why should patients be asked if they need to void before the physical examination?

_____

_____

13. What are two examples of locations for placing a paper-based patient record (PPR) for review by the provider?

_____

_____

14. What is the purpose for measuring weight?

_____

_____

15. Why is it important to use proper body mechanics?

_____

_____

16. What are the four curvatures of the vertebral column, and what is their purpose?

_____

_____

17. What body mechanics principles should be followed for each of the following?

a. Physical condition of the body

_____

_____

b. Reaching for something

_____

_____

c. Working height

_____

_____

d. Storing heavy and lighter items on shelves

_____

_____

e. Retrieving an item from an overhead shelf

_____

_____

f. Lifting an object

_____

_____

g. Transferring a patient

_____

_____

h. Patient who starts to fall

_____

_____

i. You are unsure about your ability to lift a heavy object

_____

_____

18. What is the purpose of positioning and draping?

_____

_____

_____

19. Indicate three types of examinations for which the supine position is used.

_____

_____

20. Indicate two types of examinations for which the lithotomy position is used.

_____

_____

21. Indicate one type of examination for which the knee-chest position is used.

_____

_____

22. What is the purpose of a wheelchair?

_____

_____

23. What is the purpose of a transfer belt for both the patient and the medical assistant?

_____

_____

24. What should the medical assistant do if he or she does not think it is possible to transfer a patient from a wheelchair to the examining table?

_____

_____

25. What is performed during a complete physical examination?

_____

_____

26. What is the advantage of using EMR software to document the results of a physical examination?

_____

_____

27. What are four types of assessments that can be made through inspection?

_____

_____

28. What are four types of assessments that can be made through palpation?

_____

_____

29. What can be assessed through the use of percussion?

_____

_____

30. What types of assessments can be made using auscultation?

_____

_____

31. What type of stethoscope chest piece should be used to assess the heart?

_____

CRITICAL THINKING ACTIVITIES

A. Preparation of the Examining Room

For each of the following examining room preparation guidelines, indicate the problems that may result if the guideline is not followed.

	Preparation	Problems If Not Performed
1.	Ensure the examining room is well lit.	
2.	Restock supplies that are getting low.	
3.	Empty waste containers frequently.	
4.	Replace biohazard containers as necessary.	

	Preparation	Problems If Not Performed
5.	Make sure room is well ventilated.	
6.	Maintain room temperature that is comfortable for the patient.	
7.	Clean and disinfect examining table daily.	
8.	Change the examining table paper after each patient.	
9.	Check equipment and instruments to make sure they are in proper working condition.	
10.	Know how to operate and care for each piece of equipment and instrument.	

B. Reading Weight Measurements

The diagram is an illustration of a portion of the calibration bar of an upright balance beam scale. In the spaces provided, document the weight measurements indicated on the calibration bar. In all cases, assume that the lower weight is resting in the 100-lb notched groove.

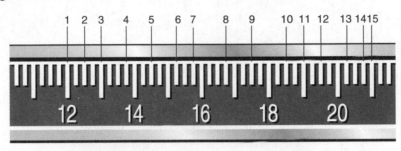

1. _____

2. _____

3. _____

4. _____

5. _____

6. _____

7. _____

8. _____

9. _____

10. _____

11. _____

12. _____

13. _____

14. _____

15. _____

167

C. Reading Height Measurements

The diagram is an illustration of a portion of the calibration rod of an upright balance beam scale. In the spaces provided, indicate the height measurements in feet and inches indicated on the calibration rod.

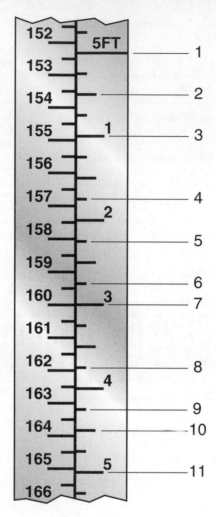

1. _____

2. _____

3. _____

4. _____

5. _____

6. _____

7. _____

8. _____

9. _____

10. _____

11. _____

D. Calculating Body Mass Index

1. Using the Highlight on Body Mass Index box on page 151 of your textbook, determine your BMI. Interpret your BMI using Table 5-2: Interpretation of Body Mass Index (BMI) in your textbook. Document the results below.

   _____

2. Determine the BMI of the following individuals and document the value in the space provided. Interpret each BMI value according to the information indicated in Table 5-2 in your textbook.

	Weight	Height	BMI	Interpretation of BMI
1.	146	5 ft 5 in		
2.	175	5 ft 6 in		
3.	110	5 ft 9 in		
4.	122	5 ft 1 in		
5.	260	6 ft		
6.	180	6 ft 8 in		
7.	330	5 ft 11 in		
8.	150	5 ft 4 in		
9.	170	5 ft 2 in		
10.	151	6 ft 4 in		

3. List the diseases that an individual with an above-normal BMI has an increased chance of developing.

   _____

   _____

   _____

   _____

E. Patient Positions

In which position would you place the patient for the following examinations or procedures?

1. Measurement of rectal temperature of an adult _____

2. Examination of the back _____

3. Measurement of vital signs _____

4. Pelvic examination _____

5. Examination of the upper extremities _____

6. Examination of the eyes, ears, nose, and throat _____

7. Examination of the breasts _____

8. Flexible sigmoidoscopy _____

9. Administration of an enema _____

10. Examination of the upper body of a patient with emphysema _____

F. Examination Techniques

List the examination technique (e.g., inspection, palpation, percussion, auscultation) that is used in each of the following situations.

1. A patient with a stutter _____

2. Taking the radial pulse _____

3. Finding the location of the apical pulse _____

4. Taking the apical pulse _____

5. Taking respiration (may be two answers, depending on method) _____

6. A patient with cracked lips _____

7. Checking for lumps in the breast _____

8. Checking reflexes _____

9. Obtaining the fetal heart rate _____

10. A patient with a fever (may be several methods) _____

G. Crossword Puzzle: The Physical Examination

Directions: Complete the crossword puzzle using the clues provided.

Across

1. Eye examiner
5. Ear examiner
7. BMI: 16 to 18.49
9. BMI: 25 to 29.9
10. "Listen to heart" position
14. Measuring the patient
16. I am listening
20. Metric unit of height
22. Metric unit of weight
23. Curative procedure
24. Reflex tester
25. Can cause premature death

Down

2. Hearing tester
3. Flex sigmoid position
4. Face-down
6. Orifice opener
8. What is the probable outcome?
11. What is wrong with you?
12. Before you measure weight
13. GYN position
15. Five feet in inches
17. Severe and intense condition
18. Provides warmth and modesty
19. Long-time illness
21. Face-up

171

Notes

PRACTICE FOR COMPETENCY

Procedure 5-1: Weight and Height
Take weight and height measurements. Document results in the chart provided.

Procedure 5-A: Body Mechanics
Demonstrate proper body mechanics while standing, sitting, and lifting an object.

Procedures 5-2 to 5-9: Positioning and Draping
Position and drape an individual in each of the following positions: sitting, supine, prone, dorsal recumbent, lithotomy, Sims, knee-chest, and Fowler.

Procedure 5-10: Wheelchair Transfer
Transfer a patient from a wheelchair to the examining table and from the examining table to a wheelchair.

Procedure 5-11: Assisting with the Physical Examination
Prepare the patient and assist with a physical examination. In the chart provided, document the results of the procedures you performed while assisting with the examination (e.g., vital signs, height, and weight).

CHART	
Date	

CHART	
Date	

Procedure 5-1: Measuring Weight and Height

Name: _____   Date: _____

Evaluated by: _____   Score: _____

Performance Objective

Outcome:	Measure weight and height.
Conditions:	Given a paper towel.
	Using an upright balance scale.
Standards:	Time: 5 minutes. Student completed procedure in _____ minutes.
	Accuracy: Satisfactory score on the Performance Evaluation Checklist.

Performance Evaluation Checklist

Trial 1	Trial 2	Point Value	Performance Standards
			Weight
		•	Sanitized hands.
			Checked the balance scale for accuracy
		•	Verified that the upper and lower weights were on zero.
		•	Looked at the indicator point to make sure the scale is balanced.
		▷	Stated what will be observed if the scale is balanced.
		▷	Explained what to do if the indicator point rests below the center.
		▷	Explained what to do if the indicator point rests above the center.
		▷	Stated what occurs if the scale is not balanced.
		•	Greeted the patient and introduced yourself.
		•	Identified the patient and explained the procedure.
		•	Instructed the patient to remove shoes and heavy outer clothing.
		•	Placed paper towel on the scale.
		•	Assisted the patient onto the scale.
		•	Instructed the patient not to move.
			Balanced the scale
		•	Moved the lower weight to the groove that did not cause the indicator point to drop to the bottom of the balance area.
		▷	Stated why the lower weight should be seated firmly in its groove.
		•	Slid the upper weight slowly until the indicator point came to a rest at the center of the balance area.

175

Trial 1	Trial 2	Point Value	Performance Standards
		•	Read the results to the nearest quarter pound. Jotted down this value or made a mental note of it.
		★	The reading was identical to the evaluator's reading.
		•	Asked the patient to step off the scale.
			Height
		•	Slid the calibration rod until it was above the patient's height.
		•	Opened the measuring bar to its horizontal position.
		•	Instructed the patient to step onto the scale platform with his or her back to the scale.
		•	Instructed the patient to stand erect and to look straight ahead.
		•	Carefully lowered the measuring bar until it rested gently on top of the patient's head.
		•	Verified that the bar was in a horizontal position.
		•	Instructed the patient to step down and put on his or her shoes.
		•	Read the marking to the nearest quarter inch. Jotted down this value or made a mental note of it.
		★	The reading was identical to the evaluator's reading.
		•	Returned the measuring bar to its vertical position.
		•	Slid the calibration rod to its lowest position.
		•	Returned the weights to zero.
		•	Sanitized hands.
			Demonstrated the following affective behavior(s) during this procedure:
		Ⓐ	Documented the results correctly.
		Ⓐ	Demonstrated (a) empathy (b) active listening (c) nonverbal communication.
		•	Demonstrated the principles of self-boundaries.
		★	Completed the procedure within 5 minutes.
			Totals

CHART	
Date	

Evaluation of Student Performance

EVALUATION CRITERIA			COMMENTS
Symbol	**Category**	**Point Value**	
★	Critical Step	16 points	
•	Essential Step	6 points	
Ⓐ	Affective Competency	6 points	
▷	Theory Question	2 points	

Score calculation: 100 points
−_____ points missed
_____ Score

Satisfactory score: 85 or above

CAAHEP Competencies Achieved

Psychomotor (Skills)

☑ I. 1. e. Measure and record height.

☑ I. 1. f. Measure and record weight.

Affective (Behavior)

☑ V. 1. Demonstrate (a) empathy (b) active listening (c) nonverbal communication.

☑ V. 2. Demonstrate the principles of self-boundaries.

ABHES Competencies Achieved

☑ 7. g. Display professionalism through written and verbal communication.

☑ 8. c. Assist provider with general/physical examination.

Notes

Procedure 5-A: Body Mechanics

Name: _____   Date: _____

Evaluated by: _____   Score: _____

Performance Objective

Outcome:	Demonstrate proper body mechanics while standing, sitting, and lifting an object.
Conditions:	Given the following: object for lifting.
	Using a chair.
Standards:	Time: 10 minutes. Student completed procedure in _____ minutes.
	Accuracy: Satisfactory score on the Performance Evaluation Checklist.

Performance Evaluation Checklist

Trial 1	Trial 2	Point Value	Performance Standards
			Standing
		•	Wore comfortable low-heeled shoes that provide good support.
		•	Held the head erect at the midline of the body.
		•	Maintained the back as straight as possible with the pelvis tucked inward.
		•	The chest is forward with the shoulders back and the abdomen drawn in and kept flat.
		▷	Stated the purpose of standing correctly.
		•	Knees are slightly flexed.
		•	Feet are pointing forward and parallel to each other about 3 inches apart.
		▷	Explained the reason for proper positioning of the feet.
		•	Arms are positioned comfortably at the side.
		•	Weight of the body is evenly distributed over both feet.
			Sitting
		•	Sat in a chair with a firm back.
		•	Back and buttocks are supported against the back of the chair.
		•	Body weight is evenly distributed over the buttocks and thighs.
		•	A small pillow or rolled towel is used.
		▷	Stated the use of the pillow or rolled towel.
		•	Feet are flat on the floor.
		•	Knees are level with the hips.

Trial 1	Trial 2	Point Value	Performance Standards
		▷	Explained what to do if prolonged sitting is required.
			Lifting
		•	Determined the weight of the object.
		▷	Stated the purpose of determining the weight of an object before lifting it.
		•	Stood in front of the object with the feet 6 to 8 inches apart.
		•	The toes are pointed outward and one foot is slightly forward.
		•	Tightened the stomach and gluteal muscles in preparation for the lift.
		•	Bent the body at the knees and hips.
		▷	Stated the purpose of bending the body at the knees and hips.
		•	Grasped the object firmly with both hands.
		•	Lifted the object smoothly with the leg muscles while keeping the back straight.
		▷	Stated why the leg muscles and not the back muscles should be used to lift the object.
		•	Held the object as close to the body as possible at waist level.
		▷	Stated why the object should not be lifted higher than the chest.
		•	Turned by pivoting the whole body.
		•	Made sure the area of transport of the object is dry and free of clutter.
		•	Lowered the object slowly while bending from the knees.
		★	Completed the procedures within 10 minutes.
			Totals

Evaluation of Student Performance

EVALUATION CRITERIA			COMMENTS
Symbol	**Category**	**Point Value**	
★	Critical Step	16 points	
•	Essential Step	6 points	
Ⓐ	Affective Competency	6 points	
▷	Theory Question	2 points	

Score calculation: 100 points
     − _____ points missed
       _____ Score

Satisfactory score: 85 or above

CAAHEP Competencies Achieved

Psychomotor (Skills)
☑ XII. 3. Use proper body mechanics.

ABHES Competencies Achieved

☑ 4. e. Perform risk management procedures.

Notes

Procedure 5-2: Sitting Position

Name: _____   Date: _____

Evaluated by: _____   Score: _____

Performance Objective

Outcome:	Position and drape an individual in the sitting position.
Conditions:	Given the following: a patient gown and a drape.
	Using an examining table.
Standards:	Time: 5 minutes. Student completed procedure in _____ minutes.
	Accuracy: Satisfactory score on the Performance Evaluation Checklist.

Performance Evaluation Checklist

Trial 1	Trial 2	Point Value	Performance Standards
		•	Sanitized hands.
		•	Greeted the patient and introduced yourself.
		•	Identified the patient.
		•	Explained what type of examination or procedure will be performed.
		•	Provided the patient with a patient gown.
		•	Instructed the patient to remove clothing and to put on a patient gown with the opening in front.
		▷	Stated what qualities the disrobing facility should have.
		•	Pulled out the footrest and assisted the patient into a sitting position.
		•	The patient's buttocks and thighs were firmly supported on the edge of the table.
		•	Placed a drape over the patient's thighs and legs.
		•	Assisted the patient off the table after the examination.
		•	Returned the footrest to its normal position.
		•	Instructed the patient to get dressed.
		•	Discarded the gown and drape in a waste container.
		▷	Stated one use of the sitting position.
			Demonstrated the following affective behavior(s) during this procedure:
		Ⓐ	Demonstrated the principles of self-boundaries.
		★	Completed the procedure within 5 minutes.
			Totals

Evaluation of Student Performance

EVALUATION CRITERIA			COMMENTS
Symbol	**Category**	**Point Value**	
★	Critical Step	16 points	
•	Essential Step	6 points	
Ⓐ	Affective Competency	6 points	
▷	Theory Question	2 points	

Score calculation: 100 points
     −   _____ points missed
        _____ Score

Satisfactory score: 85 or above

CAAHEP Competencies Achieved

Psychomotor (Skills)

☑ I. 8. Instruct and prepare a patient for a procedure or a treatment.

☑ XII. 3. Use proper body mechanics.

Affective (Behavior)

☑ V. 2. Demonstrate the principles of self-boundaries.

ABHES Competency Achieved

☑ 8. c. Assist provider with general/physical examination.

Procedure 5-3: Supine Position

Name: _____   Date: _____

Evaluated by: _____   Score: _____

Performance Objective

Outcome:	Position and drape an individual in the supine position.
Conditions:	Given the following: a patient gown and a drape.
	Using an examining table.
Standards:	Time: 5 minutes. Student completed procedure in _____ minutes.
	Accuracy: Satisfactory score on the Performance Evaluation Checklist.

Performance Evaluation Checklist

Trial 1	Trial 2	Point Value	Performance Standards
		•	Sanitized hands.
		•	Greeted the patient and introduced yourself.
		•	Identified the patient.
		•	Explained what type of examination or procedure will be performed.
		•	Provided the patient with a patient gown.
		•	Instructed the patient to remove clothing and to put on a patient gown with the opening in front.
		•	Pulled out the footrest and assisted the patient into a sitting position.
		•	Placed a drape over the patient's thighs and legs.
		•	Asked the patient to move back on the table.
		•	Pulled out the table extension while supporting the patient's lower legs.
		•	Asked the patient to lie down on his or her back with the legs together.
		•	Placed the patient's arms above the head or alongside the body.
		•	Positioned the drape lengthwise over the patient.
		▷	Stated the purpose of the drape.
		•	Moved the drape according to the body parts being examined.
		•	Assisted the patient back into a sitting position after the examination.
		•	Slid the table extension back into place while supporting the patient's lower legs.
		•	Assisted the patient from the examining table.
		•	Returned the footrest to its normal position.

Trial 1	Trial 2	Point Value	Performance Standards
		•	Instructed the patient to get dressed.
		•	Discarded the gown and drape in a waste container.
		▷	Stated one use of the supine position.
			Demonstrated the following affective behavior(s) during this procedure:
		Ⓐ	Demonstrated the principles of self-boundaries.
		★	Completed the procedure within 5 minutes.
			Totals

Evaluation of Student Performance

EVALUATION CRITERIA			COMMENTS
Symbol	**Category**	**Point Value**	
★	Critical Step	16 points	
•	Essential Step	6 points	
Ⓐ	Affective Competency	6 points	
▷	Theory Question	2 points	

Score calculation: 100 points
− _____ points missed
_____ Score

Satisfactory score: 85 or above

CAAHEP Competencies Achieved

Psychomotor (Skills)
☑ I. 8. Instruct and prepare a patient for a procedure or a treatment.
☑ XII. 3. Use proper body mechanics.

Affective (Behavior)
☑ V. 2. Demonstrate the principles of self-boundaries.

ABHES Competency Achieved

☑ 8. c. Assist provider with general/physical examination.

Procedure 5-4: Prone Position

Name: _____   Date: _____

Evaluated by: _____   Score: _____

Performance Objective

Outcome:	Position and drape an individual in the prone position.
Conditions:	Given the following: a patient gown and a drape.
	Using an examining table.
Standards:	Time: 5 minutes. Student completed procedure in _____ minutes.
	Accuracy: Satisfactory score on the Performance Evaluation Checklist.

Performance Evaluation Checklist

Trial 1	Trial 2	Point Value	Performance Standards
		•	Sanitized hands.
		•	Greeted the patient and introduced yourself.
		•	Identified the patient.
		•	Explained what type of examination or procedure will be performed.
		•	Provided the patient with a patient gown.
		•	Instructed the patient to remove clothing and to put on a patient gown with the opening in back.
		•	Pulled out the footrest and assisted the patient into a sitting position.
		•	Placed a drape over the patient's thighs and legs.
		•	Asked the patient to move back on the table.
		•	Pulled out the table extension while supporting the patient's lower legs.
		•	Asked the patient to lie down on his or her back.
		•	Positioned the drape lengthwise over the patient.
		•	Asked the patient to turn onto his or her stomach by rolling toward you.
		•	Provided assistance.
		▷	Stated the reason for providing assistance.
		•	Positioned the patient with his or her legs together and the head turned to one side.
		•	Placed the patient's arms above the head or alongside the body.
		•	Adjusted the drape as needed.
		•	Moved the drape according to the body parts being examined.

187

Trial 1	Trial 2	Point Value	Performance Standards
		•	Assisted the patient into the supine position after the examination.
		•	Assisted the patient into a sitting position.
		•	Slid the table extension back into place while supporting the patient's lower legs.
		•	Assisted the patient from the examining table.
		•	Returned the footrest to its normal position.
		•	Instructed the patient to get dressed.
		•	Discarded the gown and drape in a waste container.
		▷	Stated one use of the prone position.
			Demonstrated the following affective behavior(s) during this procedure:
		Ⓐ	Demonstrated the principles of self-boundaries.
		★	Completed the procedure within 5 minutes.
			Totals

Evaluation of Student Performance

EVALUATION CRITERIA			COMMENTS
Symbol	**Category**	**Point Value**	
★	Critical Step	16 points	
•	Essential Step	6 points	
Ⓐ	Affective Competency	6 points	
▷	Theory Question	2 points	

Score calculation: 100 points
− _____ points missed
_____ Score

Satisfactory score: 85 or above

CAAHEP Competencies Achieved

Psychomotor (Skills)
☑ I. 8. Instruct and prepare a patient for a procedure or a treatment.
☑ XII. 3. Use proper body mechanics.

Affective (Behavior)
☑ V. 2. Demonstrate the principles of self-boundaries.

ABHES Competency Achieved

☑ 8. c. Assist provider with general/physical examination.

EVALUATION OF COMPETENCY

Procedure 5-5: Dorsal Recumbent Position

Name: _____   Date: _____

Evaluated by: _____   Score: _____

Performance Objective

Outcome:	Position and drape an individual in the dorsal recumbent position.
Conditions:	Given the following: a patient gown and a drape.
	Using an examining table.
Standards:	Time: 5 minutes. Student completed procedure in _____ minutes.
	Accuracy: Satisfactory score on the Performance Evaluation Checklist.

Performance Evaluation Checklist

Trial 1	Trial 2	Point Value	Performance Standards
		•	Sanitized hands.
		•	Greeted the patient and introduced yourself.
		•	Identified the patient.
		•	Explained what type of examination or procedure will be performed.
		•	Provided the patient with a patient gown.
		•	Instructed the patient to remove clothing and to put on a patient gown with the opening in front.
		•	Pulled out the footrest and assisted the patient into a sitting position.
		•	Placed a drape over the patient's thighs and legs.
		•	Asked the patient to move back on the table.
		•	Pulled out the table extension while supporting the patient's lower legs.
		•	Asked the patient to lie down on his or her back.
		•	Placed the patient's arms above the head or alongside the body.
		•	Positioned the drape diagonally over the patient.
		•	Asked the patient to bend the knees and place each foot at the edge of the table with the soles of the feet flat on the table.
		•	Provided assistance.
		•	Pushed in the table extension and the footrest.
		•	Adjusted the drape as needed.
		•	Folded back the center corner of the drape when the provider was ready to examine the patient.

Trial 1	Trial 2	Point Value	Performance Standards
		•	Pulled out the footrest and the table extension after the examination.
		•	Assisted the patient back into a supine position and then into a sitting position.
		•	Slid the table extension back into place while supporting the patient's lower legs.
		•	Assisted the patient from the examining table.
		•	Returned the footrest to its normal position.
		•	Instructed the patient to get dressed.
		•	Discarded the gown and drape in a waste container.
		▷	Stated one use of the dorsal recumbent position.
			Demonstrated the following affective behavior(s) during this procedure:
		Ⓐ	Demonstrated the principles of self-boundaries.
		★	Completed the procedure within 5 minutes.
			Totals

Evaluation of Student Performance

EVALUATION CRITERIA			COMMENTS
Symbol	**Category**	**Point Value**	
★	Critical Step	16 points	
•	Essential Step	6 points	
Ⓐ	Affective Competency	6 points	
▷	Theory Question	2 points	

Score calculation: 100 points
−_____ points missed
_____ Score

Satisfactory score: 85 or above

CAAHEP Competencies Achieved

Psychomotor (Skills)
☑ I. 8. Instruct and prepare a patient for a procedure or a treatment.
☑ XII. 3. Use proper body mechanics.

Affective (Behavior)
☑ V. 2. Demonstrate the principles of self-boundaries.

ABHES Competency Achieved

☑ 8 c. Assist provider with general/physical examination.

Procedure 5-6: Lithotomy Position

Name: _____   Date: _____

Evaluated by: _____   Score: _____

Performance Objective

Outcome:	Position and drape an individual in the lithotomy position.
Conditions:	Given the following: a patient gown and a drape.
	Using an examining table.
Standards:	Time: 5 minutes. Student completed procedure in _____ minutes.
	Accuracy: Satisfactory score on the Performance Evaluation Checklist.

Performance Evaluation Checklist

Trial 1	Trial 2	Point Value	Performance Standards
		•	Sanitized hands.
		•	Greeted the patient and introduced yourself.
		•	Identified the patient.
		•	Explained what type of examination or procedure will be performed.
		•	Provided the patient with a patient gown.
		•	Instructed the patient to remove clothing and to put on a patient gown with the opening in front.
		•	Pulled out the footrest and assisted the patient into a sitting position.
		•	Placed a drape over the patient's thighs and legs.
		•	Asked the patient to move back on the table.
		•	Pulled out the table extension while supporting the patient's lower legs.
		•	Asked the patient to lie down on his or her back.
		•	Placed the patient's arms above the head or alongside the body.
		•	Positioned the drape diagonally over the patient.
		•	Pulled out the stirrups and positioned them at an angle.
		•	Positioned the stirrups so that they were level with the examining table and pulled out approximately 1 foot from the edge of the table.
		•	Asked the patient to bend the knees and place each foot into a stirrup.
		•	Provided assistance.
		•	Pushed in the table extension and the footrest.

Trial 1	Trial 2	Point Value	Performance Standards
		•	Instructed the patient to slide buttocks to the edge of the table and to rotate thighs outward as far as is comfortable.
		•	Repositioned the drape as needed.
		•	Folded back the center corner of the drape when the provider was ready to examine the genital area.
		•	After completion of the examination, pulled out the footrest and the table extension.
		•	Asked the patient to slide the buttocks back from the end of the table.
		•	Lifted the patient's legs out of the stirrups at the same time and placed them on the table extension.
		▷	Stated why both legs should be lifted at the same time.
		•	Returned stirrups to the normal position.
		•	Assisted the patient back into a sitting position.
		•	Slid the table extension back into place while supporting the patient's lower legs.
		•	Assisted the patient from the examining table.
		•	Returned the footrest to its normal position.
		•	Instructed the patient to get dressed.
		•	Discarded the gown and drape in a waste container.
		▷	Stated one use of the lithotomy position.
			Demonstrated the following affective behavior(s) during this procedure:
		Ⓐ	Demonstrated the principles of self-boundaries.
		★	Completed the procedure within 5 minutes.
			Totals

Evaluation of Student Performance

EVALUATION CRITERIA			COMMENTS
Symbol	**Category**	**Point Value**	
★	Critical Step	16 points	
•	Essential Step	6 points	
Ⓐ	Affective Competency	6 points	
▷	Theory Question	2 points	

Score calculation: 100 points
− _____ points missed
_____ Score

Satisfactory score: 85 or above

CAAHEP Competencies Achieved

Psychomotor (Skills)

☑ I. 8. Instruct and prepare a patient for a procedure or a treatment.

☑ XII. 3. Use proper body mechanics.

Affective (Behavior)

☑ V. 2. Demonstrate the principles of self-boundaries.

ABHES Competency Achieved

☑ 8. c. Assist provider with general/physical examination.

Notes

Procedure 5-7: Sims Position

Name: _____   Date: _____

Evaluated by: _____   Score: _____

Performance Objective

Outcome:	Position and drape an individual in the Sims position.
Conditions:	Given the following: a patient gown and a drape.
	Using an examining table.
Standards:	Time: 5 minutes. Student completed procedure in _____ minutes.
	Accuracy: Satisfactory score on the Performance Evaluation Checklist.

Performance Evaluation Checklist

Trial 1	Trial 2	Point Value	Performance Standards
		•	Sanitized hands.
		•	Greeted the patient and introduced yourself.
		•	Identified the patient.
		•	Explained what type of examination or procedure will be performed.
		•	Provided the patient with a patient gown.
		•	Instructed the patient to remove clothing and to put on a patient gown with the opening in back.
		•	Pulled out the footrest and assisted the patient into a sitting position.
		•	Placed a drape over the patient's thighs and legs.
		•	Asked the patient to move back on the table.
		•	Pulled out the table extension while supporting the patient's lower legs.
		•	Asked the patient to lie down on his or her back.
		•	Positioned the drape lengthwise over the patient.
		•	Asked the patient to turn onto the left side.
		•	Provided assistance.
		•	Positioned the left arm behind the body and the right arm forward with the elbow bent.
		•	Assisted the patient in flexing the legs with the right leg flexed sharply and the left leg flexed slightly.
		•	Adjusted the drape by folding back the drape to expose the anal area when the provider was ready to examine the patient.

Trial 1	Trial 2	Point Value	Performance Standards
		•	Assisted the patient into a supine position and then into a sitting position following the examination.
		•	Slid the table extension back into place while supporting the patient's lower legs.
		•	Assisted the patient from the examining table.
		•	Returned the footrest to its normal position.
		•	Instructed the patient to get dressed.
		•	Discarded the gown and drape in a waste container.
		▷	Stated one use of the Sims position.
			Demonstrated the following affective behavior(s) during this procedure:
		Ⓐ	Demonstrated the principles of self-boundaries.
		★	Completed the procedure within 5 minutes.
			Totals

Evaluation of Student Performance

EVALUATION CRITERIA			COMMENTS
Symbol	**Category**	**Point Value**	
★	Critical Step	16 points	
•	Essential Step	6 points	
Ⓐ	Affective Competency	6 points	
▷	Theory Question	2 points	

Score calculation: 100 points

    − _____ points missed

    _____ Score

Satisfactory score: 85 or above

CAAHEP Competencies Achieved

Psychomotor (Skills)

☑ I. 8. Instruct and prepare a patient for a procedure or a treatment.

☑ XII. 3. Use proper body mechanics.

Affective (Behavior)

☑ V. 2. Demonstrate the principles of self-boundaries.

ABHES Competency Achieved

☑ 8. c. Assist provider with general/physical examination.

Procedure 5-8: Knee-Chest Position

Name: _____   Date: _____

Evaluated by: _____   Score: _____

Performance Objective

Outcome:	Position and drape an individual in the knee-chest position.
Conditions:	Given the following: a patient gown and a drape.
	Using an examining table.
Standards:	Time: 5 minutes. Student completed procedure in _____ minutes.
	Accuracy: Satisfactory score on the Performance Evaluation Checklist.

Performance Evaluation Checklist

Trial 1	Trial 2	Point Value	Performance Standards
		•	Sanitized hands.
		•	Greeted the patient and introduced yourself.
		•	Identified the patient.
		•	Explained what type of examination or procedure will be performed.
		•	Provided the patient with a patient gown.
		•	Instructed the patient to remove clothing and to put on a patient gown with the opening in back.
		•	Pulled out the footrest and assisted the patient into a sitting position.
		•	Placed a drape over the patient's thighs and legs.
		•	Asked the patient to move back on the table.
		•	Pulled out the table extension while supporting the patient's lower legs.
		•	Assisted the patient into the supine position and then into the prone position.
		•	Positioned the drape diagonally over the patient.
		•	Asked the patient to bend the arms at the elbows and rest them alongside the head.
		•	Asked the patient to elevate the buttocks while keeping the back straight.
		•	Turned the patient's head to one side, with the weight of the body supported by the chest.
		•	Used a pillow for additional support, if needed.
		•	Separated the knees and lower legs approximately 12 inches.
		•	Adjusted the drape diagonally as needed.

Trial 1	Trial 2	Point Value	Performance Standards
		•	Folded back a small portion of the drape to expose the anal area when the provider was ready to examine the patient.
		•	Assisted the patient into a prone position and then into a supine position after the examination.
		•	Allowed the patient to rest in a supine position before sitting up.
		▷	Stated why the patient should be allowed to rest.
		•	Assisted the patient into a sitting position.
		•	Slid the table extension back into place while supporting the patient's lower legs.
		•	Assisted the patient from the examining table.
		•	Returned the footrest to its normal position.
		•	Instructed the patient to get dressed.
		•	Discarded the gown and drape in a waste container.
		▷	Stated one use of the knee-chest position.
			Demonstrated the following affective behavior(s) during this procedure:
		Ⓐ	Demonstrated the principles of self-boundaries.
		★	Completed the procedure within 5 minutes.
			Totals

Evaluation of Student Performance

EVALUATION CRITERIA			COMMENTS
Symbol	**Category**	**Point Value**	
★	Critical Step	16 points	
•	Essential Step	6 points	
Ⓐ	Affective Competency	6 points	
▷	Theory Question	2 points	

Score calculation: 100 points

− _____ points missed

_____ Score

Satisfactory score: 85 or above

CAAHEP Competencies Achieved

Psychomotor (Skills)

☑ I. 8. Instruct and prepare a patient for a procedure or a treatment.

☑ XII. 3. Use proper body mechanics.

Affective (Behavior)

☑ V. 2. Demonstrate the principles of self-boundaries.

ABHES Competency Achieved

☑ 8. c. Assist provider with general/physical examination.

e Procedure 5-9: Fowler Position

Name: _____   Date: _____

Evaluated by: _____   Score: _____

Performance Objective

Outcome: Position and drape an individual in the Fowler position.

Conditions: Given the following: a patient gown and a drape.

Using an examining table.

Standards: Time: 5 minutes.   Student completed procedure in _____ minutes.

Accuracy: Satisfactory score on the Performance Evaluation Checklist.

Performance Evaluation Checklist

Trial 1	Trial 2	Point Value	Performance Standards
		•	Sanitized hands.
		•	Greeted the patient and introduced yourself.
		•	Identified the patient.
		•	Explained what type of examination or procedure will be performed.
		•	Provided the patient with a patient gown.
		•	Instructed the patient to remove clothing and to put on a patient gown with the opening in front.
		•	Positioned the head of the table at a 45-degree angle for a semi-Fowler position or at a 90-degree angle for a full Fowler position.
		•	Pulled out the footrest and assisted the patient into a sitting position.
		•	Placed a drape over the patient's thighs and legs.
		•	Pulled out the table extension while supporting the patient's lower legs.
		•	Asked the patient to lean back against the table head.
		•	Provided assistance.
		•	Positioned the drape lengthwise over the patient.
		•	Moved the drape according to the body parts being examined.
		•	Assisted the patient into a sitting position after the examination.
		•	Slid the table extension back into place while supporting the patient's lower legs.
		•	Assisted the patient from the examining table.
		•	Instructed the patient to get dressed.
		•	Returned the head of the table and the footrest to their normal positions.

Trial 1	Trial 2	Point Value	Performance Standards
		•	Discarded the gown and drape in a waste container.
		▷	Stated one use of the Fowler position.
			Demonstrated the following affective behavior(s) during this procedure:
		Ⓐ	Demonstrated the principles of self-boundaries.
		★	Completed the procedure within 5 minutes.
			Totals

Evaluation of Student Performance

EVALUATION CRITERIA			COMMENTS
Symbol	**Category**	**Point Value**	
★	Critical Step	16 points	
•	Essential Step	6 points	
Ⓐ	Affective Competency	6 points	
▷	Theory Question	2 points	

Score calculation: 100 points
−   _____ points missed
_____ Score

Satisfactory score: 85 or above

CAAHEP Competencies Achieved

Psychomotor (Skills)
☑ I. 8. Instruct and prepare a patient for a procedure or a treatment.
☑ XII. 3. Use proper body mechanics.

Affective (Behavior)
☑ V. 2. Demonstrate the principles of self-boundaries.

ABHES Competency Achieved

☑ 8. c. Assist provider with general/physical examination.

Procedure 5-10: Wheelchair Transfer

Name: _____   Date: _____

Evaluated by: _____   Score: _____

Performance Objective

Outcome:	Transfer a patient from a wheelchair to the examining table and from the examining table to a wheelchair.
Conditions:	Given the following: transfer belt.
	Using an examining table and a wheelchair.
Standards:	Time: 10 minutes. Student completed procedure in _____ minutes.
	Accuracy: Satisfactory score on the Performance Evaluation Checklist.

Performance Evaluation Checklist

Trial 1	Trial 2	Point Value	Performance Standards
			Transferring to the examining table:
		•	Sanitized hands.
		•	Greeted the patient and introduced yourself.
		•	Identified the patient and explained the procedure.
		•	Determined whether the patient has the mental and physical capability to perform the transfer.
		•	Estimated the weight of the patient and whether he or she can assist in the transfer.
		•	Assessed your ability to safely make the transfer.
		▷	Stated factors that would prevent you from making the transfer.
		•	Wrapped the transfer belt around the patient's waist and fastened it.
		•	The belt was snug with just enough space to allow the fingers to be inserted comfortably.
		▷	Stated why the belt should be snug.
		•	With the patient's stronger side next to the table, positioned the wheelchair at a 45-degree angle to the end of the examining table.
		•	If the table is height-adjustable, adjusted it to the same height as the wheelchair or slightly lower.
		•	If the table is not height-adjustable, pulled out the footrest.
		•	Locked the brakes of the wheelchair.
		▷	Stated why the brakes should be locked.

Trial 1	Trial 2	Point Value	Performance Standards
		•	Folded back the wheelchair footrests.
		•	Informed the patient what to do during the transfer.
		•	Made sure the patient's feet were flat on the floor.
		•	Stood in front of the patient with the feet 6 to 8 inches apart, with one foot slightly forward and the knees bent.
		•	Asked the patient to place his or her arms on the armrests of the wheelchair and to lean forward.
		•	Grasped the transfer belt on either side of the patient's waist using an underhand grasp.
		▷	Stated the purpose of the transfer belt.
		•	Instructed the patient to push off the armrests and into a standing position on the count of 3.
		•	Straightened the knees and assisted the patient to a standing position by pulling upward on the transfer belt.
		•	Kept the back straight and lifted with the knees, arms, and legs, and not the back.
		•	Pivoted and positioned the patient's buttocks and back of the legs toward the examining table.
		•	Instructed the patient to step backward onto the footrest, one foot at a time.
		•	Gradually lowered the patient into a sitting position on the examining table.
		•	Removed the transfer belt.
		•	Unlocked the wheelchair and moved it out of the way.
		•	Pushed in the footrest of the examining table.
		•	Stayed with the patient to prevent falls.
			Transferring to the wheelchair:
		•	Wrapped the transfer belt snugly around the patient's waist and fastened it.
		•	Positioned the wheelchair at a 45-degree angle to the end of the examining table.
		•	If the table is height-adjustable, adjusted it to the same height as the wheelchair or slightly lower.
		•	If the table is not height-adjustable, pulled out the footrest.
		•	Locked the wheelchair in place and folded back the footrests, if needed.
		•	Informed the patient of what to do during the transfer.
		•	Stood in front of the patient with the feet 6 to 8 inches apart, with one foot slightly forward and the knees bent.

Trial 1	Trial 2	Point Value	Performance Standards
		•	Asked the patient to place his or her arms on your shoulders.
		•	Did not allow the patient to place his or her arms around your neck.
		•	Grasped the transfer belt on either side of the patient's waist using an underhand grasp.
		•	Instructed the patient to stand on the count of 3.
		•	Straightened your knees and assisted the patient to a standing position by pulling upward on the transfer belt.
		•	Instructed the patient to step down from the footrest, one foot at a time.
		•	Pivoted the patient until the back of the legs are against the seat of the wheelchair.
		•	Asked the patient to grasp the armrests of the wheelchair.
		•	Gradually lowered the patient into the wheelchair by bending at the knees.
		•	Removed the transfer belt and made sure the patient was comfortable.
		•	Repositioned the wheelchair footrests and assisted the patient in placing his or her feet in them.
		•	Unlocked the wheelchair.
		•	Pushed in the footrest of the examining table.
			Demonstrated the following affective behavior(s) during this procedure:
		Ⓐ	Demonstrated the principles of self-boundaries.
		★	Completed the procedure within 10 minutes.
			Totals

Evaluation of Student Performance

EVALUATION CRITERIA			COMMENTS
Symbol	**Category**	**Point Value**	
★	Critical Step	16 points	
•	Essential Step	6 points	
Ⓐ	Affective Competency	6 points	
▷	Theory Question	2 points	

Score calculation: 100 points
−_____ points missed
_____ Score

Satisfactory score: 85 or above

CAAHEP Competencies Achieved

Psychomotor (Skills)

☑ I. 8. Instruct and prepare a patient for a procedure or a treatment.

☑ XII. 3. Use proper body mechanics.

Affective (Behavior)

☑ V. 2. Demonstrate the principles of self-boundaries.

ABHES Competencies Achieved

☑ 8. c. Assist provider with general/physical examination.

☑ 8. j. Make adaptations for patients with special needs (psychological or physical limitations).

Procedure 5-11: Assisting with the Physical Examination

Name: _____ Date: _____

Evaluated by: _____ Score: _____

Performance Objective

Outcome:	Prepare the patient and assist with a physical examination.
Conditions:	Given the following: equipment for the type of examination to be performed, patient examination gown, and drapes.
	Using an examining table.
Standards:	Time: 20 minutes. Student completed procedure in _____ minutes.
	Accuracy: Satisfactory score on the Performance Evaluation Checklist.

Performance Evaluation Checklist

Trial 1	Trial 2	Point Value	Performance Standards
		•	Prepared examination room.
		•	Sanitized hands.
		•	Assembled all necessary equipment.
		•	Arranged instruments in a neat and orderly manner.
		•	Obtained the patient's medical record.
		•	Went to the waiting room, and asked the patient to come back.
		•	Escorted the patient to the examination room.
		•	Asked the patient to be seated.
		•	Greeted the patient and introduced yourself.
		•	Identified the patient by full name and date of birth.
		▷	Stated why a calm and friendly manner should be used.
		•	Seated yourself facing the patient at a distance of 3 to 4 feet.
		•	Obtained and documented essential patient information on patient allergies, current medications, and patient symptoms.
		•	Measured vital signs and documented results.
		▷	Stated the adult normal range for temperature (97° F to 99° F), pulse (60 to 100 beats/min), respiration (12 to 20 breaths/min), and blood pressure (<120/80 mm Hg).
		•	Measured weight and height, and documented results.
		•	Asked the patient if he or she needs to void.
		▷	Stated why the patient should be asked to void.

Trial 1	Trial 2	Point Value	Performance Standards
		•	Instructed the patient to remove all clothing and put on an examining gown.
		•	Informed the patient that the provider will be in soon.
		•	Left the room to provide the patient with privacy.
		•	Made the patient's medical record available to the provider (if using a PPR).
		•	Checked to make sure the patient is ready to be seen.
		•	Informed provider that the patient is ready.
			Assisted the provider:
		•	Ensured the patient was in a sitting position on examination table.
		•	Handed the ophthalmoscope to the provider when requested.
		•	Dimmed the lights when the provider was ready to use the ophthalmoscope.
		▷	Stated why the lights are dimmed.
		▷	Stated the proper use of the ophthalmoscope.
		•	Handed the otoscope to the examiner when requested.
		▷	Stated the proper use of the otoscope.
		•	Is able to change the speculum and bulb in the otoscope.
		•	Handed the tongue depressor to the examiner when requested.
		•	Offered reassurance to the patient as needed.
		•	Positioned the patient as required for examination of the remaining body systems.
			Assisted and instructed the patient:
		•	Allowed the patient to rest in a sitting position before getting off the examining table.
		▷	Stated why the patient should be allowed to rest before getting off the table.
		•	Assisted the patient off the examining table.
		•	Instructed the patient to get dressed.
		•	Provided the patient with any necessary instructions.
		▷	Stated what type of instructions may need to be relayed to the patient.
		•	Sanitized hands and documented any instructions given to the patient.
		•	Escorted the patient to the reception area.
			Cleaned the examination room:
		•	Discarded paper on the examining table and unrolled a fresh length.
		•	Discarded all disposable supplies into an appropriate waste container.

Trial 1	Trial 2	Point Value	Performance Standards
		•	Checked to make sure ample supplies are available.
		•	Removed reusable equipment for sanitization, sterilization, or disinfection.
			Demonstrated the following affective behavior(s) during this procedure:
		Ⓐ	Incorporated critical thinking skills when performing patient assessment.
		Ⓐ	Incorporated critical thinking skills when performing patient care.
		Ⓐ	Showed awareness of a patient's concerns related to the procedure being performed.
		Ⓐ	Demonstrated respect for individual diversity including (a) gender (b) race (c) religion (d) age (e) economic status (f) appearance.
		Ⓐ	Demonstrated sensitivity to patient rights.
		Ⓐ	Protected the integrity of the medical record.
		★	Completed the procedure within 20 minutes.
			Totals

CHART	
Date	

Evaluation of Student Performance

EVALUATION CRITERIA			COMMENTS
Symbol	**Category**	**Point Value**	
★	Critical Step	16 points	
•	Essential Step	6 points	
Ⓐ	Affective Competency	6 points	
▷	Theory Question	2 points	

Score calculation: 100 points
− _____ points missed
_____ Score
Satisfactory score: 85 or above

CAAHEP Competencies Achieved

Psychomotor (Skills)

☑ I. 3. Perform patient screening using established protocols.

☑ I. 8. Instruct and prepare a patient for a procedure or a treatment.

☑ I. 9. Assist provider with a patient exam.

☑ V. 1. Use feedback techniques to obtain patient information including: (a) reflection (b) restatement (c) clarification.

☑ V. 4. Coach patients regarding: (a) office policy (b) health maintenance (c) disease prevention (d) treatment plan.

☑ V. 9. Develop a current list of community resources related to patients' health care needs.

☑ V. 11. Report relevant information concisely and accurately.

☑ X. 1. Apply HIPAA rules in regard to: (a) privacy (b) release of information.

☑ X. 3. Document patient care accurately in the medical record.

☑ XII. 3. Use proper body mechanics.

Affective (Behavior)

☑ I. 1. Incorporate critical thinking skills when performing patient assessment.

☑ I. 2. Incorporate critical thinking skills when performing patient care.

☑ I. 3. Show awareness of a patient's concerns related to the procedure being performed.

☑ V. 1. Demonstrate (a) empathy (b) active listening (c) nonverbal communication.

☑ V. 3. Demonstrate respect for individual diversity including (a) gender (b) race (c) religion (d) age (e) economic status (f) appearance.

☑ X. 1. Demonstrate sensitivity to patient rights.

☑ X. 2. Protect the integrity of the medical record.

ABHES Competencies Achieved

☑ 4. a. Follow documentation guidelines.

☑ 5. e. Analyze the effect of hereditary and environmental influences on behavior.

☑ 7. f. Maintain inventory of equipment and supplies.

☑ 7. g. Display professionalism through written and verbal communications.

☑ 9. b. Obtain vital signs, obtain patient history, and formulate chief complaint.

☑ 9. c. Assist provider with general/physical examination.

☑ 9. h. Teach self-examination, disease management and health promotion.

☑ 9. i. Identify community resources and Complementary and Alternative Medicine practices (CAM).

Eye and Ear Assessment and Procedures

CHAPTER ASSIGNMENTS

√ After Completing	Date Due	Study Guide Pages	STUDY GUIDE ASSIGNMENTS (CTA = Critical Thinking Activity)	Possible Points	Points You Earned
		215	Pretest	10	
		216	Term Key Term Assessment		
		216	A. Definitions	13	
		216	B. Word Parts (Add 1 point for each key term)	11	
		217-220	Evaluation of Learning questions	32	
		220	CTA A: Measuring Distance Visual Acuity	6	
		220	CTA B: Interpreting Visual Acuity Results	4	
		221	CTA C: Documenting Visual Acuity Results	4	
		221-222	CTA D: Ear Procedures	8	
		222	CTA E: Dear Gabby	10	
		223	CTA F: Crossword Puzzle	18	
		224	CTA G: Eye and Ear Conditions	40	
			Evolve Site: Can You Hear Me Now? (Record points earned)		
			Evolve Site: Eye-dentify (Record points earned)		
			Evolve Site: Apply Your Knowledge questions	10	
			Evolve Site: Video Evaluation	70	
		215	Posttest	10	

			ADDITIONAL ASSIGNMENTS		
			Total points		

√ When Assigned by Your Instructor	Study Guide Pages	Practices Required	LABORATORY ASSIGNMENTS (Procedure Number and Name)	Score*
	227	5	**Practice for Competency** 6-1: Assessing Distance Visual Acuity—Snellen Chart Textbook reference: pp. 187-188	
	229-231		**Evaluation of Competency** 6-1: Assessing Distance Visual Acuity—Snellen Chart	*
	227-228	3	**Practice for Competency** 6-2: Assessing Color Vision: Ishihara Test Textbook reference: pp. 188-189	
	233-235		**Evaluation of Competency** 6-2: Assessing Color Vision: Ishihara Test	*
	227	3	**Practice for Competency** 6-3: Performing an Eye Irrigation Textbook reference: pp. 191-192	
	237-239		**Evaluation of Competency** 6-3: Performing an Eye Irrigation	*
	227	3	**Practice for Competency** 6-4: Performing an Eye Instillation Textbook reference: pp. 193-194	
	241-243		**Evaluation of Competency** 6-4: Performing an Eye Instillation	*
	227	3	**Practice for Competency** 6-5: Performing an Ear Irrigation Textbook reference: pp. 201-203	
	245-247		**Evaluation of Competency** 6-5: Performing an Ear Irrigation	*
	227	3	**Practice for Competency** 6-6: Performing an Ear Instillation Textbook reference: pp. 203-204	
	249-251		**Evaluation of Competency** 6-6: Performing an Ear Instillation	*
			ADDITIONAL ASSIGNMENTS	

Notes

Name: _____   Date: _____

True or False

_____ 1. Refraction refers to the bending of light rays so that they can be focused on the retina.

_____ 2. A person who is farsighted has a condition known as myopia.

_____ 3. An optometrist can perform eye surgery.

_____ 4. The Snellen eye test is conducted at a distance of 20 feet.

_____ 5. The Snellen eye chart should be positioned at the medical assistant's eye level.

_____ 6. An eye instillation may be performed to treat an eye infection.

_____ 7. Conjunctivitis caused by a bacterium is not contagious.

_____ 8. The most specific type of hearing test is the tuning fork test.

_____ 9. Serous otitis media can result in a conductive hearing loss.

_____ 10. An ear instillation may be performed to treat an ear infection.

POSTTEST

True or False

_____ 1. A person who cannot see objects close up has a condition known as amblyopia.

_____ 2. Visual acuity refers to sharpness of vision.

_____ 3. Presbyopia is a decrease in the elasticity of the lens due to the aging process.

_____ 4. An optician fills prescriptions for eyeglasses.

_____ 5. The Snellen Big E chart is used with school-aged children.

_____ 6. The most common color vision defects are congenital in nature.

_____ 7. The external auditory canal of an adult is straightened by pulling the ear downward and backward.

_____ 8. The range of frequencies for normal speech is 300 to 4000 Hz.

_____ 9. Intense noise can result in a sensorineural hearing loss.

_____ 10. Tympanometry is used to diagnose patients with auditory nerve damage.

A. Definitions

Directions: Match each key term with its definition.

_____ 1. Astigmatism

_____ 2. Audiometer

_____ 3. Canthus

_____ 4. Cerumen

_____ 5. Hyperopia

_____ 6. Impacted

_____ 7. Instillation

_____ 8. Irrigation

_____ 9. Myopia

_____ 10. Otoscope

_____ 11. Presbyopia

_____ 12. Refraction

_____ 13. Tympanic membrane

A. The washing of a body canal with a flowing solution

B. A decrease in the elasticity of the lens that occurs with aging, resulting in a decreased ability to focus on close objects

C. Farsightedness

D. The deflection or bending of light rays by a lens

E. The junction of the eyelids at either corner of the eye

F. Nearsightedness

G. The dropping of a liquid into a body cavity

H. An instrument for examining the external ear canal and tympanic membrane

I. Earwax

J. An instrument used to quantitatively measure hearing acuity for the various frequencies of sound waves

K. A thin, semitransparent membrane located between the external ear canal and the middle ear that receives and transmits sound waves

L. A refractive error that causes distorted and blurred vision for both near and far objects due to a cornea that is oval shaped

M. Wedged firmly together so as to be immovable

B. Word Parts

Directions: Indicate the meaning of each word part in the space provided. List as many medical terms as possible that incorporate the word part in the space provided.

Word Part	Meaning of Word Part	Medical Terms That Incorporate Word Part
1. a-		
2. stigm/a		
3. -ism		
4. audi/o		
5. -meter		
6. hyper-		
7. -opia		
8. ot/o		
9. -scope		
10. tympan/o		
11. -ic		

Directions: Fill in each blank with the correct answer.

1. What is the name of the tough white outer layer of the eye?

   _____

2. What is the function of the lens?

   _____

3. What is the function of the retina?

   _____

4. What parts of the eye are covered with conjunctiva?

   _____

5. What is visual acuity?

   _____

   _____

6. What types of symptoms might be experienced with myopia?

   _____

   _____

7. What methods can be used to correct myopia?

   _____

   _____

8. What causes an individual with astigmatism to have distorted and blurred vision?

   _____

   _____

9. Describe what each of the following eye professionals is qualified to perform.

   a. Ophthalmologist

   _____

   _____

   b. Optometrist

   _____

   _____

   c. Optician

   _____

   _____

10. What condition can be detected by measuring distance visual acuity?

_____

11. What type of patient would warrant use of the Snellen Big E eye chart? (Give two examples.)

_____

_____

12. Explain the significance of the top number and bottom number next to each line of letters on the Snellen eye chart.

_____

_____

13. List two conditions that can be detected by measuring near visual acuity.

_____

_____

14. Explain the difference between congenital and acquired color vision defects.

_____

_____

_____

15. What is a polychromatic plate?

_____

_____

_____

16. List three reasons for performing eye irrigation.

_____

_____

_____

17. List three reasons for performing eye instillation.

_____

_____

_____

18. What is the function of the ear auricle?

_____

_____

19. What is the function of cerumen?

_____

_____

20. Explain why the external auditory canal must be straightened when viewing it with an otoscope.

_____

_____

21. What is the normal appearance of the tympanic membrane?

_____

_____

22. What is the purpose of the eustachian tube?

_____

_____

23. What is the function of the semicircular canals?

_____

_____

24. What is the range of frequencies for normal speech?

_____

_____

25. List five conditions that may cause conductive hearing loss.

_____

_____

_____

26. List four conditions that may result in sensorineural hearing loss.

_____

_____

27. What information is obtained through audiometry?

_____

_____

_____

28. What information is obtained through tympanometry?

_____

_____

_____

29. List three reasons for performing ear irrigation.

_____

_____

Chapter 6 Eye and Ear Assessment and Procedures

30. List three reasons for performing ear instillation.

_____

31. Explain how impacted cerumen is removed from the ear.

_____

_____

_____

32. Explain how to straighten the external auditory canal in an adult and in children 3 years old or younger.

_____

_____

_____

CRITICAL THINKING ACTIVITIES

A. Measuring Distance Visual Acuity

For each of the following situations, write **C** if the technique is correct and **I** if the technique is incorrect.

_____ 1. The patient is not given an opportunity to study the Snellen chart before beginning the test.

_____ 2. The Snellen chart is positioned at the medical assistant's eye level.

_____ 3. The patient is instructed to use his or her hand to cover the eye that is not being tested.

_____ 4. The medical assistant instructs the patient to close the eye that is not being tested.

_____ 5. The first line that the medical assistant asks the patient to identify is the 20/20 line.

_____ 6. The medical assistant observes the patient for signs of squinting or leaning forward during the test.

B. Interpreting Visual Acuity Results

1. A patient has a distance visual acuity reading of 20/30 in the right eye. Using this information, answer the following questions:

   a. How far was the patient from the eye chart?

   _____

   b. At what distance would a person with normal acuity be able to read this line?

   _____

2. A patient has a distance visual acuity reading of 20/10 in the left eye. Using this information, answer the following questions:

   a. How far was the patient from the eye chart?

   _____

   b. At what distance would a person with normal acuity be able to read this line?

   _____

C. Documenting Visual Acuity Results

Properly document the distance visual acuity results in the spaces provided. In all cases, the line indicated is the smallest line the patient could read at a distance of 20 feet.

1. The patient read the line marked 20/30 with the right eye with two errors; with the left eye, the patient read the line marked 20/30 with one error. The patient was wearing corrective lenses.

   _____

   _____

2. The patient read the line marked 20/20 with the right eye with one error; with the left eye, the patient read the line marked 20/20 with no errors. The patient was wearing corrective lenses.

   _____

   _____

3. The patient read the line marked 20/40 with the right eye with two errors; with the left eye, the patient read the line marked 20/30 with one error. The patient exhibited squinting and frowning during the test. The patient was not wearing corrective lenses.

   _____

   _____

4. The patient read the line marked 20/15 with the right eye with no errors; with the left eye, the patient read the line marked 20/20 with one error. The patient was not wearing corrective lenses.

   _____

   _____

D. Ear Procedures

Explain the principle for each of the following procedures.

Ear Irrigation

1. Positioning the patient's head so that it is tilted toward the affected ear

   _____

   _____

2. Cleansing the outer ear before irrigating

   _____

   _____

3. Straightening the external auditory canal

   _____

   _____

4. Injecting the irrigating solution toward the roof of the ear canal

   _____

   _____

5. Making sure not to obstruct the canal opening

_____

_____

Ear Instillation

6. Positioning the patient's head so that it is tilted toward the unaffected ear

_____

_____

7. Instructing the patient to lie on the unaffected side after the instillation

_____

_____

8. Placing a cotton wick in the patient's ear

_____

_____

E. Dear Gabby

Gabby has a middle ear infection and is not feeling well. She wants you to fill in for her. In the space provided, respond to the following letter.

Dear Gabby:

I am dating the sweetest and dearest man. "Mike" has only one flaw. He likes loud music. He had those big boom boxes installed in his car. When we drive somewhere in his car, he blasts the music. Sometimes, when we are driving down a street, people even turn around to see where the loud music is coming from. The music hurts my ears, and I cannot think straight. My ears even start ringing when we go on a trip. When I am talking to Mike, he says I mumble, and I have to speak extra loud around him. I keep telling Mike that the loud music is going to damage our hearing, but he says that we are way too young for that and that only old people have trouble hearing. Please help me, Gabby, because I love going on trips with Mike, but not if my ears hurt afterward.

Signed, Ears Are Ringing

_____

_____

_____

_____

_____

_____

_____

_____

_____

_____

F. Crossword Puzzle: Eye and Ear

Directions: Complete the crossword puzzle using the clues provided.

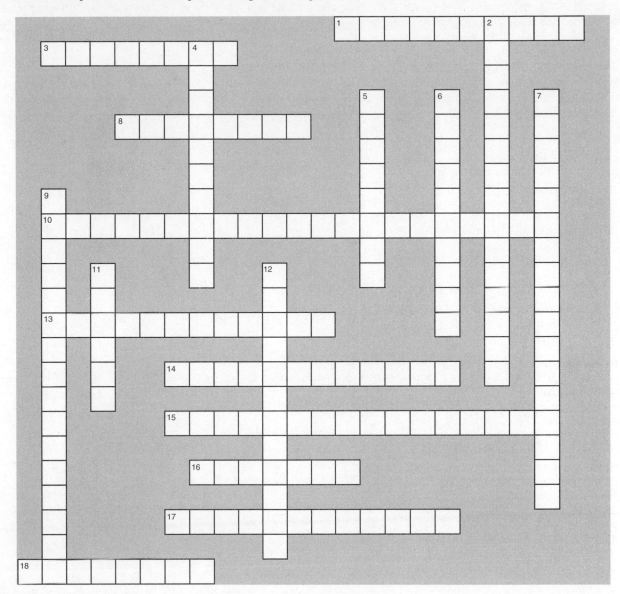

Across
1 Decreased lens elasticity
3 Fills eyeglasses prescriptions
8 Color blindness test
10 Impacted cerumen may cause this
13 Fixed stapes
14 Assesses mobility of eardrum
15 Drum in your ear
16 Earwax
17 Normal DVA
18 Straighten this before ear irrigation

Down
2 Physician who diagnoses and treats eye disorders
4 Instrument that measures hearing
5 A cause of pink eye
6 Caught it!
7 Fluid in middle ear
9 Middle ear infection
11 Cannot see far away
12 Sharpness of vision

Chapter **6** **Eye and Ear Assessment and Procedures**

G. Eye and Ear Conditions

1. You and your classmates work at a large clinic. It is National Eye and Ear Week. The providers at your clinic ask you to develop for their patients informative, creative, and colorful brochures about eye and ear conditions. Choose a condition, and design a brochure using the blank Frequently Asked Questions (FAQ) brochure provided on the following page. Each student in the class should select a different topic. On a separate sheet of paper, write three true or false questions related to the information in your brochure.

2. Present your brochure to the class. After all the brochures have been presented, each student should ask three questions to the entire class to see how well the class understands eye and ear conditions. (*Note:* You can take notes during the presentations and refer to them when answering the questions.)

Eye

1. Amblyopia (lazy eye)
2. Age-related macular degeneration
3. Astigmatism
4. Blepharitis
5. Cataracts
6. CMV retinitis
7. Corneal ulcer
8. Corneal abrasion
9. Strabismus (cross-eyed)
10. Diabetic retinopathy
11. Drooping eyelids (ptosis)
12. Dry eyes
13. Floaters and spots
14. Glaucoma
15. Keratoconus
16. Ocular hypertension
17. Retinal detachment
18. Retinitis pigmentosa
19. Stye

Ear

1. Acute mastoiditis
2. External otitis
3. Meniere's disease
4. Noise-induced hearing loss
5. Presbycusis
6. Serous otitis media

FAQ ON:

Q: A:

Q: A:

Q: A:

Q: A:

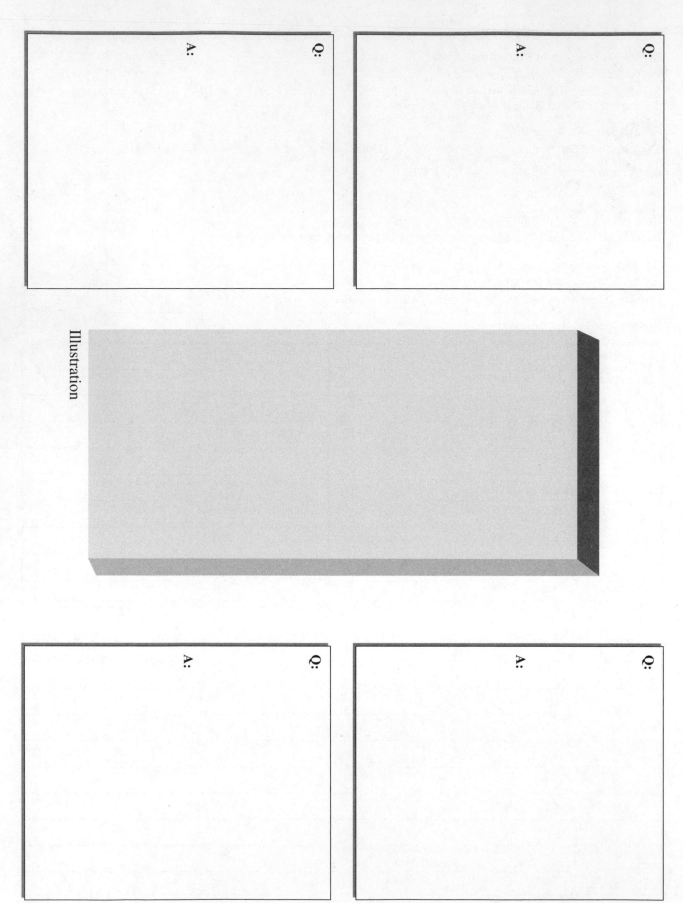

Illustration

Q:

A:

Q:

A:

Q:

A:

Q:

A:

Eye Assessment and Procedures

Procedure 6-1: Distance Visual Acuity

Assess distance visual acuity using a Snellen eye chart, and document results in the chart provided. Circle any readings that indicate distance visual acuity above or below average.

Procedure 6-2: Color Vision

Assess color vision, and document results in the Ishihara charting grid provided. Circle any abnormal results.

Procedure 6-3: Eye Irrigation

Perform an eye irrigation, and document the procedure in the chart provided.

Procedure 6-4: Eye Instillation

Perform an eye instillation, and document the procedure in the chart provided.

Ear Procedures

Procedure 6-5: Ear Irrigation

Perform an ear irrigation, and document the procedure in the chart provided.

Procedure 6-6: Ear Instillation

Perform an ear instillation, and document the procedure in the chart provided.

CHART	
Date	

227

DOCUMENTATION GRID FOR THE ISHIHARA TEST		
Plate No.	Normal Person	Results
1	12	
2	8	
3	5	
4	29	
5	74	
6	7	
7	45	
8	2	
9	X	
10	16	
11	Traceable	
Date:		
Evaluated by:		

DOCUMENTATION GRID FOR THE ISHIHARA TEST		
Plate No.	Normal Person	Results
1	12	
2	8	
3	5	
4	29	
5	74	
6	7	
7	45	
8	2	
9	X	
10	16	
11	Traceable	
Date:		
Evaluated by:		

EVALUATION OF COMPETENCY

Procedure 6-1: Assessing Distance Visual Acuity—Snellen Chart

Name: _____   Date: _____

Evaluated by: _____   Score: _____

Performance Objective

Outcome:	Assess distance visual acuity.
Conditions:	Given the following: Snellen eye chart, eye occluder, and an antiseptic wipe.
Standards:	Time: 5 minutes. Student completed procedure in _____ minutes.
	Accuracy: Satisfactory score on the Performance Evaluation Checklist.

Performance Evaluation Checklist

Trial 1	Trial 2	Point Value	Performance Standards
		•	Sanitized hands.
		•	Assembled equipment.
		•	Disinfected the eye occluder with an antiseptic wipe.
		•	Greeted the patient and introduced yourself.
		•	Identified the patient and explained the procedure.
		•	Determined whether the patient wears corrective lenses and instructed patient to leave them on during the test.
		•	Positioned patient 20 feet from the eye chart.
		•	Positioned the center of the eye chart at patient's cyc lcvcl.
		•	Instructed patient to cover the left eye with the occluder and to keep the left eye open.
		▷	Stated how the occluder should be positioned if the patient wears glasses.
		▷	Explained why the patient's left eye should remain open.
		•	Instructed patient not to squint during the test.
		▷	Explained why the patient should not squint during the test.
		•	Asked patient to identify the 20/70 line, using the right eye.
		▷	Stated why the test should begin with a line that is above the 20/20 line.
		•	Proceeded down the chart if the patient identified the 20/70 line or proceeded up the chart if the patient was unable to identify the 20/70 line.
		•	Continued until the smallest line of letters that the patient could read was reached.
		•	Observed patient for any unusual symptoms.
		•	Jotted down the numbers next to the smallest line read by the patient.
		•	Asked patient to cover the right eye and to keep the right eye open.

Chapter **6** Eye and Ear Assessment and Procedures

Trial 1	Trial 2	Point Value	Performance Standards
		•	Measured visual acuity in the left eye.
		•	Jotted down the numbers next to the smallest line read by the patient.
		★	The visual acuity measurements were identical to the evaluator's measurements.
		•	Documented the results correctly.
		•	Disinfected the occluder with an antiseptic wipe.
		•	Sanitized hands.
			Demonstrated the following affective behavior(s) during this procedure:
		Ⓐ	Incorporated critical thinking skills when performing patient assessment.
		★	Completed the procedure within 5 minutes.
			Totals

CHART	
Date	

Evaluation of Student Performance

EVALUATION CRITERIA			COMMENTS
Symbol	**Category**	**Point Value**	
★	Critical Step	16 points	
•	Essential Step	6 points	
Ⓐ	Affective Competency	6 points	
▷	Theory Question	2 points	

Score calculation: 100 points
− _____ points missed
_____ Score

Satisfactory score: 85 or above

CAAHEP Competencies Achieved

Psychomotor (Skills)

☑ I. 8. Instruct and prepare a patient for a procedure or a treatment.

Affective (Behavior)

☑ I. 1. Incorporate critical thinking skills when performing patient assessment.

ABHES Competencies Achieved

☑ 4. a. Follow documentation guidelines.

☑ 8. e. Perform specialty procedures, but not limited to minor surgery, cardiac, respiratory, OB-GYN, neurological, and gastroenterology.

Notes

e **Procedure 6-2: Assessing Color Vision—Ishihara Test**

Name: _____ Date: _____

Evaluated by: _____ Score: _____

Performance Objective

Outcome:	Assess color vision.
Conditions:	Given an Ishihara book of color plates and a cotton swab.
Standards:	Time: 10 minutes. Student completed procedure in _____ minutes.
	Accuracy: Satisfactory score on the Performance Evaluation Checklist.

Performance Evaluation Checklist

Trial 1	Trial 2	Point Value	Performance Standards
		•	Sanitized hands.
		•	Assembled equipment.
		•	Conducted the test in a quiet room illuminated by natural daylight.
		▷	Stated why natural daylight should be used.
		•	Greeted the patient and introduced yourself.
		•	Identified the patient.
		•	Explained the procedure using the practice plate.
		▷	Stated the purpose of the practice plate.
		•	Held the first plate 30 inches from the patient at a right angle to the patient's line of vision.
		•	Instructed patient to keep both eyes open.
		•	Told patient that he or she would have 3 seconds to identify each plate.
		•	Asked the patient to identify the number on the plate.
		•	Asked the patient to trace plates that have a winding line with a cotton swab.
		▷	Stated why a cotton swab should be used to make the tracing.
		•	Documented the results after identification of each plate.
		•	Continued until the patient viewed all plates.
		•	Documented the results correctly.
		★	The results were identical to the evaluator's results.
		•	Returned the Ishihara book to its proper place, storing it in a closed position.
		▷	Explained why the book should be stored in a closed position.

Trial 1	Trial 2	Point Value	Performance Standards
			Demonstrated the following affective behavior(s) during this procedure:
		Ⓐ	Incorporated critical thinking skills when performing patient assessment.
		★	Completed the procedure within 10 minutes.
			Totals

CHART		
Plate No.	**Normal Person**	**Results**
1	12	
2	8	
3	5	
4	29	
5	74	
6	7	
7	45	
8	2	
9	X	
10	16	
11	Traceable	
Date:		
Evaluated by:		

Evaluation of Student Performance

EVALUATION CRITERIA			COMMENTS
Symbol	**Category**	**Point Value**	
★	Critical Step	16 points	
•	Essential Step	6 points	
Ⓐ	Affective Competency	6 points	
▷	Theory Question	2 points	

Score calculation: 100 points
−_____ points missed
_____ Score
Satisfactory score: 85 or above

CAAHEP Competencies Achieved

Psychomotor (Skills)
☑ I. 8. Instruct and prepare a patient for a procedure or a treatment.

Affective (Behavior)
☑ I. 1. Incorporate critical thinking skills when performing patient assessment.

ABHES Competencies Achieved

☑ 4. a. Follow documentation guidelines.
☑ 8. e. Perform specialty procedures, but not limited to minor surgery, cardiac, respiratory, OB-GYN, neurological, and gastroenterology.

Chapter **6 Eye and Ear Assessment and Procedures**

Procedure 6-3: Performing an Eye Irrigation

Name: _____ Date: _____

Evaluated by: _____ Score: _____

Performance Objective

Outcome:	Perform an eye irrigation.
Conditions:	Given the following: disposable (nonpowdered) gloves, irrigating solution, solution container, disposable rubber bulb syringe, basin, moisture-resistant towel, and sterile gauze pads.
Standards:	Time: 5 minutes. Student completed procedure in _____ minutes.
	Accuracy: Satisfactory score on the Performance Evaluation Checklist.

Performance Evaluation Checklist

Trial 1	Trial 2	Point Value	Performance Standards
		•	Sanitized hands.
		•	Assembled equipment.
		•	Checked the solution label with the provider's instructions.
		•	Checked expiration date of the solution.
		▷	Stated the reason for checking the expiration date.
		•	Warmed the irrigating solution to body temperature.
		▷	Explained why the solution should be at body temperature.
		•	Checked the label a second time and poured the solution into a basin.
		•	Checked the label a third time before returning the container to storage.
		•	Greeted the patient and introduced yourself.
		•	Identified the patient and explained the procedure.
		•	Asked patient to remove glasses or contact lenses.
		•	Positioned patient in a lying or sitting position.
		•	Placed a moisture-resistant towel on the patient's shoulder.
		•	Positioned a basin tightly against the patient's cheek under the affected eye.
		•	Asked the patient to tilt head in the direction of the affected eye and hold the basin in place.
		▷	Explained why the patient's head is turned in the direction of the affected eye.
		•	Applied nonpowdered gloves.
		▷	Stated why nonpowdered gloves should be used.
		•	Cleansed the eyelids from inner to outer canthus.

Trial 1	Trial 2	Point Value	Performance Standards
		▷	Stated why eyelids are cleansed.
		•	Filled irrigating syringe.
		•	Instructed patient to keep both eyes open and to look at a focal point.
		▷	Stated the reason for looking at a focal point.
		•	Separated eyelids.
		•	Held tip of syringe 1 inch above the eye at the inner canthus.
		•	Allowed solution to flow over the eye at a moderate rate from the inner canthus to the outer canthus and directed solution to the lower conjunctiva.
		▷	Explained why the syringe should be directed toward the lower conjunctiva.
		•	Did not allow syringe to touch the eye.
		•	Refilled the syringe and continued irrigating until the desired results were obtained or all the solution was used.
		•	Dried the eyelids with a gauze pad from inner to outer canthus.
		•	Removed gloves and sanitized hands.
		•	Documented the procedure correctly.
		•	Returned equipment.
			Demonstrated the following affective behavior(s) during this procedure:
		Ⓐ	Incorporated critical thinking skills when performing patient care.
		Ⓐ	Showed awareness of a patient's concerns related to the procedure being performed.
		Ⓐ	Explained to a patient the rationale for performance of a procedure.
		★	Completed the procedure within 5 minutes.
			Totals

CHART	
Date	

Evaluation of Student Performance

EVALUATION CRITERIA			COMMENTS
Symbol	**Category**	**Point Value**	
★	Critical Step	16 points	
•	Essential Step	6 points	
Ⓐ	Affective Competency	6 points	
▷	Theory Question	2 points	

Score calculation: 100 points

$-$ _____ points missed

____ Score

Satisfactory score: 85 or above

CAAHEP Competencies Achieved

Psychomotor (Skills)

☑ I. 8. Instruct and prepare a patient for a procedure or a treatment.

☑ II. 1. Calculate proper dosages of medication for administration.

☑ X.3. Document patient care accurately in the medical record.

Affective (Behavior)

☑ I. 2. Incorporate critical thinking skills when performing patient care.

☑ I. 3. Show awareness of a patient's concerns related to the procedure being performed.

☑ V. 4. Explain to a patient the rationale for performance of a procedure.

ABHES Competencies Achieved

☑ 2. c. Identify diagnostic and treatment modalities as they relate to each body system.

☑ 4. a. Follow documentation guidelines.

☑ 8. e. Perform specialty procedures, but not limited to minor surgery, cardiac, respiratory, OB-GYN, neurological, and gastroenterology.

Notes

Chapter **6 Eye and Ear Assessment and Procedures**

Procedure 6-4: Performing an Eye Instillation

Name: _____ Date: _____

Evaluated by: _____ Score: _____

Performance Objective

Outcome:	Perform an eye instillation.
Conditions:	Given the following: disposable (nonpowdered) gloves, ophthalmic medication, tissues, and gauze pads.
Standards:	Time: 5 minutes. Student completed procedure in _____ minutes.
	Accuracy: Satisfactory score on the Performance Evaluation Checklist.

Performance Evaluation Checklist

Trial 1	Trial 2	Point Value	Performance Standards
		•	Sanitized hands.
		•	Assembled equipment.
		•	Checked the drug label when removing it from storage.
		▷	Stated what word must appear on the medication label.
		•	Checked drug label and dosage against the provider's instructions.
		•	Checked the expiration date of the medication.
		•	Greeted the patient and introduced yourself.
		•	Identified the patient and explained the procedure.
		•	Positioned patient in a sitting or supine position.
		•	Applied nonpowdered gloves.
		•	Prepared the medication.
		•	Checked the drug label and removed the cap.
		•	Asked patient to look up and exposed the lower conjunctival sac.
		▷	Explained the reason for asking patient to look up.
		•	Drew the skin of the cheek downward and exposed the conjunctival sac.
		•	Inserted the medication correctly.
		▷	Explained how to instill eyedrops and ointment.
		•	Instructed the patient to close his or her eyes gently and move the eyeballs.
		▷	Stated the reason for closing the eyes and moving the eyeballs.
		•	Told the patient that the instillation may temporarily blur vision.
		•	Dried the eyelids with a gauze pad from inner to outer canthus.

241

Trial 1	Trial 2	Point Value	Performance Standards
		•	Removed gloves and sanitized hands.
		•	Documented the procedure correctly.
		•	Returned equipment.
			Demonstrated the following affective behavior(s) during this procedure:
		Ⓐ	Incorporated critical thinking skills when performing patient care.
		Ⓐ	Showed awareness of a patient's concerns related to the procedure being performed.
		Ⓐ	Explained to a patient the rationale for performance of a procedure.
		★	Completed the procedure within 5 minutes.
			Totals
CHART			
Date			

Evaluation of Student Performance

EVALUATION CRITERIA			COMMENTS
Symbol	**Category**	**Point Value**	
★	Critical Step	16 points	
•	Essential Step	6 points	
Ⓐ	Affective Competency	6 points	
▷	Theory Question	2 points	

Score calculation: 100 points
− _____ points missed
_____ Score

Satisfactory score: 85 or above

CAAHEP Competencies Achieved

Psychomotor (Skills)

☑ I. 8. Instruct and prepare a patient for a procedure or a treatment.

☑ II. 1. Calculate proper dosages of medication for administration.

☑ X.3. Document patient care accurately in the medical record.

Affective (Behavior)

☑ I. 2. Incorporate critical thinking skills when performing patient care.

☑ I. 3. Show awareness of a patient's concerns related to the procedure being performed.

☑ V. 4. Explain to a patient the rationale for performance of a procedure.

ABHES Competencies Achieved

☑ 2. c. Identify diagnostic and treatment modalities as they relate to each body system.

☑ 4. a. Follow documentation guidelines.

☑ 8. e. Perform specialty procedures, but not limited to minor surgery, cardiac, respiratory, OB-GYN, neurological, and gastroenterology.

Notes

Procedure 6-5: Performing an Ear Irrigation

Name: _____   Date: _____

Evaluated by: _____   Score: _____

Performance Objective

Outcome:	Perform an ear irrigation.
Conditions:	Given the following: disposable gloves, irrigating solution, solution container, irrigating syringe, ear basin, moisture-resistant towel, gauze pads, and ear wick.
Standards:	Time: 10 minutes. Student completed procedure in _____ minutes.
	Accuracy: Satisfactory score on the Performance Evaluation Checklist.

Performance Evaluation Checklist

Trial 1	Trial 2	Point Value	Performance Standards
		•	Sanitized hands.
		•	Assembled equipment.
		•	Checked the label of the irrigating solution with the provider's instructions.
		•	Checked expiration date of the solution.
		•	Warmed the irrigating solution to body temperature.
		▷	Stated the reason for warming the irrigating solution.
		•	Checked the label a second time and poured the solution into a basin.
		•	Checked the label a third time before returning the container to storage.
		•	Greeted the patient and introduced yourself.
		•	Identified the patient and explained the procedure.
		•	Positioned the patient in a sitting position.
		•	Placed a towel on the patient's shoulder under the ear to be irrigated.
		•	Positioned a basin under the affected ear and asked the patient to hold it in place.
		•	Asked the patient to tilt his or her head toward the affected ear.
		▷	Explained why the head should be tilted toward the affected ear.
		•	Applied gloves.
		•	Cleansed the outer ear.
		▷	Explained why the outer ear should be cleansed.
		•	Filled the irrigating syringe.
		•	Expelled air from the syringe.

Trial 1	Trial 2	Point Value	Performance Standards
		▷	Explained why air should be expelled from the syringe.
		•	Properly straightened the ear canal.
		▷	Stated why the canal must be straightened.
		•	Inserted the syringe tip into the ear.
		•	Did not insert the syringe too deeply.
		•	Made sure that the tip of the syringe did not obstruct the canal opening.
		▷	Stated why the canal should not be obstructed.
		•	Injected the irrigating solution toward the roof of the ear canal.
		▷	Stated why solution should be injected toward the roof of the canal.
		•	Refilled the syringe and continued irrigating until the desired results were obtained or all the solution was used.
		•	Observed the returning solution to note the material present and the amount.
		•	Dried outside of the ear with a gauze pad.
		•	Informed the patient that the ear will feel sensitive.
		•	Instructed the patient to lie on the affected side on the treatment table.
		▷	Explained why the patient should lie on the affected side.
		•	Inserted a cotton wick loosely in the ear canal for 15 minutes.
		▷	Stated the purpose of the cotton wick.
		•	Removed gloves and sanitized hands.
		•	Documented the procedure correctly.
		•	Returned equipment.
			Demonstrated the following affective behavior(s) during this procedure:
		Ⓐ	Incorporated critical thinking skills when performing patient care.
		Ⓐ	Showed awareness of a patient's concerns related to the procedure being performed.
		Ⓐ	Explained to a patient the rationale for performance of a procedure.
		★	Completed the procedure within 10 minutes.
			Totals

CHART

Date	

Evaluation of Student Performance

EVALUATION CRITERIA			COMMENTS
Symbol	**Category**	**Point Value**	
★	Critical Step	16 points	
•	Essential Step	6 points	
Ⓐ	Affective Competency	6 points	
▷	Theory Question	2 points	

Score calculation: 100 points
−_____ points missed
____ Score

Satisfactory score: 85 or above

CAAHEP Competencies Achieved

Psychomotor (Skills)

☑ I. 8. Instruct and prepare a patient for a procedure or a treatment.

☑ II. 1. Calculate proper dosages of medication for administration.

☑ X.3. Document patient care accurately in the medical record.

Affective (Behavior)

☑ I. 2. Incorporate critical thinking skills when performing patient care.

☑ I. 3. Show awareness of a patient's concerns related to the procedure being performed.

☑ V. 4. Explain to a patient the rationale for performance of a procedure.

ABHES Competencies Achieved

☑ 2. c. Identify diagnostic and treatment modalities as they relate to each body system.

☑ 4. a. Follow documentation guidelines.

☑ 8. e. Perform specialty procedures, but not limited to minor surgery, cardiac, respiratory, OB-GYN, neurological, and gastroenterology.

Chapter **6 Eye and Ear Assessment and Procedures**

Procedure 6-6: Performing an Ear Instillation

Name: _____   Date: _____

Evaluated by: _____   Score: _____

Performance Objective

Outcome:	Perform an ear instillation.
Conditions:	Given the following: disposable gloves, otic medication, and gauze pad.
Standards:	Time: 5 minutes. Student completed procedure in _____ minutes.
	Accuracy: Satisfactory score on the Performance Evaluation Checklist.

Performance Evaluation Checklist

Trial 1	Trial 2	Point Value	Performance Standards
		•	Sanitized hands.
		•	Assembled equipment.
		•	Checked the drug label when removing the medication from storage.
		▷	Stated what word must appear on the medication label.
		•	Checked the drug label and dosage against the provider's instructions.
		•	Checked the expiration date of the medication.
		▷	Explained what might occur if the medication is outdated.
		•	Greeted the patient and introduced yourself.
		•	Identified the patient and explained the procedure.
		•	Positioned patient in a sitting position.
		•	Warmed the eardrops with your hands.
		•	Applied gloves.
		•	Mixed medication if required, by shaking the container.
		•	Checked the drug label and removed the cap.
		•	Asked the patient to tilt the head in the direction of the unaffected ear.
		•	Properly straightened the ear canal.
		▷	Stated the reason for straightening the canal.
		•	Placed tip of dropper at the opening of the ear canal and inserted the proper amount of medication.
		•	Instructed the patient to lie on the unaffected side for 2 to 3 minutes.
		▷	Explained why the patient should lie on the unaffected side.
		•	Placed a moistened cotton wick loosely in the ear canal for 15 minutes.

249

Trial 1	Trial 2	Point Value	Performance Standards
		▷	Stated the reason for moistening the wick.
		•	Removed gloves and sanitized hands.
		•	Documented the procedure correctly.
		•	Returned equipment.
			Demonstrated the following affective behavior(s) during this procedure:
		Ⓐ	Incorporated critical thinking skills when performing patient care.
		Ⓐ	Showed awareness of a patient's concerns related to the procedure being performed.
		Ⓐ	Explained to a patient the rationale for performance of a procedure.
		★	Completed the procedure within 5 minutes.
			Totals

CHART	
Date	

Evaluation of Student Performance

EVALUATION CRITERIA			COMMENTS
Symbol	**Category**	**Point Value**	
★	Critical Step	16 points	
•	Essential Step	6 points	
Ⓐ	Affective Competency	6 points	
▷	Theory Question	2 points	

Score calculation: 100 points
− _____ points missed
_____ Score

Satisfactory score: 85 or above

CAAHEP Competencies Achieved

Psychomotor (Skills)

☑ I. 8. Instruct and prepare a patient for a procedure or a treatment.

☑ II. 1. Calculate proper dosages of medication for administration.

☑ X.3. Document patient care accurately in the medical record.

Affective (Behavior)

☑ I. 2. Incorporate critical thinking skills when performing patient care.

☑ I. 3. Show awareness of a patient's concerns related to the procedure being performed.

☑ V. 4. Explain to a patient the rationale for performance of a procedure.

ABHES Competencies Achieved

☑ 2. c. Identify diagnostic and treatment modalities as they relate to each body system.

☑ 4. a. Follow documentation guidelines.

☑ 8. e. Perform specialty procedures, but not limited to minor surgery, cardiac, respiratory, OB-GYN, neurological, and gastroenterology.

7 Physical Agents to Promote Tissue Healing

CHAPTER ASSIGNMENTS

√ After Completing	Date Due	Study Guide Pages	STUDY GUIDE ASSIGNMENTS (CTA = Critical Thinking Activity)	Possible Points	Points You Earned
		257	Pretest	10	
		258	Key Term Assessment	15	
		258-261	Evaluation of Learning questions	28	
		262	CTA A: Dear Gabby	10	
		262-263	CTA B: Cast Care	20	
		265	CTA C: Crutch Guidelines	8	
		266	CTA D: Accessibility for Physical Disabilities	7	
		267	CTA E: Crossword Puzzle	26	
		268	CTA F: Bone and Joint Conditions	40	
			Evolve Site: Quiz Show (Record points earned)		
			Evolve Site: Apply Your Knowledge questions	10	
			Evolve Site: Video Evaluation	63	
		257	Posttest	10	
			ADDITIONAL ASSIGNMENTS		
			Total points		

√ When Assigned by Your Instructor	Study Guide Page(s)	Practices Required	LABORATORY ASSIGNMENTS (Procedure Number and Name)	Score*
	271	3	**Practice for Competency** 7-1: Applying a Heating Pad Textbook reference: p. 212-213	
	273-274		**Evaluation of Competency** 7-1: Applying a Heating Pad	*
	271	3	**Practice for Competency** 7-2: Applying a Hot Soak Textbook reference: p. 213-214	
	275-277		**Evaluation of Competency** 7-2: Applying a Hot Soak	*
	271	3	**Practice for Competency** 7-3: Applying a Hot Compress Textbook reference: pp. 214-215	
	279-281		**Evaluation of Competency** 7-3: Applying a Hot Compress	*
	271	3	**Practice for Competency** 7-4: Applying an Ice Bag Textbook reference: pp. 216-217	
	283-284		**Evaluation of Competency** 7-4: Applying an Ice Bag	*
	271	3	**Practice for Competency** 7-5: Applying a Cold Compress Textbook reference: pp. 217-218	
	285-286		**Evaluation of Competency** 7-5: Applying a Cold Compress	*
	271	3	**Practice for Competency** 7-6: Applying a Chemical Pack Textbook reference: p. 218	
	287-288		**Evaluation of Competency** 7-6: Applying a Chemical Pack	*
	271	3	**Practice for Competency** 7-7: Measuring for Axillary Crutches Textbook reference: p. 227	
	289-290		**Evaluation of Competency** 7-7: Measuring for Axillary Crutches	*
	271	3 × for each gait	**Practice for Competency** 7-8: Instructing a Patient in Crutch Gaits Textbook reference: pp. 228-230	
	291-293		**Evaluation of Competency** 7-8: Instructing a Patient in Crutch Gaits	*

√ When Assigned by Your Instructor	Study Guide Page(s)	Practices Required	LABORATORY ASSIGNMENTS (Procedure Number and Name)	Score*
	271	Cane: 3 Walker: 3	**Practice for Competency** 7-9 and 7-10: Instructing a Patient in the Use of a Cane and Walker Textbook reference: p. 231	
	295-296		**Evaluation of Competency** 7-9 and 7-10: Instructing a Patient in the Use of a Cane and Walker	*
			ADDITIONAL ASSIGNMENTS	

Name: _____ Date: _____

True or False

_____ 1. A hot compress is an example of moist heat.

_____ 2. Erythema is redness of the skin caused by dilation of superficial blood vessels.

_____ 3. The local application of cold may be used to relieve muscle spasms.

_____ 4. Chemical cold packs should be stored in the refrigerator.

_____ 5. An orthodontist is a physician who specializes in the diagnosis and treatment of disorders of the musculoskeletal system.

_____ 6. The most frequent reason for applying a cast is to aid in the nonsurgical correction of a deformity.

_____ 7. Numbness of the fingers or toes may indicate that a cast is too tight.

_____ 8. A coat hanger can be used to scratch under a cast if itching occurs.

_____ 9. Ambulation refers to the inability to walk.

_____ 10. A patient using crutches should be instructed to support his or her weight against the axilla.

? POSTTEST

True or False

_____ 1. The recommended time for the application of heat is 15 to 30 minutes.

_____ 2. The local application of heat results in constriction of blood vessels in the area to which it is applied.

_____ 3. The most frequent cause of low back pain is poor posture.

_____ 4. An ice bag should be filled with large pieces of ice.

_____ 5. If axillary crutches have been fitted properly, the elbow will be flexed at an angle of 30 degrees.

_____ 6. A wet cast can cause a pressure area to occur.

_____ 7. The purpose of cast padding is to prevent pressure areas.

_____ 8. It usually takes 10 to 12 weeks for a fracture to heal.

_____ 9. Incorrectly fitted crutches may cause crutch palsy.

_____ 10. A cane should be held on the strong side of the body.

Directions: Match each key term with its definition.

D	1. Ambulation	A. A discharge produced by the body's tissues
G	2. Brace	B. An overstretching of a muscle caused by trauma
C	3. Compress	C. A soft, moist, absorbent cloth that is folded in several layers and applied to a part of the body in the local application of heat or cold
F	4. Edema	D. Walking or moving from one place to another
I	5. Erythema	E. The direct immersion of a body part in water or a medicated solution
A	6. Exudate	F. The retention of fluid in the tissues, resulting in swelling
H	7. Long arm cast	G. An orthopedic device used to support and hold a part of the body in the correct position to allow functioning and healing
M	8. Maceration	H. A cast that extends from the axilla to the fingers
L	9. Orthopedist	I. Reddening of the skin caused by dilation of superficial blood vessels in the skin
N	10. Short leg cast	J. Trauma to a joint that causes injury to the ligaments
E	11. Soak	K. The process of pus formation
O	12. Splint	L. A physician who specializes in the diagnosis and treatment of disorders of the musculoskeletal system
J	13. Sprain	M. The softening and breaking down of the skin as a result of prolonged exposure to moisture
B	14. Strain	N. A cast that begins just below the knee and extends to the toes
K	15. Suppuration	O. An orthopedic device used to support and immobilize a part of the body

EVALUATION OF LEARNING

Directions: Fill in each blank with the correct answer.

1. State whether the following is an example of dry heat, moist heat, dry cold, or moist cold.

   a. Hot compress

   _____

   b. Ice bag

   _____

   c. Heating pad

   _____

   d. Chemical hot pack

   _____

   e. Cold compress

   _____

2. List three factors that must be taken into consideration when applying heat or cold.

   _____

   _____

3. How does the local application of heat to an affected area for a short period of time influence the following?

a. The diameter of the blood vessels in the affected area

_____

b. The blood supply to the affected area

_____

c. Tissue metabolism in the affected area

_____

4. What happens to the diameter of blood vessels if heat is applied for a prolonged period (more than 1 hour)?

_____

_____

5. List three reasons for applying heat locally.

_____

_____

_____

6. How does the local application of cold for a short period of time to an affected area influence the following?

a. The diameter of the blood vessels in the affected area

_____

b. The blood supply to the affected area

_____

_____

c. Tissue metabolism in the affected area

_____

_____

7. List two reasons for applying cold locally.

_____

_____

8. What are three reasons for applying a cast?

_____

_____

_____

9. What causes a pressure area?

_____

_____

10. What are the symptoms of a pressure area?

_____

11. What are the complications of a pressure ulcer?

_____

_____

12. What is the purpose of covering the body part with a stockinette before applying a cast?

_____

_____

13. What is the purpose of applying cast padding during cast application?

_____

_____

14. Why should each of the following precautions be taken when applying a cast?

    a. Removing synthetic casting particles using an alcohol swab

    _____

    b. Checking the circulation, sensation, and movement of the extremity

    _____

15. Why is it important to dry a synthetic cast as soon as possible after it gets wet?

_____

16. What symptoms may indicate that a cast is too tight and an infection is developing?

_____

17. How is a cast removed?

_____

_____

18. What will the affected extremity look like after a cast has been removed?

_____

19. List two examples of conditions for which a splint may be applied.

_____

_____

20. List one example of a condition for which a brace may be applied.

_____

_____

21. What factors does the provider take into consideration when prescribing an ambulatory assistive device?

_____

_____

22. Describe one advantage of the forearm crutch.

_____

23. What may occur if axillary crutches are not fitted properly?

_____

_____

24. List eight guidelines that must be followed during crutch use to ensure safety.

_____

_____

_____

_____

_____

_____

_____

_____

25. List one use for each of the following crutch gaits:

a. Four-point gait _____

b. Three-point gait _____

c. Swing-to gait _____

26. List and describe the three types of canes.

_____

_____

27. List two reasons for prescribing a cane.

_____

_____

28. List two reasons for prescribing a walker.

_____

_____

A. Dear Gabby

Gabby was called out of town unexpectedly and wants you to fill in for her. In the space provided, respond to the following letter.

Dear Gabby:

I am 15 years old and in the 10th grade. I need your help. I have a backpack; my dad weighed it and said it was 40 pounds. I only weigh 105 pounds. My back and neck hurt from lugging it around. I have to walk almost one-half mile to the bus stop. I do not have time to use my locker between classes because it is down a flight of stairs and at the end of the hall. Once, when I started using my locker, my science teacher got mad at me because I was late getting to class. Gabby, what should I do?

Signed,
Pain in the Neck

_____

_____

_____

_____

_____

_____

_____

_____

_____

_____

B. Cast Care

1. You are employed by a pediatric orthopedic surgeon. She is concerned because many of her school-aged patients do not follow proper guidelines for the care of their fiberglass casts, even with their parents' constant reminders. She asks you to develop a creative and colorful instruction sheet in the shape of a cast that presents cast care instructions at a level that can be understood by this age group (6 to 12 years old). Use the illustration of the cast on page 263 to design your instruction sheet.

2. After developing your instruction sheet, get into a group of three or four students and share your sheets. Have the group decide whether the instructions on each sheet are appropriate for a school-aged child and whether the sheet would be visually appealing to this age group.

Instruction Sheet for Cast Care

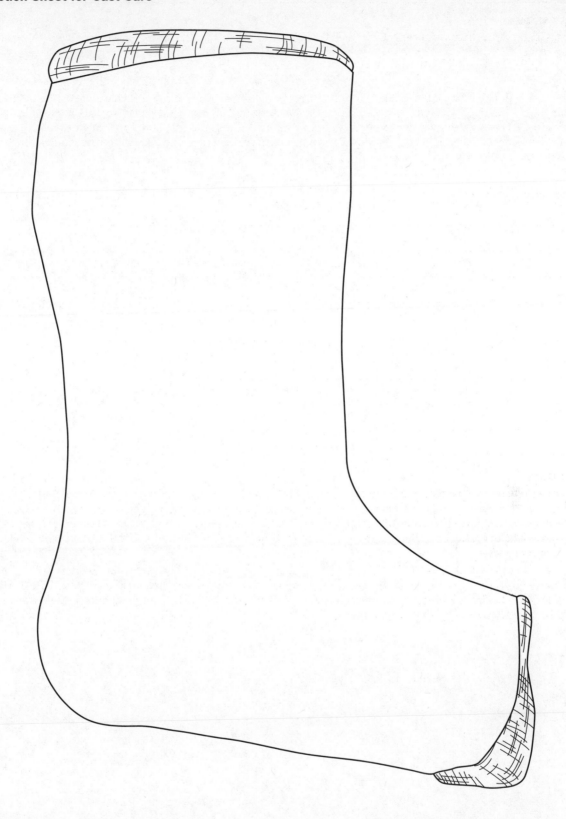

C. Crutch Guidelines

Each of the following patients is wearing a long leg cast because of a broken tibia and is using wooden axillary crutches to ambulate. Evaluate the crutch technique being practiced by each patient. Write **C** if the technique is correct and **I** if the technique is incorrect. If the technique is correct, explain why it should be performed this way. If incorrect, indicate what may happen from performing the technique in this manner.

1. Andy Morris wears Nike sports shoes when ambulating with his crutches.

   _____

   _____

2. Juliet Wright does not stand up straight when using her crutches.

   _____

   _____

3. Miguel Saldivia puts his weight on the axilla when getting around on his crutches.

   _____

   _____

4. Lindy Campbell has a lot of decorative throw rugs in her house, and she does not want to remove them.

   _____

   _____

5. Andrew Spence likes to move quickly on his crutches, so he advances them forward about 20 inches with each step when using the swing-through gait.

   _____

   _____

6. Hanna Romes has tingling in her hands but thinks it is just part of what happens when one uses crutches.

   _____

   _____

7. Tamra Hetrick pads both the shoulder rests and the handgrips of her crutches.

   _____

   _____

8. Erica Anderson's crutch tips get wet, but she does not take the time to dry them before going into a shopping mall.

   _____

   _____

D. Accessibility for Physical Disabilities

Next to each of the following facilities, list the features you have observed that facilitate accessibility of individuals with a physical disability.

1. Schools

_____

_____

2. Grocery stores

_____

_____

3. Shopping malls

_____

_____

4. Movie theaters

_____

_____

5. Restaurants

_____

_____

6. Doctors' offices

_____

_____

7. Community parks

_____

_____

E. Crossword Puzzle: Physical Agents to Promote Tissue Healing

Directions: Complete the crossword puzzle using the clues presented below.

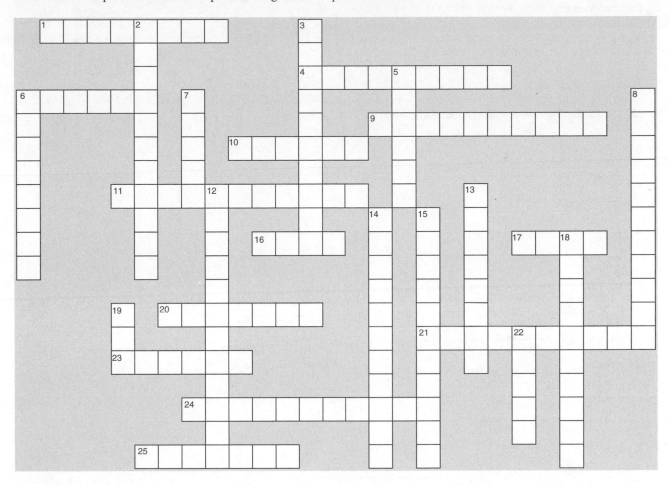

Across
1 Transfers weight from legs to arms
4 Cold blood vessels do this
6 Removable immobilizer
9 Popular synthetic cast
10 Warm blood vessels do this
11 Prevents pressure areas
16 Examples: standard, tripod, or quad
17 Takes 4 to 6 weeks for fracture to do this
20 Discharge
21 Purpose of a cast
23 Needed after knee replacement
24 Bone doctor
25 Cuts cast in half

Down
2 "Too long" crutches may cause this
3 Soft and broken down skin
5 Maximum minutes for heat application
6 Elevate cast to prevent this
7 Do not bend here to lift!
8 Prevents LBP
12 Cast is rubbing against the skin
13 Red skin
14 Pus formation
15 Located between skin and cast padding
18 Walking
19 Blow-dry a cast on this setting
22 Holds body part in correct position

F. Bone and Joint Conditions

1. It is National Bone and Joint Week. The mayor has asked you and your classmates to develop informative, creative, and colorful brochures for the community about bone and joint conditions. Choose a condition below and design a brochure using the blank Frequently Asked Questions (FAQs) brochure provided on the following page. Each student in the class should select a different topic. On a separate sheet of paper, write three true or false questions relating to the information in your brochure.

2. Present your brochure to the class. After all the brochures have been presented, each student should ask the three questions to the entire class to see how well the class understands bone and joint conditions. (*Note:* You can take notes during the presentations and refer to them when answering the questions.)

   1. Bursitis

   2. Congenital hip dysplasia

   3. Epicondylitis

   4. Fibromyalgia

   5. Gout

   6. Hammer toe

   7. Herniated disk

   8. Juvenile rheumatoid arthritis

   9. Knee replacement surgery

   10. Kyphosis

   11. Osteoarthritis

   12. Osteomyelitis

   13. Osteoporosis

   14. Paget's disease

   15. Rheumatoid arthritis

   16. Scoliosis

   17. Sprain

   18. Strain

   19. Tendinitis

FAQ ON:

Q:

A:

Q:

A:

Q:

A:

Q:

A:

Chapter **7** **Physical Agents to Promote Tissue Healing**

Q:

A:

Q:

A:

Illustration

Q:

A:

Q:

A:

Chapter **7 Physical Agents to Promote Tissue Healing**

Local Application of Heat and Cold

Procedures 7-1, 7-2, and 7-3: Application of Heat

Apply the following heat treatments, and document the procedure in the chart provided: heating pad, hot soak, hot compress, and chemical hot pack.

Procedures 7-4, 7-5, and 7-6: Application of Cold

Apply the following cold treatments, and document the results in the chart provided: ice bag, cold compress, and chemical cold pack.

Ambulatory Aids

Procedure 7-7: Axillary Crutch Measurement

Measure an individual for axillary crutches, and document the procedure in the chart provided.

Procedure 7-8: Crutch Gaits

Instruct an individual in mastering the following crutch gaits: four-point, two-point, three-point, swing-to, and swing-through. Document the procedure in the chart provided.

Procedure 7-9: Cane

Instruct an individual in the use of a cane, and document the procedure in the chart provided.

Procedure 7-10: Walker

Instruct an individual in the use of a walker, and document the procedure in the chart provided.

CHART	
Date	

CHART	
Date	

Procedure 7-1: Applying a Heating Pad

Name: _____   Date: _____

Evaluated by: _____   Score: _____

Performance Objective

Outcome:	Apply a heating pad.
Conditions:	Given a heating pad with a protective covering.
Standards:	Time: 5 minutes. Student completed procedure in _____ minutes.
	Accuracy: Satisfactory score on the Performance Evaluation Checklist.

Performance Evaluation Checklist

Trial 1	Trial 2	Point Value	Performance Standards
		•	Sanitized hands.
		•	Assembled the equipment.
		•	Greeted the patient and introduced yourself.
		•	Identified the patient and explained the procedure.
		•	Placed the heating pad in a protective covering.
		•	Connected the plug to an electrical outlet and set the selector switch to the proper setting.
		•	Placed the heating pad on patient's affected body area and asked how the temperature felt.
		•	Instructed the patient not to lie on the pad or turn the temperature setting higher.
		▷	Stated why the patient should be instructed not to lie on the heating pad.
		▷	Explained why the patient may want to increase the temperature.
		•	Checked the patient's skin periodically.
		•	Administered treatment for the proper length of time as designated by the provider.
		•	Sanitized hands.
		•	Documented the procedure correctly.
		•	Properly cared for and returned the equipment to its storage place.
			Demonstrated the following affective behavior(s) during this procedure:
		Ⓐ	Incorporated critical thinking skills when performing patient assessment.
		Ⓐ	Incorporated critical thinking skills when performing patient care.
		★	Completed the procedure within 5 minutes.
			Totals

Evaluation of Student Performance

EVALUATION CRITERIA			COMMENTS
Symbol	**Category**	**Point Value**	
★	Critical Step	16 points	
•	Essential Step	6 points	
Ⓐ	Affective Competency	6 points	
▷	Theory Question	2 points	

Score calculation: 100 points
  − _____ points missed
  _____ Score

Satisfactory score: 85 or above

CAAHEP Competencies Achieved

Psychomotor (Skills)

☑ I. 8. Instruct and prepare a patient for a procedure or a treatment.

☑ V. 11. Report relevant information concisely and accurately.

Affective (Behavior)

☑ I. 1. Incorporate critical thinking skills when performing patient assessment.

☑ I. 2. Incorporate critical thinking skills when performing patient care.

ABHES Competencies Achieved

☑ 2. c. Identify diagnostic and treatment modalities as they relate to each body system.

☑ 8. e. Display professionalism through written and verbal communications.

☑ 9. e. Perform specialty procedures including but not limited to minor surgery, cardiac, respiratory, OB-GYN, neurological and gastroenterology.

Procedure 7-2: Applying a Hot Soak

Name: _____   Date: _____

Evaluated by: _____   Score: _____

Performance Objective

Outcome:	Apply a hot soak.
Conditions:	Given the following: soaking solution, bath thermometer, basin, and bath towels.
Standards:	Time: 10 minutes. Student completed procedure in _____ minutes.
	Accuracy: Satisfactory score on the Performance Evaluation Checklist.

Performance Evaluation Checklist

Trial 1	Trial 2	Point Value	Performance Standards
		•	Sanitized hands.
		•	Assembled the equipment.
		•	Checked the label on the solution container.
		•	Warmed the soaking solution.
		•	Greeted the patient and introduced yourself.
		•	Identified the patient and explained the procedure.
		•	Filled a basin one-half to two-thirds full with the warmed soaking solution.
		•	Checked the temperature of the solution with a bath thermometer.
		▷	Stated the safe temperature range that should be used for an adult patient (105° F to 110° F).
		•	Assisted the patient into a comfortable position and padded the side of the basin with a towel.
		•	Slowly and gradually immersed the affected body part into the solution and asked the patient how the temperature felt.
		•	Kept the solution at a constant temperature by removing cooler solution and adding hot solution.
		•	Placed a hand between the patient and the solution when adding more solution.
		•	Stirred the solution with your hand while pouring it.
		•	Checked the patient's skin periodically.
		•	Applied the hot soak for the proper length of time as designated by the provider.
		•	Completely dried the affected part.
		•	Sanitized hands.
		•	Documented the procedure correctly.

Trial 1	Trial 2	Point Value	Performance Standards
		•	Properly cared for and returned the equipment to its storage place.
			Demonstrated the following affective behavior(s) during this procedure:
		Ⓐ	Incorporated critical thinking skills when performing patient assessment.
		Ⓐ	Incorporated critical thinking skills when performing patient care.
		★	Completed the procedure within 10 minutes.
			Totals

CHART	
Date	

Evaluation of Student Performance

EVALUATION CRITERIA			COMMENTS
Symbol	**Category**	**Point Value**	
★	Critical Step	16 points	
•	Essential Step	6 points	
Ⓐ	Affective Competency	6 points	
▷	Theory Question	2 points	

Score calculation: 100 points
−_____ points missed
_____ Score

Satisfactory score: 85 or above

CAAHEP Competencies Achieved

Psychomotor (Skills)

☑ I. 8. Instruct and prepare a patient for a procedure or a treatment.

☑ V. 11. Report relevant information concisely and accurately.

Affective (Behavior)

☑ I. 1. Incorporate critical thinking skills when performing patient assessment.

☑ I. 2. Incorporate critical thinking skills when performing patient care.

ABHES Competencies Achieved

☑ 2. c. Identify diagnostic and treatment modalities as they relate to each body system.

☑ 7. g. Display professionalism through written and verbal communications.

☑ 8. e. Perform specialty procedures including but not limited to minor surgery, cardiac, respiratory, OB-GYN, neurological, and gastroenterology.

Notes

e **Procedure 7-3: Applying a Hot Compress**

Name: _____ Date: _____

Evaluated by: _____ Score: _____

Performance Objective

Outcome:	Apply a hot compress.
Conditions:	Given the following: solution for the compresses, bath thermometer, basin, washcloths, and a towel.
Standards:	Time: 10 minutes. Student completed procedure in _____ minutes.
	Accuracy: Satisfactory score on the Performance Evaluation Checklist.

Performance Evaluation Checklist

Trial 1	Trial 2	Point Value	Performance Standards
		•	Sanitized hands.
		•	Assembled the equipment.
		•	Checked the label on the solution container.
		•	Warmed the soaking solution.
		•	Greeted the patient and introduced yourself.
		•	Identified the patient and explained the procedure.
		•	Filled the basin half full with the warmed solution.
		•	Checked the temperature of the solution with a bath thermometer.
		▷	Stated the safe temperature range that should be used for an adult patient (105° F to 110° F).
		•	Completely immersed the compress in the solution.
		•	Squeezed excess solution from the compress.
		•	Applied the compress to the affected body part and asked the patient how the temperature felt.
		•	Placed additional compresses in the solution.
		•	Repeated the application every 2 to 3 minutes for the duration of time specified by the provider.
		•	Checked the patient's skin periodically.
		•	Checked the temperature of the solution periodically, removed cooler fluid, and added hot fluid if needed.
		•	Administered the treatment for the proper length of time as designated by a provider.
		•	Thoroughly dried the affected part.

Trial 1	Trial 2	Point Value	Performance Standards
		•	Sanitized hands.
		•	Documented the procedure correctly.
		•	Properly cared for and returned the equipment to its storage place.
			Demonstrated the following affective behavior(s) during this procedure:
		Ⓐ	Incorporated critical thinking skills when performing patient assessment.
		Ⓐ	Incorporated critical thinking skills when performing patient care.
		★	Completed the procedure within 10 minutes.
			Totals

CHART

Date	

Evaluation of Student Performance

EVALUATION CRITERIA			COMMENTS
Symbol	**Category**	**Point Value**	
★	Critical Step	16 points	
•	Essential Step	6 points	
Ⓐ	Affective Competency	6 points	
▷	Theory Question	2 points	

Score calculation: 100 points
− _____ points missed
_____ Score

Satisfactory score: 85 or above

CAAHEP Competencies Achieved

Psychomotor (Skills)

☑ I. 8. Instruct and prepare a patient for a procedure or a treatment.

☑ V. 11. Report relevant information concisely and accurately.

Affective (Behavior)

☑ I. 1. Incorporate critical thinking skills when performing patient assessment.

☑ I. 2. Incorporate critical thinking skills when performing patient care.

ABHES Competencies Achieved

☑ 2. c. Identify diagnostic and treatment modalities as they relate to each body system.

☑ 7. g. Display professionalism through written and verbal communications.

☑ 8. e. Perform specialty procedures including but not limited to minor surgery, cardiac, respiratory, OB-GYN, neurological, and gastroenterology.

Chapter **7** **Physical Agents to Promote Tissue Healing**

e Procedure 7-4: Applying an Ice Bag

Name: _____   Date: _____

Evaluated by: _____   Score: _____

Performance Objective

Outcome:	Apply an ice bag.
Conditions:	Given the following: ice bag and protective covering, and small pieces of ice.
Standards:	Time: 10 minutes. Student completed procedure in _____ minutes.
	Accuracy: Satisfactory score on the Performance Evaluation Checklist.

Performance Evaluation Checklist

Trial 1	Trial 2	Point Value	Performance Standards
		•	Sanitized hands.
		•	Assembled the equipment.
		•	Greeted the patient and introduced yourself.
		•	Identified the patient and explained the procedure.
		•	Checked the ice bag for leakage.
		•	Filled the bag one-half to two-thirds full with small pieces of ice.
		▷	Explained why small pieces of ice are used.
		•	Expelled air from the bag.
		▷	Explained the reason for expelling air from bag.
		•	Placed the bag in a protective covering.
		▷	Stated the purpose of placing the bag in a protective covering.
		•	Placed the bag on the affected body area and asked the patient how the temperature felt.
		•	Checked the patient's skin periodically.
		▷	Listed skin changes that would warrant removal of the bag.
		•	Refilled the bag with ice and changed the protective covering when needed.
		•	Administered the treatment for the proper length of time as designated by the provider.
		•	Sanitized hands.
		•	Documented the procedure correctly.
		•	Properly cared for and returned the equipment to its storage place.
			Demonstrated the following affective behavior(s) during this procedure:
		Ⓐ	Incorporated critical thinking skills when performing patient assessment.
		Ⓐ	Incorporated critical thinking skills when performing patient care.
		★	Completed the procedure within 10 minutes.
			Totals

Chapter **7 Physical Agents to Promote Tissue Healing**

CHART	
Date	

Evaluation of Student Performance

EVALUATION CRITERIA			COMMENTS
Symbol	**Category**	**Point Value**	
★	Critical Step	16 points	
•	Essential Step	6 points	
Ⓐ	Affective Competency	6 points	
▷	Theory Question	2 points	

Score calculation: 100 points
− _____ points missed
_____ Score

Satisfactory score: 85 or above

CAAHEP Competencies Achieved

Psychomotor (Skills)

☑ I. 8. Instruct and prepare a patient for a procedure or a treatment.

☑ V. 11. Report relevant information concisely and accurately.

Affective (Behavior)

☑ I. 1. Incorporate critical thinking skills when performing patient assessment.

☑ I. 2. Incorporate critical thinking skills when performing patient care.

ABHES Competencies Achieved

☑ 2. c. Identify diagnostic and treatment modalities as they relate to each body system.

☑ 7. g. Display professionalism through written and verbal communications.

☑ 8. e. Perform specialty procedures including but not limited to minor surgery, cardiac, respiratory, OB-GYN, neurological, and gastroenterology.

Procedure 7-5: Applying a Cold Compress

Name: _____   Date: _____

Evaluated by: _____   Score: _____

Performance Objective

Outcome:	Apply a cold compress.
Conditions:	Given the following: ice cubes, a basin, and washcloths.
Standards:	Time: 10 minutes. Student completed procedure in _____ minutes.
	Accuracy: Satisfactory score on the Performance Evaluation Checklist.

Performance Evaluation Checklist

Trial 1	Trial 2	Point Value	Performance Standards
		•	Sanitized hands.
		•	Assembled the equipment.
		•	Checked the label on the solution.
		•	Greeted the patient and introduced yourself.
		•	Identified the patient and explained the procedure.
		•	Placed large ice cubes in the basin and added the solution until the basin is half full.
		▷	Explained why larger pieces of ice are used.
		•	Completely immersed the compress in the solution.
		•	Squeezed excess solution from the compress.
		•	Applied the compress to the affected body part and asked the patient how the temperature felt.
		•	Placed additional compresses in the solution.
		•	Repeated the application every 2 to 3 minutes for the duration of time specified by the provider.
		•	Checked the patient's skin periodically.
		•	Added ice if needed to keep the solution cold.
		•	Administered the treatment for the proper length of time as designated by the provider.
		•	Thoroughly dried the affected part.
		•	Sanitized hands.
		•	Documented the procedure correctly.
		•	Properly cared for and returned the equipment to its storage place.
			Demonstrated the following affective behavior(s) during this procedure:
		Ⓐ	Incorporated critical thinking skills when performing patient assessment.
		Ⓐ	Incorporated critical thinking skills when performing patient care.
		★	Completed the procedure within 10 minutes.
			Totals

Chapter **7** **Physical Agents to Promote Tissue Healing**

CHART	
Date	

Evaluation of Student Performance

EVALUATION CRITERIA			COMMENTS
Symbol	**Category**	**Point Value**	
★	Critical Step	16 points	
•	Essential Step	6 points	
Ⓐ	Affective Competency	6 points	
▷	Theory Question	2 points	

Score calculation: 100 points
− _____ points missed
_____ Score

Satisfactory score: 85 or above

CAAHEP Competencies Achieved

Psychomotor (Skills)

☑ I. 8. Instruct and prepare a patient for a procedure or a treatment.
☑ V. 11. Report relevant information concisely and accurately.

Affective (Behavior)

☑ I. 1. Incorporate critical thinking skills when performing patient assessment.
☑ I. 2. Incorporate critical thinking skills when performing patient care.

ABHES Competencies Achieved

☑ 2. c. Identify diagnostic and treatment modalities as they relate to each body system.
☑ 7. g. Display professionalism through written and verbal communications.
☑ 8. e. Perform specialty procedures including but not limited to minor surgery, cardiac, respiratory, OB-GYN, neurological, and gastroenterology.

Procedure 7-6: Applying a Chemical Pack

Name: _____ Date: _____

Evaluated by: _____ Score: _____

Performance Objective

Outcome:	Apply a chemical cold and hot pack.
Conditions:	Given a chemical cold and hot pack.
Standards:	Time: 5 minutes. Student completed procedure in _____ minutes.
	Accuracy: Satisfactory score on the Performance Evaluation Checklist.

Performance Evaluation Checklist

Trial 1	Trial 2	Point Value	Performance Standards
		•	Sanitized hands.
		•	Assembled the equipment.
		•	Greeted the patient and introduced yourself.
		•	Identified the patient and explained the procedure.
		•	Shook the crystals to the bottom of bag.
		•	Squeezed the bag firmly to break the inner water bag.
		•	Shook the bag vigorously to mix the contents.
		•	Covered the bag with a protective covering.
		•	Applied the bag to the affected area.
		•	Checked the patient's skin periodically.
		•	Administered the treatment for the proper length of time.
		•	Discarded the bag in an appropriate receptacle.
		•	Sanitized hands.
		•	Documented the procedure correctly.
			Demonstrated the following affective behavior(s) during this procedure:
		Ⓐ	Incorporated critical thinking skills when performing patient assessment.
		Ⓐ	Incorporated critical thinking skills when performing patient care.
		★	Completed the procedure within 5 minutes.
			Totals

Chapter **7** **Physical Agents to Promote Tissue Healing**

Evaluation of Student Performance

EVALUATION CRITERIA			COMMENTS
Symbol	**Category**	**Point Value**	
★	Critical Step	16 points	
•	Essential Step	6 points	
Ⓐ	Affective Competency	6 points	
▷	Theory Question	2 points	

Score calculation: 100 points
− _____ points missed
____ Score

Satisfactory score: 85 or above

CAAHEP Competencies Achieved

Psychomotor (Skills)

☑ I. 8. Instruct and prepare a patient for a procedure or a treatment.
☑ V. 11. Report relevant information concisely and accurately.

Affective (Behavior)

☑ I. 1. Incorporate critical thinking skills when performing patient assessment.
☑ I. 2. Incorporate critical thinking skills when performing patient care.

ABHES Competencies Achieved

☑ 2. c. Identify diagnostic and treatment modalities as they relate to each body system.
☑ 7. g. Display professionalism through written and verbal communications.
☑ 8. e. Perform specialty procedures including but not limited to minor surgery, cardiac, respiratory, OB-GYN, neurological, and gastroenterology.

Procedure 7-7: Measuring for Axillary Crutches

Name: _____   Date: _____

Evaluated by: _____   Score: _____

Performance Objective

Outcome:	Measure an individual for axillary crutches.
Conditions:	Given the following: axillary crutches and a tape measure.
Standards:	Time: 10 minutes. Student completed procedure in _____ minutes.
	Accuracy: Satisfactory score on the Performance Evaluation Checklist.

Performance Evaluation Checklist

Trial 1	Trial 2	Point Value	Performance Standards
		•	Asked the patient to stand erect.
		•	Positioned the crutches with the tips at a distance of 2 inches in front of, and 4 to 6 inches to the side of, each foot.
		•	Adjusted crutch length so that the shoulder rests were approximately 1½ to 2 inches below the axilla.
		•	Asked the patient to support his or her weight by the handgrips.
		•	Adjusted the handgrips so that the patient's elbow was flexed approximately 30 degrees.
		•	Checked the fit of the crutches by placing two fingers between the top of the crutch and the patient's axilla.
		•	Documented the procedure correctly.
			Demonstrated the following affective behavior(s) during this procedure:
		Ⓐ	Incorporated critical thinking skills when performing patient assessment.
		Ⓐ	Incorporated critical thinking skills when performing patient care.
		★	Completed the procedure within 10 minutes.
			Totals

CHART	
Date	

Evaluation of Student Performance

EVALUATION CRITERIA			COMMENTS
Symbol	**Category**	**Point Value**	
★	Critical Step	16 points	
•	Essential Step	6 points	
Ⓐ	Affective Competency	6 points	
▷	Theory Question	2 points	

Score calculation: 100 points
        − _____ points missed
          ____ Score

Satisfactory score: 85 or above

CAAHEP Competencies Achieved

Psychomotor (Skills)

☑ I. 8. Instruct and prepare a patient for a procedure or a treatment.

Affective (Behavior)

☑ I. 1. Incorporate critical thinking skills when performing patient assessment.
☑ I. 2. Incorporate critical thinking skills when performing patient care.

ABHES Competencies Achieved

☑ 7. g. Display professionalism through written and verbal communications.
☑ 8. j. Make adaptations for patients with special needs (psychological or physical limitations).

e Procedure 7-8: Instructing a Patient in Crutch Gaits

Name: _____   Date: _____

Evaluated by: _____   Score: _____

Performance Objective

Outcome:	Instruct an individual in the following crutch gaits: four-point, two-point, three-point, swing-to, and swing-through.
Conditions:	Given axillary crutches.
Standards:	Time: 15 minutes. Student completed procedure in _____ minutes.
	Accuracy: Satisfactory score on the Performance Evaluation Checklist.

Performance Evaluation Checklist

Trial 1	Trial 2	Point Value	Performance Standards
			Tripod Position
			Instructed the patient:
		•	Stand erect and face straight ahead.
		•	Place the tips of crutches 4 to 6 inches in front of, and 4 to 6 inches to side of, each foot.
		▷	Stated one use of the tripod position.
			Four-Point Gait
			Instructed the patient:
		•	Begin in the tripod position.
		•	Move the right crutch forward.
		•	Move the left foot forward to the level of the left crutch.
		•	Move the left crutch forward.
		•	Move the right foot forward to the level of the right crutch.
		•	Repeat the above sequence.
		▷	Stated one use of the four-point gait.
			Two-Point Gait
			Instructed the patient:
		•	Begin in the tripod position.
		•	Move the left crutch and the right foot forward at the same time.
		•	Move the right crutch and the left foot forward at the same time.
		•	Repeat the above sequence.
		▷	Stated one use of the two-point gait.

Chapter **7** Physical Agents to Promote Tissue Healing

Trial 1	Trial 2	Point Value	Performance Standards
			Three-Point Gait
			Instructed the patient:
		•	Begin in the tripod position.
		•	Move both crutches and the affected leg forward.
		•	Move the unaffected leg forward while balancing weight on both crutches.
		•	Repeat the above sequence.
		▷	Stated two uses of the three-point gait.
			Swing-To Gait
			Instructed the patient:
		•	Begin in the tripod position.
		•	Move both crutches forward together.
		•	Lift and swing body to the crutches.
		•	Repeat the above sequence.
		▷	Stated one use of the swing-to gait.
			Swing-Through Gait
			Instructed the patient:
		•	Begin in the tripod position.
		•	Move both crutches forward together.
		•	Lift and swing the body past the crutches.
		•	Repeat the above sequence.
		▷	Stated one use of the swing-through gait.
			Demonstrated the following affective behavior(s) during this procedure:
		Ⓐ	Demonstrated: (a) empathy (b) active listening (c) nonverbal communication.
		★	Completed the procedure within 15 minutes.
			Totals

CHART	
Date	

292

Evaluation of Student Performance

EVALUATION CRITERIA			COMMENTS
Symbol	**Category**	**Point Value**	
★	Critical Step	16 points	
•	Essential Step	6 points	
Ⓐ	Affective Competency	6 points	
▷	Theory Question	2 points	

Score calculation: 100 points
− _____ points missed
_____ Score

Satisfactory score: 85 or above

CAAHEP Competencies Achieved

Psychomotor (Skills)
☑ I. 8. Instruct and prepare a patient for a procedure or a treatment.
☑ V. 4. Coach patients regarding: (a) office policies (b) health maintenance (c) disease prevention (d) treatment plans.

Affective (Behavior)
☑ V. 1. Demonstrate: (a) empathy (b) active listening (c) nonverbal communication.

ABHES Competencies Achieved

☑ 7. g. Display professionalism through written and verbal communications.
☑ 8. j. Make adaptations for patients with special needs (psychological or physical limitations).

Notes

Chapter **7** **Physical Agents to Promote Tissue Healing**

Procedures 7-9 and 7-10: Instructing a Patient in Use of a Cane and Walker

Name: _____ Date: _____

Evaluated by: _____ Score: _____

Performance Objective

Outcome:	Instruct an individual in the use of a cane and walker.
Conditions:	Given the following: a cane and a walker.
Standards:	Time: 10 minutes. Student completed procedure in _____ minutes.
	Accuracy: Satisfactory score on the Performance Evaluation Checklist.

Performance Evaluation Checklist

Trial 1	Trial 2	Point Value	Performance Standards
			Cane
			Instructed the patient:
		•	Hold the cane on the strong side of body.
		•	Place the tip of the cane 4 to 6 inches to the side of foot.
		•	Move the cane forward approximately 12 inches.
		•	Move the affected leg forward to the level of the cane.
		•	Move the strong leg forward and ahead of the cane and weak leg.
		•	Repeat the above sequence.
		▷	Stated one condition for which a cane is used.
			Walker
			Instructed the patient:
		•	Pick up the walker and move it forward approximately 6 inches.
		•	Move the right foot and then the left foot up to the walker.
		•	Repeat the above sequence.
		▷	Stated one condition for which a walker is used.
			Demonstrated the following affective behavior(s) during this procedure:
		Ⓐ	Demonstrated: (a) empathy (b) active listening (c) nonverbal communication.
		★	Completed the procedure within 10 minutes.
			Totals

CHART	
Date	

Evaluation of Student Performance

EVALUATION CRITERIA			COMMENTS
Symbol	**Category**	**Point Value**	
★	Critical Step	16 points	
•	Essential Step	6 points	
Ⓐ	Affective Competency	6 points	
▷	Theory Question	2 points	

Score calculation: 100 points

−_____ points missed

_____ Score

Satisfactory score: 85 or above

CAAHEP Competencies Achieved

Psychomotor (Skills)

☑ I. 8. Instruct and prepare a patient for a procedure or a treatment.

☑ V. 4. Coach patients regarding: (a) office policies (b) health maintenance (c) disease prevention (d) treatment plans.

Affective (Behavior)

☑ V. 1. Demonstrate: (a) empathy (b) active listening (c) nonverbal communication.

ABHES Competencies Achieved

☑ 7. g. Display professionalism through written and verbal communications.

☑ 8. j. Make adaptations for patients with special needs (psychological or physical limitations).

8 The Gynecologic Examination and Prenatal Care

√ After Completing	Date Due	Study Guide Pages	STUDY GUIDE ASSIGNMENTS (CTA = Critical Thinking Activity)	Possible Points	Points You Earned
			e Evolve Site: Road to Recovery: OB/GYN Terminology (Record points earned)		
			e Evolve Site: Apply Your Knowledge questions	12	
			e Evolve Site: Video Evaluation	48	
		301	[?] Posttest	10	
			ADDITIONAL ASSIGNMENTS		
			Total points		

√ When Assigned by Your Instructor	Study Guide Pages	Practices Required	LABORATORY ASSIGNMENTS (Procedure Number and Name)	Score*
	333-334	5	**Practice for Competency** 8-1: Breast Self-Examination Instructions Textbook reference: pp. 246-248	
	343-346		**Evaluation of Competency** 8-1: Breast Self-Examination Instructions	*
	335-336	5	**Practice for Competency** 8-2: Assisting with a Gynecologic Examination Textbook reference: pp. 249-252	
	347-351		**Evaluation of Competency** 8-2: Assisting with a Gynecologic Examination	*
	337-342	5	**Practice for Competency** 8-3: Assisting with a Return Prenatal Examination Textbook reference: pp. 274-277	
	353-356		**Evaluation of Competency** 8-3: Assisting with a Return Prenatal Examination	*
			ADDITIONAL ASSIGNMENTS	

Notes

Name: _____   Date: _____

True or False

_____ 1. A complete gynecologic examination consists of a breast examination and a pelvic examination.

_____ 2. The American College of Obstetricians and Gynecologists recommends that a woman perform a breast self-examination weekly.

_____ 3. The purpose of the Pap test is for the early detection of cervical cancer.

_____ 4. The patient should be instructed to douche before having a Pap test.

_____ 5. Trichomoniasis produces a profuse, frothy vaginal discharge.

_____ 6. Another name for candidiasis is a yeast infection.

_____ 7. Prenatal refers to the care of the pregnant woman before delivery of the infant.

_____ 8. During each return prenatal visit, the mother's urine is tested for glucose and protein.

_____ 9. The normal range for the fetal pulse rate is between 120 and 160 beats per minute.

_____ 10. Amniocentesis can be used to diagnose certain genetically transmitted conditions.

? POSTTEST

True or False

_____ 1. The patient position for a breast examination is the lithotomy position.

_____ 2. Most breast lumps are discovered by the physician.

_____ 3. Trichomoniasis is caused by a virus.

_____ 4. Chlamydia often occurs in association with syphilis.

_____ 5. In the absence of complications, the first prenatal visit should be scheduled after a woman misses her first period.

_____ 6. True labor pains are referred to as Braxton Hicks contractions.

_____ 7. The purpose of measuring fundal height is to determine the degree of cervical dilation and effacement.

_____ 8. The fetal heart tones can first be detected between 4 and 6 weeks of gestation using a Doppler fetal pulse detector.

_____ 9. Obstetric ultrasound scanning is used to assess fetal lung maturity.

_____ 10. The perineum is the period of time in which the body systems are returning to their prepregnant state.

Chapter **8** **The Gynecologic Examination and Prenatal Care**

A. Definitions

Gynecologic Examination

Directions: Match each key term with its definition.

_E_ 1. Adnexal

_F_ 2. Amenorrhea

_C_ 3. Atypical

_Q_ 4. Cervix

_N_ 5. Colposcopy

_H_ 6. Cytology

_R_ 7. Dysmenorrhea

_M_ 8. Dyspareunia

_K_ 9. Dysplasia

_B_ 10. Endocervix

_A_ 11. External os

_I_ 12. Gynecology

_S_ 13. Menopause

_P_ 14. Menorrhagia

_O_ 15. Metrorrhagia

_L_ 16. Perimenopause

_D_ 17. Perineum

_J_ 18. Risk factor

_G_ 19. Vulva

A. The opening of the cervical canal of the uterus into the vagina

B. The mucous membrane lining the cervical canal

C. Deviation from the normal

D. The external region between the vaginal orifice and the anus in a female and between the scrotum and the anus in a male

E. Adjacent

F. The absence or cessation of the menstrual period

G. The region of the female external genital organs

H. The science that deals with the study of cells, including their origin, structure, function, and pathology

I. The branch of medicine that deals with the diseases of the reproductive organs of women

J. Anything that increases an individual's chance of developing a disease

K. The growth of abnormal cells

L. Before the onset of menopause, the phase during which a woman with regular periods changes to irregular cycles and increased periods of amenorrhea

M. Pain in the vagina or pelvis experienced by a woman during sexual intercourse

N. Examination of the cervix using a lighted instrument with a magnifying lens

O. Bleeding between menstrual periods

P. Excessive bleeding during a menstrual period

Q. The lower narrow end of the uterus that opens into the vagina

R. Pain associated with the menstrual period

S. The permanent cessation of menstruation

Prenatal Care

Directions: Match each key term with its definition.

_G_ 1. Abortion
_X_ 2. Braxton Hicks contractions
_O_ 3. Dilation (of the cervix)
_M_ 4. EDD
_R_ 5. Effacement
_BB_ 6. Embryo
_B_ 7. Engagement
_I_ 8. Fetal heart rate
_Z_ 9. Fetal heart tones
_BB_ 10. Fetus
_H_ 11. Fundus
_P_ 12. Gestation
_CC_ 13. Gestational age
_S_ 14. Gravidity
_AA_ 15. Infant
_Q_ 16. Lochia
_L_ 17. Multigravida
_A_ 18. Multipara
_T_ 19. Nullipara
_U_ 20. Obstetrics
_E_ 21. Parity
_Y_ 22. Position
_W_ 23. Postpartum
_DD_ 24. Preeclampsia
_C_ 25. Prenatal
_EE_ 26. Presentation
_FF_ 27. Preterm birth
_V_ 28. Primigravida
_N_ 29. Primipara
_F_ 30. Puerperium
_J_ 31. Quickening
_GG_ 32. Term birth
_HH_ 33. Toxemia
_D_ 34. Trimester

A. A woman who has completed two or more pregnancies to the age of viability, regardless of whether they ended in live infants or stillbirths
B. The entrance of the fetal head or the presenting part into the pelvic inlet
C. Before birth
D. Three months, or one third, of the gestational period of pregnancy
E. The condition of having borne offspring regardless of the outcome
F. The period, usually 4 to 6 weeks, after delivery, in which the uterus and the body systems are returning to normal
G. The termination of the pregnancy before the fetus reached the age of viability (20 weeks)
H. The dome-shaped upper portion of the uterus between the fallopian tubes
I. The number of times per minute the fetal heart beats
J. The first movements of the fetus in utero as felt by the mother
K. The child in utero, from the third month after conception to birth
L. A woman who has been pregnant more than once
M. Projected birth date of the infant
N. A woman who has carried a pregnancy to fetal viability for the first time, regardless of whether the infant was stillborn or alive at birth
O. The stretching of the external os from an opening a few millimeters wide to an opening large enough to allow the passage of an infant (approximately 10 cm)
P. The period of intrauterine development from conception to birth
Q. A discharge from the uterus after delivery consisting of blood, tissue, white blood cells, and some bacteria
R. The thinning and shortening of the cervical canal from its normal length of 1 to 2 cm to a structure with paper-thin edges in which there is no canal at all
S. The total number of pregnancies a woman has had regardless of duration, including a current pregnancy
T. A woman who has not carried a pregnancy to the point of viability (20 weeks of gestation)
U. The branch of medicine concerned with the care of the woman during pregnancy, childbirth, and the postpartal period
V. A woman who is pregnant for the first time
W. Occurring after childbirth
X. Intermittent and irregular painless uterine contractions that occur throughout pregnancy
Y. The relation of the presenting part of the fetus to the maternal pelvis
Z. The sounds of the heartbeat of the fetus heard through the mother's abdominal wall
AA. A child from birth to 12 months of age
BB. The child in utero from the time of conception to the beginning of the first trimester
CC. The age of the fetus between conception and birth
DD. A major complication of pregnancy characterized by increasing hypertension, albuminuria, and edema
EE. Indication of the part of the fetus that is closest to the cervix and will be delivered first
FF. Delivery occurring between 20 and 37 weeks, regardless of whether the child was born alive or stillborn
GG. Delivery occurring after 37 weeks, regardless of whether the child was born alive or stillborn
HH. A condition occurring in pregnant women that includes preeclampsia and eclampsia

303

B. Word Parts

Directions: Indicate the meaning of each word part in the space provided. List as many medical terms as possible that incorporate the word part in the space provided.

Word Part	Meaning of Word Part	Medical Terms That Incorporate Word Part
1. a-		
2. men/o		
3. -orrhea		
4. colp/o		
5. -scopy		
6. cyt/o		
7. -ology		
8. dys-		
9. -plasia		
10. ecto-		
11. endo-		
12. gynec/o		
13. multi-		
14. par/o		
15. nulli-		
16. peri-		
17. post-		
18. pre-		
19. nat/o		
20. -al		
21. prim/i		
22. tri-		

Gynecologic Examination

Directions: Fill in each blank with the correct answer.

1. What is the purpose of the gynecologic examination?

_____

_____

_____

2. What is the purpose of performing a breast examination?

_____

_____

_____

3. What should a woman do if a lump or other change is discovered during a breast self-examination?

_____

_____

4. What are the components of the pelvic examination?

_____

_____

5. What position is generally used for the pelvic examination?

_____

6. How can the medical assistant help the patient to relax during the pelvic examination?

_____

_____

7. What is the function of a vaginal speculum?

_____

_____

8. What is the purpose of performing a visual examination of the vagina and the cervix?

_____

_____

9. What are three examples of vaginal infections that cause a discharge?

_____

10. What is the purpose of performing a Pap test?

_____

_____

11. What causes most cervical cancers?

_____

12. Describe the schedule for having a Pap test as recommended by the American Cancer Society.

_____

_____

_____

13. Why should the medical assistant instruct the patient not to douche or insert vaginal medications for 2 days before coming to the medical office to have a Pap test?

_____

_____

_____

_____

14. What are the three types of specimens that may be obtained for a Pap test? Where is each collected?

_____

_____

_____

15. Why must the slides be fixed immediately after collection of a specimen for the direct-smear Pap test method?

_____

_____

_____

16. What are the advantages of using the liquid-based Pap test method?

_____

_____

_____

_____

17. List three conditions that the maturation index can help to evaluate.

_____

_____

_____

18. Why is the Bethesda system recommended for reporting the results of the Pap test?

_____

_____

_____

19. Describe the information included in each of the following categories of a cytology report:

   a. Specimen type

   _____

   _____

   b. Satisfactory for evaluation

   _____

   _____

   c. Unsatisfactory for evaluation

   _____

   _____

   d. Negative for intraepithelial lesion or malignancy

   _____

   _____

   e. Epithelial cell abnormality

   _____

   _____

   f. Interpretation or result

   _____

   _____

   g. Automated review

   _____

   _____

   h. Ancillary testing

20. What is the purpose of performing the bimanual pelvic examination?

   _____

   _____

21. What is the purpose of the rectal-vaginal examination?

   _____

   _____

22. Describe the laboratory procedure that can be used to identify *Trichomonas vaginalis* in the medical office.

_____

_____

_____

23. What medication is used to treat trichomoniasis? Why must the patient's sexual partner also be treated?

_____

_____

24. Describe the laboratory procedure that can be used to identify *Candida albicans* in the medical office.

_____

_____

_____

25. What medications are used to treat candidiasis?

_____

_____

26. What are the symptoms of PID? What complications can occur from PID?

_____

_____

27. How are chlamydial and gonorrheal infections usually diagnosed?

_____

_____

28. List the symptoms of each of the following sexually transmitted diseases:

a. Trichomoniasis in the female

_____

_____

_____

b. Candidiasis in the female

_____

_____

_____

_____

c. Chlamydia

Female:

_____

_____

Male:

_____

_____

d. Gonorrhea

Female:

_____

_____

Male:

_____

_____

Prenatal Care

Directions: Fill in each blank with the correct answer.

1. What is the purpose of prenatal care?

_____

_____

2. List the three categories of medical office visits for provision of prenatal and postnatal care to the pregnant woman.

_____

_____

_____

3. List the four components of the first prenatal visit.

_____

_____

_____

_____

4. What is the purpose of the prenatal record?

_____

_____

5. List two types of information included in the past medical history (of the prenatal record).

_____

_____

_____

6. List three types of information included in the present pregnancy history.

_____

_____

_____

7. What are the warning signs of a spontaneous abortion?

_____

_____

8. What are the warning signs of preeclampsia?

_____

_____

9. What is the purpose of the interval prenatal history?

_____

_____

10. Explain the importance of performing a physical examination on the prenatal patient.

_____

_____

_____

11. What is the importance of making sure a pregnant woman does not have gonorrhea before delivery of the infant?

_____

_____

12. Why is a pregnant woman tested for group B streptococcus (GBS)? When is the woman tested for GBS?

_____

_____

13. What is the purpose of performing a hemoglobin and hematocrit evaluation on a prenatal patient?

_____

_____

14. What is the importance of assessing the Rh factor and ABO blood type of a pregnant woman?

_____

_____

15. What is the purpose of performing a glucose challenge test on a pregnant woman?

_____

_____

16. What is the purpose of performing a rubella titer test on a pregnant woman?

_____

_____

17. Why does the Centers for Disease Control and Prevention recommend that pregnant women have a blood test to screen for exposure to the hepatitis B virus?

_____

_____

18. What is the purpose of the return prenatal visit? List the usual schedule for return prenatal visits.

_____

_____

_____

19. What tests are performed on the patient's urine specimen at each return visit, and why is each performed?

_____

_____

_____

_____

20. List two purposes of measuring the fundal height.

_____

_____

21. What is the normal range for the fetal heart rate?

_____

22. What is the purpose of performing a vaginal examination as the patient nears term?

_____

_____

23. What is the purpose of performing each of the following special tests and procedures?

a. Multiple marker test _____

_____

b. Obstetric ultrasound scan _____

_____

c. Amniocentesis _____

_____

d. Fetal heart rate monitoring _____

_____

311

24. What type of patient preparation is required for a transabdominal ultrasound scan?

_____

_____

25. What conditions might warrant performing an amniocentesis?

_____

_____

_____

26. What is the difference between the following fetal heart rate monitoring tests: nonstress test and contraction stress test?

_____

_____

_____

27. What occurs during the puerperium?

_____

_____

28. Explain the changes in the lochia that should normally occur during the puerperium.

_____

_____

_____

_____

29. List the procedures generally included in the 6-week postpartum examination.

_____

_____

_____

_____

CRITICAL THINKING ACTIVITIES

A. Breast Cancer

Select three of the following questions that interest you the most. Using the following Internet sites, answer these questions in the space provided.

National Cancer Institute: www.cancer.gov
American Cancer Society: www.cancer.org
Cancer Treatment Centers of America: www.cancercenter.com

1. Can a male develop breast cancer? Elaborate on your answer.
2. How does tamoxifen work in treating breast cancer?
3. What are the pros and cons of being tested for the breast cancer gene?
4. What methods are used to reconstruct the breast after a mastectomy?
5. What new diagnostic methods are being explored to detect breast cancer?
6. What complementary and alternative therapies are being used in the treatment of breast cancer?

Question # _____

_____

_____

_____

_____

_____

_____

Question # _____

_____

_____

_____

_____

_____

_____

Question # _____

_____

_____

_____

_____

_____

B. Methods of Contraception

Patients coming to the medical office for gynecologic examinations frequently ask the medical assistant questions regarding methods of contraception. The medical assistant should have knowledge of the various types of contraceptives, how they work to prevent pregnancy, and the advantages and disadvantages of each. A list of common contraceptive methods is provided. List the information requested for each in the spaces provided. Internet sites on the topic of contraception can be used to complete this activity.

Contraceptive Method	Mode of Action	Advantages	Disadvantages
Oral contraceptives			
Contraceptive injections			
Contraceptive patch			

Contraceptive Method	Mode of Action	Advantages	Disadvantages
Birth control implant			
Male condom			
Female condom			

Contraceptive Method	Mode of Action	Advantages	Disadvantages
Spermicide			
Diaphragm			
Cervical cap			

Contraceptive Method	Mode of Action	Advantages	Disadvantages
Vaginal sponge			
Vaginal ring			
Intrauterine device (IUD)			

Contraceptive Method	Mode of Action	Advantages	Disadvantages
Fertility awareness-based method			
Surgical sterilization			
Emergency contraception			

C. Herpesvirus and Human Papillomavirus

You are working for an obstetrics and gynecology (OB/GYN) office. Your physician is concerned about the increase in the number of patients contracting herpesvirus and human papillomavirus (HPV) infections. He or she asks you to design a colorful, creative, and informative brochure on herpesvirus and HPV infections using the brochures provided on the following pages. These brochures will be published and placed in the waiting room to educate patients about these sexually transmitted infections (STIs). STI Internet sites can be used to complete this activity.

Notes

HERPES

How common is herpes?

How can herpes be prevented?

Chapter **8** **The Gynecologic Examination and Prenatal Care**

What is herpes?

How do you get herpes?

How is herpes diagnosed?

What are the symptoms?

What causes herpes to recur?

How is herpes treated?

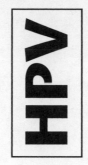

How common is HPV?

What are the complications of HPV?

Chapter **8** **The Gynecologic Examination and Prenatal Care**

What is HPV?

How do you get HPV?

How is HPV tested?

What are the symptoms?

How is HPV diagnosed?

How can HPV be prevented?

D. Signs and Symptoms of Pregnancy

Listed here are the common signs and symptoms of pregnancy. Define each of them and, if possible, explain what causes the sign or symptom to occur. Pregnancy and childbirth Internet sites can be used to obtain information to complete this activity.

1. Amenorrhea

   The absence of monthly menstrual periods due to e, pregnancy, birth control

2. Fatigue

   extremely tired resulting in mental or physical exertion or illness

3. Urinary frequency

   It's due to increase of hormones progesterone and human chorionic gonadotropin. And added pressure on the bladder.

4. Quickening

   Mother feeling baby move as early as 13-16 weeks during pregnancy.

5. Goodell's sign

   is indication of pregnancy, Positive pregnancy test abd getting bigger.

6. Hegar's sign

7. Braxton Hicks contractions

   contractions in the uterus during pregnancy.

8. Skin changes: striae gravidarum, chloasma, linea nigra

   Stretch marks during pregnancy, enlarged breast and abd.

E. Calculation of the Expected Date of Delivery

Calculate the expected date of delivery (EDD) for the following patients using Nägele's rule. The first day of each patient's last menstrual period (LMP) is listed.

1. February 10, 2019 ___11-17-2020___
2. April 28, 2019 ___2-05-2020___
3. July 20, 2019 ___4-27-2020___
4. October 2, 2019 ___7-9-2020___
5. December 22, 2019 ___9-29-2020___

F. Documenting Gravidity and Parity

The following patients are in your medical office for their first prenatal visit. In the space provided, document the following information in terms of gravidity and parity.

1. Melissa Turner is pregnant for the third time. Her first pregnancy resulted in the birth of a baby boy, now alive and well. She lost her second pregnancy at 16 weeks' gestation.

   G: _3_   T: _1_   P: ___   A: _1_   L: _1_

2. Amanda Schuster is pregnant for the third time. Her first pregnancy resulted in the birth of twin girls, now alive and well. Her second pregnancy resulted in the birth of a baby girl, now alive and well.

   G: _3_   T: _3_   P: ___   A: ___   L: _3_

3. Leah Morrow is pregnant for the fourth time. She lost her first pregnancy at 2 months' gestation. Her second pregnancy was carried to term but resulted in the birth of a stillborn. Her third pregnancy resulted in the birth of a baby girl, now alive and well.

   G: _4_   T: _1_   P: _1_   A: _1_   L: _1_

4. Rose Samson is pregnant for the fifth time. She carried her first pregnancy to 24 weeks and delivered a stillborn baby. Her second pregnancy resulted in the birth of a baby girl, now alive and well. She lost her third pregnancy at 12 weeks' gestation. Her fourth pregnancy resulted in the birth of a baby boy, now alive and well.

   G: _5_   T: _2_   P: _1_   A: _1_   L: _2_

G. Nutrition During Pregnancy

1. Brianna Flint is in your medical office for her first prenatal visit. This is her first pregnancy, and she is concerned about adequate nutrition during her pregnancy. Explain why the following nutrients are of particular importance during pregnancy, and provide good food sources of each. Pregnancy and childbirth Internet sites can be used to obtain information to complete this activity.

2. In a classroom situation, select a partner. In a role-playing situation, one student takes the role of the medical assistant, and the other plays the role of the patient. Explain to the patient the importance of these nutrients, and list good food sources of each.

Nutrient	Importance During Pregnancy	Food Sources
Iron		
Calcium		
Protein		
Folic acid		

327

H. Minor Discomforts of Pregnancy

1. Listed here are the minor discomforts that a prenatal patient may experience during pregnancy. Indicate measures the patient can take to help prevent or relieve each discomfort. Pregnancy and childbirth Internet sites can be used to obtain information to complete this activity.

2. In a classroom situation, select a partner. In a role-playing situation, one student takes the role of the medical assistant, and the other plays the role of the patient. The patient should indicate that she has a problem with each of these discomforts, and the medical assistant should respond by describing measures the patient can take to help prevent or relieve each problem.

a. Nausea (morning sickness)

_____

_____

b. Heartburn

_____

_____

c. Fatigue

_____

_____

d. Constipation

_____

_____

e. Backache

_____

_____

f. Breathing difficulties

_____

_____

g. Varicose veins

_____

_____

h. Hemorrhoids

_____

_____

i. Leg cramps

_____

_____

j. Swelling of the lower legs and feet

_____

_____

I. Health Promotion During Pregnancy

1. Obtain a prenatal guidebook, and list the guidelines the patient should follow with respect to each of the areas provided. Pregnancy and childbirth Internet sites can be used to obtain information to complete this activity.

2. In a classroom situation, select a partner. In a role-playing situation, one student takes the role of the medical assistant, and the other plays the role of the patient. The patient should ask for guidance regarding each of these areas, and the medical assistant should respond with appropriate information.

   a. Nutrition

   _____

   _____

   b. Employment

   _____

   _____

   c. Exercise

   _____

   _____

   d. Travel

   _____

   _____

   e. Smoking

   _____

   _____

   f. Alcohol

   _____

   _____

   g. Medication

   _____

   _____

J. Breast-feeding

1. Lucy Clark asks you for information regarding the advantages and disadvantages of breast-feeding and bottle-feeding. List these in the following chart. Pregnancy and childbirth Internet sites can be used to obtain information to complete this activity.

2. In a classroom situation, select a partner. In a role-playing situation, one student takes the role of the medical assistant, and the other plays the role of the patient. The patient should ask for information regarding the advantages and disadvantages of both methods, and the medical assistant should respond with appropriate information.

Bottle-feeding	
Advantages	*Disadvantages*

Breast-feeding	
Advantages	*Disadvantages*

K. Prenatal Ultrasound

View obstetric ultrasound scans at the following Internet sites:

www.ob-ultrasound.net/frames.htm

www.layyous.com/ultasound/ultrasound_video.htm

The following scans can be viewed at these sites:

1. Gestational sac

2. Fetus at various gestational ages

3. Fetal measurements

4. Fetal organs

5. Three-dimensional (3D) and four-dimensional (4D) images of the fetus

330

L. Crossword Puzzle: Gynecology and Obstetrics

Directions: Complete the crossword puzzle using the clues presented below.

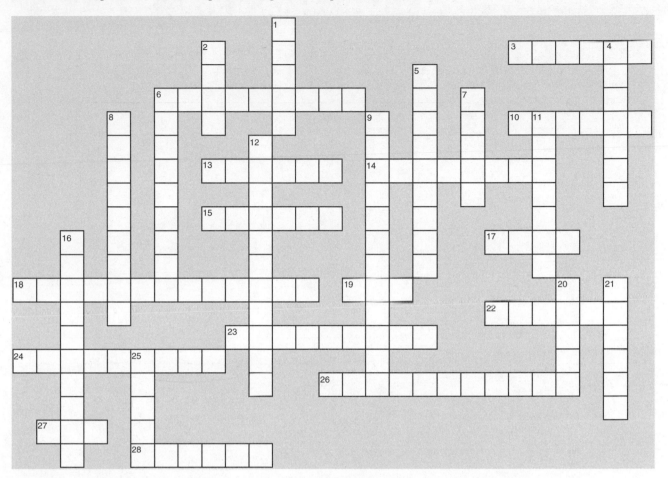

Across

3 STI preventer
6 Breast radiograph
10 Malignant or benign?
13 What most breast lumps are
14 May not occur with STI, especially in females?
15 Age to begin BSE
17 Definite minor Pap changes
18 Abnormal reported as normal
19 Screening test for GDM
22 Breast exam position
23 Pelvic exam position
24 STI symptom
26 Freezes the cervix
27 Cause of most cervical cancers
28 How cervical cancer develops

Down

1 Birth size of macrosomia baby
2 Warning sign of breast cancer
4 Risk factor for GDM
5 Antibiotics cure this STI
6 Menstrual cycle ceases
7 HPV symptom
8 What all STIs can be
9 Cervical cancer surgery
11 What a GDM mother may need
12 Serious STI complication
16 Examination of the cervix
20 Breast cancer increases (age)
21 A viral STI
25 Slightly abnormal Pap cells

Chapter **8** The Gynecologic Examination and Prenatal Care

Notes

Procedure 8-1: Breast Self-Examination

Instruct an individual about the procedure for performing a breast self-examination and document the procedure in the chart provided.

CHART	
Date	

CHART	
Date	

Procedure 8-2: Gynecologic Examination

1. Complete the cytology request form provided using a female classmate as the patient.

2. Practice the procedure for assisting with a gynecologic examination. Document the vital signs and height and weight in the chart provided.

	CHART
Date	

GYN CYTOLOGY REQUISITION

THOMAS WOODSIDE, MD
501 MAIN ST
ST. LOUIS, MO 63146
(314) 883–0093

PATIENT INFO

Patient's Name (Last)	(First)	(MI)	Date of Birth MO | DAY | YR	Collection Time : AM PM	Collection Date MO | DAY | YR	Patient's ID #

Patient's Address   Phone

City   State   ZIP

RESP. PARTY

Name of Responsible Party (if different from patient)

Address of Responsible Party   APT #

City   State   ZIP

INSURANCE

Patient's Relationship to Responsible Party ☐ 1. Self   ☐ 2. Spouse   ☐ 3. Child   ☐ 4. Other

Insurance Company Name	Plan	Carrier Code
Subscriber/Member #	Location	Group #
Insurance Address		Physician's Provider #
City	State	ZIP
Employer's Name or Number	Insured SSN	

Diagnosis/Signs/Symptoms in ICD-9 Format (Highest Specificity)

REQUIRED

ICD-9 codes are the internationally accepted method of describing the clinical picture of the patient. All diagnoses should be provided by the ordering physician or his or her authorized designee. The following is a partial list of common diagnoses in ICD-9 format. Most third party payers require an ICD-9 code to indicate the medical necessity of the test(s) and/or profile(s) ordered. For a complete list of all ICD-9 codes, please refer to a current ICD-9 manual.

V76.2	Routine Cervical Pap Smear	616.0	Cervicitis	626.8	Abnormal Bleeding
V15.89	High Risk Cervical Screening	616.10	Vaginitis	627.1	Postmenopausal Bleeding
V22.2	Pregnancy	617.0	Endometriosis, Uterus	627.3	Atrophic Vaginitis
079.4	Human Papillomavirus	622.1	Dysplasia, Cervix	795.0	Abnormal Cervical Pap Smear
180.0	Malignant Neoplasm, Cervix	623.0	Dysplasia, Vagina		

COLLECTION METHOD

Liquid-Based Prep

192055 ☐ Thin Prep Pap Test

192039 ☐ Thin Prep Pap Test w/reflex to HPV
Hybrid Capture when ASC-US or SIL

192047 ☐ Thin Prep Pap Test w/reflex to high-risk only
HPV Hybrid Capture when ASC-US

Pap Smear

009100 ☐ 1 Slide   009191 ☐ 2 Slides

Pap Smear and Maturation Index

009209 ☐ 1 Slide   190074 ☐ 2 Slides

SOURCE OF SPECIMEN

☐ Cervical

☐ Endocervical

☐ Vaginal

Date LMP

____ / ____ / ____
Mo   Day   Year

COLLECTION TECHNIQUE

☐ Spatula

☐ Brush

☐ Broom

☐ Other
_____

PATIENT HISTORY

☐ Pregnant
☐ Lactating
☐ Oral Contraceptives
☐ Postmenopausal
☐ Hormone Replacement Therapy

☐ PMP Bleeding
☐ Postpartum
☐ IUD
☐ Postcoital Bleeding
☐ DES Exposure
☐ Previous Abnormal Pap Test

☐ Other _____

PREVIOUS TREATMENT   Date/Results

☐ None
☐ Colposcopy and Bx   _____
☐ Cryosurgery   _____
☐ LEEP   _____
☐ Laser Vaporization   _____
☐ Conization   _____
☐ Hysterectomy   _____
☐ Radiation   _____
☐ Chemotherapy   _____

Procedure 8-3: Return Prenatal Examination

1. Complete the prenatal health history form provided using a female classmate as the patient.

2. Prepare the patient and assist with a return prenatal examination. Document the results of procedures you performed on the chart provided.

	CHART
Date	

CHART	
Date	

PRENATAL HEALTH HISTORY

PATIENT INFORMATION

Date: _____ EDD: _____   Referred By: _____
Name: _____   Phone (home): _____
        LAST   FIRST   MIDDLE   Phonc (work): _____
Address: _____   Emergency Contact: _____
           CITY   STATE   ZIP   Phone: _____

Date of Birth: ___/___/___   Age: ____   Marital Status: _____
Occupation: _____
Education: ☐ High School   ☐ College   ☐ Post-graduate

PAST MEDICAL HISTORY

	○ Neg + Pos	DETAIL POSITIVE REMARKS INCLUDE DATE AND TREATMENT			○ Neg + Pos	DETAIL POSITIVE REMARKS INCLUDE DATE AND TREATMENT
1. DIABETES				16. D (Rh) SENSITIZED		
2. HYPERTENSION				17. PULMONARY (TB, ASTHMA)		
3. HEART DISEASE				18. RHEUMATIC FEVER		
4. AUTOIMMUNE DISORDER				19. BLEEDING TENDENCY		
5. KIDNEY DISEASE/UTI				20. GYN SURGERY		
6. NEUROLOGIC/EPILEPSY						
7. PSYCHIATRIC				21. OPERATIONS/HOSPITALIZATIONS (YEAR AND REASON)		
8. HEPATITIS/LIVER DISEASE						
9. VARICOSITIES/PHLEBITIS						
10. THYROID DYSFUNCTION				22. ANESTHETIC COMPLICATIONS		
11. TRAUMA/DOMESTIC VIOLENCE				23. HISTORY OF ABNORMAL PAP		
12. BLOOD TRANSFUSION				24. UTERINE ANOMALY/DES		

	AMT/DAY PREPREG.	AMT/DAY PREG.	# YEARS USE			
				25. INFERTILITY		
13. TOBACCO				26. SEXUALLY TRANSMITTED DISEASE		
14. ALCOHOL						
15. STREET DRUGS				27. OTHER		

IMMUNIZATIONS:

Mark an X next to those you have had.

☐ Influenza   ☐ Chickenpox
☐ Hepatitis B   ☐ Pneumococcal
☐ Hib   ☐ Tuberculin Test
☐ Polio   ☐ Tetanus Booster
☐ MMR

ALLERGIES:

List all allergies (foods, drugs, environment).   ☐ None

_____
_____
_____
_____
_____
_____

MENSTRUAL HISTORY

Menarche: Age of Onset _____
Frequency: Q _____ Days
Duration: _____ Days
Amount of Flow: ☐ Small   ☐ Moderate   ☐ Large

GYN Disorders (List): _____
_____
_____

On contraceptive at conception?   ☐ Yes   ☐ No

Chapter **8** **The Gynecologic Examination and Prenatal Care**

OBSTETRIC HISTORY

G _____ T _____ P _____ A _____ L _____
(Total Pregnancies) (Term) (Preterm) (Abortions) (Living Children)

PREVIOUS PREGNANCIES:

DATE MONTH/ YEAR	WEEKS GEST.	LENGTH OF LABOR	BIRTH WEIGHT	SEX M/F	TYPE DELIVERY	ANES.	MATERNAL COMPLICATIONS	INFANT COMPLICATIONS

PRESENT PREGNANCY HISTORY

NAUSEA			ABDOMINAL PAIN	
VOMITING			URINARY COMPLAINTS	
FATIGUE			VAGINAL BLEEDING	
BREAST CHANGES			VAGINAL DISCHARGE	
INDIGESTION			PRURITUS	
CONSTIPATION			ACCIDENTS	
PERSISTENT HEADACHES			SURGERY	
DIZZINESS			X-RAYS	
VISUAL DISTURBANCE			RUBELLA EXPOSURE	
EDEMA (SPECIFY AREA)			OTHER VIRAL INFECTIONS	

LMP _____ / _____ / _____
     Mo   Day   Year

Amount of Flow: ☐ Small   ☐ Moderate   ☐ Large

CURRENT MEDICATIONS: (Include prescription, OTC, herbal, and vitamins). ☐ None

Medication _____   **Frequency** _____

_____

_____

INITIAL PHYSICAL EXAMINATION

DATE ___ / ___ / ___

1. HEENT	☐ NORMAL	☐ ABNORMAL	12. VULVA	☐ NORMAL	☐ CONDYLOMA	☐ LESIONS
2. FUNDI	☐ NORMAL	☐ ABNORMAL	13. VAGINA	☐ NORMAL	☐ INFLAMMATION	☐ DISCHARGE
3. TEETH	☐ NORMAL	☐ ABNORMAL	14. CERVIX	☐ NORMAL	☐ INFLAMMATION	☐ LESIONS
4. THYROID	☐ NORMAL	☐ ABNORMAL	15. UTERUS SIZE	_____ WEEKS		☐ FIBROIDS
5. BREASTS	☐ NORMAL	☐ ABNORMAL	16. ADNEXA	☐ NORMAL	☐ MASS	
6. LUNGS	☐ NORMAL	☐ ABNORMAL	17. RECTUM	☐ NORMAL	☐ ABNORMAL	
7. HEART	☐ NORMAL	☐ ABNORMAL	18. DIAGONAL CONJUGATE	☐ REACHED	☐ NO	_____CM
8. ABDOMEN	☐ NORMAL	☐ ABNORMAL	19. SPINES	☐ AVERAGE	☐ PROMINENT	☐ BLUNT
9. EXTREMITIES	☐ NORMAL	☐ ABNORMAL	20. SACRUM	☐ CONCAVE	☐ STRAIGHT	☐ ANTERIOR
10. SKIN	☐ NORMAL	☐ ABNORMAL	21. SUBPUBIC ARCH	☐ NORMAL	☐ WIDE	☐ NARROW
11. LYMPH NODES	☐ NORMAL	☐ ABNORMAL	22. GYNECOID PELVIC TYPE	☐ YES	☐ NO	

COMMENTS (Number and explain abnormals): _____

_____

_____

_____ **EXAM BY** _____

INTERVAL PRENATAL HISTORY

Date 20___	Weeks Gestation	Height of Fundus (cm)	Weight	B/P	Urine Glucose	Urine Protein	FHT	Vaginal Examination	Presentation	Edema	Discharge	Bleeding	Contractions	Fetal Activity	NST	Next Appt.	Initials

PLANS/EDUCATION (COUNSELED ✓)

☐ ANESTHESIA PLANS _____

☐ TOXOPLASMOSIS PRECAUTIONS (CATS/RAW MEAT) ____ ___

☐ CHILDBIRTH CLASSES _____

☐ PHYSICAL/SEXUAL ACTIVITY _____

☐ LABOR SIGNS _____

☐ NUTRITION COUNSELING _____

☐ BREAST OR BOTTLE FEEDING _____

☐ NEWBORN CAR SEAT _____

☐ POSTPARTUM BIRTH CONTROL _____

☐ ENVIRONMENTAL/WORK HAZARDS _____

☐ TUBAL STERILIZATION _____

☐ VBAC COUNSELING _____

☐ CIRCUMCISION _____

☐ TRAVEL _____

☐ LIFESTYLE, TOBACCO, ALCOHOL _____

REQUESTS _____

_____

_____

TUBAL STERILIZATION DATE INITIALS

CONSENT SIGNED ___/___/___ _____

LABORATORY		PATIENT'S NAME _____			
INITIAL LABS	DATE	RESULTS		REVIEWED	COMMENTS
BLOOD TYPE	/ /	A B AB O			
Rh FACTOR	/ /	☐ Pos ☐ Neg			
Rh ANTIBODY SCREEN	/ /	☐ Pos ☐ Neg			
HCT/HGB	/ /	_____ % _____ g/dL			
RUBELLA ANTIBODY TITER	/ /	Immune Nonimmune			
VDRL	/ /	☐ NR ☐ R			
HBsAg (HEPATITIS B)	/ /	☐ Pos ☐ Neg			
HIV	/ /	☐ Pos ☐ Neg ☐ Declined			
URINE CULTURE/SCREEN	/ /				
PAP TEST	/ /	☐ Normal ☐ Abnormal			
CHLAMYDIA (DNA PROBE)	/ /	☐ Pos ☐ Neg			
GONORRHEA (DNA PROBE)	/ /	☐ Pos ☐ Neg			
7–20 WEEK LABS (WHEN INDICATED/ELECTED)	DATE	RESULTS		REVIEWED	COMMENTS
ULTRASOUND #1 (7–13 WEEKS)	/ /	EDD:			
ULTRASOUND #2 (18–20 WEEKS)	/ /	EFW:			
TRIPLE SCREEN (15–20 WEEKS)	/ /				
CVS	/ /				
AMNIOCENTESIS	/ /				
24–28 WEEK LABS (WHEN INDICATED)	DATE	RESULTS		REVIEWED	COMMENTS
HCT/HGB	/ /	_____ % _____ g/dL			
GCT (24–28 WKS)	/ /	1 Hour _____			
GTT (IF SCREEN ABNORMAL)	/ /	_____ FBS _____ 1 Hour			
		_____ 2 Hour _____ 3 Hour			
D (Rh) ANTIBODY SCREEN	/ /				
D IMMUNE GLOBULIN (RhIG) GIVEN (28 WKS)	/ /	SIGNATURE			
32–36 WEEK LABS	DATE	RESULTS		REVIEWED	COMMENTS
HCT/HGB (32 WKS)	/ /	_____ % _____ g/dL			
ULTRASOUND #3 (34 WKS)	/ /	EFW:			
GROUP B STREP (35–37 WKS)	/ /	☐ Pos ☐ Neg			
ADDITIONAL LAB TESTS	DATE	RESULTS		REVIEWED	COMMENTS
	/ /				
	/ /				
	/ /				
	/ /				
	/ /				

e Procedure 8-1: Breast Self-Examination Instructions

Name: _____   Date: _____

Evaluated by: _____   Score: _____

Performance Objective

Outcome:	Instruct a patient in the procedure for performing a breast self-examination.
Conditions:	Using a small pillow.
Standards:	Time: 10 minutes. Student completed procedure in _____ minutes.
	Accuracy: Satisfactory score on the Performance Evaluation Checklist.

Performance Evaluation Checklist

Trial 1	Trial 2	Point Value	Performance Standards
		•	Greeted the patient and introduced yourself.
		•	Identified the patient and explained that you will be instructing the patient in a BSE.
		•	Explained the purpose of the exam, when to perform it, and the three methods of examination.
		▷	Explained why three methods are used to examine the breasts.
			Instructed the patient:
			1. Before a mirror
		•	Remove clothing from the waist up.
		•	Place arms at the sides and inspect the breasts.
		•	Inspect for a change in size or shape; swelling, puckering, or dimpling; change in skin texture; nipple retraction; change in nipple size or position compared with the other breast.
		▷	Described what may cause puckering or dimpling of the skin.
		•	Slowly raise arms over the head and inspect the breasts.
		▷	Stated what should normally occur when the arms are moved at the same time.
		•	Rest palms on the hips, press down firmly, and inspect the breasts.
		▷	Stated the purpose of flexing the chest muscles.
		•	Gently squeeze each nipple and look for a discharge.
			2. Lying down
		•	Place a pillow (or folded towel) under the right shoulder.
		•	Place the right hand behind the head.
		▷	Stated the purpose of the pillow and hand placement.

Trial 1	Trial 2	Point Value	Performance Standards
		•	Use the finger pads of the middle three fingers of the left hand.
		▷	Explained why the finger pads should be used.
		•	Use small, rotating motions and continuous firm pressure.
		•	Use one of the following patterns to move around the breast: circular, vertical strip, or wedge.
		▷	Stated why a pattern is used.
			Circular pattern:
		•	Visualize the breast as a clock face.
		•	Start at the outside edge of the breast.
		•	Proceed clockwise until you return to the starting point.
		•	Move in 1 inch, and repeat the circle.
		•	Continue until the nipple is reached.
			Vertical strip:
		•	Divide the breast into strips.
		•	Start at the underarm.
		•	Slowly move fingers down until they are below the breast.
		•	Move fingers 1 inch toward middle and move back up.
		•	Repeat until the entire breast has been examined.
			Wedge:
		•	Divide the breasts into wedges.
		•	Start at the outer edge of the breast.
		•	Move fingers toward the nipple and back to edge of breast.
		•	Repeat until the entire breast has been examined.
			Use the following techniques during the examination:
		•	Press firmly enough to feel the different breast tissues.
		•	Palpate for lumps, hard knots, or thickening.
		▷	Explained how normal breast tissue feels.
		•	Examine the entire chest area from your collarbone to the base of a properly fitted bra and from the breastbone to the underarm.
		•	Pay special attention to the area between the breast and underarm, including the underarm itself.
		▷	Explained why the underarm should be examined.

Trial 1	Trial 2	Point Value	Performance Standards
		•	Continue the examination until every part of the right breast has been examined, including the nipple.
		•	Repeat the procedure on the left breast, with a pillow or rolled towel under the left shoulder with the left hand behind the head, and using the right hand to palpate.
			3. In the shower
		•	Gently lather each breast.
		▷	Explained why the breasts should be examined in the shower.
		•	Place the right hand behind the head.
		•	Use the finger pads of the middle three fingers of the left hand.
		•	Use small, rotating motions and continuous, firm pressure.
		•	Use your preferred pattern to thoroughly examine the right breast and underarm for lumps, hard knots, or thickening.
		•	Repeat the procedure on the left breast by using the pads of your right fingers.
		•	Instructed the patient to report any lumps or changes to the physician immediately.
		▷	Explained why it is important to report changes immediately.
		•	Documented the procedure correctly.
			Demonstrated the following affective behavior(s) during this procedure:
		Ⓐ	Showed awareness of a patient's concerns related to the procedure being performed.
		Ⓐ	Explained to a patient the rationale for performance of a procedure.
		★	Completed the procedure within 10 minutes.
			Totals

CHART

Date	

Chapter **8** **The Gynecologic Examination and Prenatal Care**

Evaluation of Student Performance

EVALUATION CRITERIA			COMMENTS
Symbol	**Category**	**Point Value**	
★	Critical Step	16 points	
•	Essential Step	6 points	
Ⓐ	Affective Competency	6 points	
▷	Theory Question	2 points	

Score calculation: 100 points
            −_____ points missed
            ____ Score

Satisfactory score: 85 or above

CAAHEP Competencies Achieved

Psychomotor (Skills)

☑ V. 4. Coach patients regarding: (a) office policies (b) health maintenance (c) disease prevention (d) treatment plan.

☑ X. 3. Document patient care accurately in the medical record.

Affective (Behavior)

☑ I. 3. Show awareness of a patient's concerns related to the procedure being performed.

☑ V. 4. Explain to a patient the rationale for performance of a procedure.

ABHES Competencies Achieved

☑ 4. a. Follow documentation guidelines.

☑ 7. g. Display professionalism through written and verbal communications.

☑ 8. h. Teach self-examination, disease management and health promotion.

Procedure 8-2: Assisting with a Gynecologic Examination

Name: _____ Date: _____

Evaluated by: _____ Score: _____

Performance Objective

Outcome:	Assist with a gynecologic examination.
Conditions:	Using an examining table.
	Given the following: disposable gloves, examining gown and drape, disposable vaginal speculum, lubricant, gauze pads, collection vial, plastic spatula and endocervical brush or cytology broom, Hemoccult slide and developing solution, tissues, biohazard waste container, cytology request form, biohazard specimen transport bag.
Standards:	Time: 15 minutes. Student completed procedure in _____ minutes.
	Accuracy: Satisfactory score on the Performance Evaluation Checklist.

Performance Evaluation Checklist

Trial 1	Trial 2	Point Value	Performance Standards
		•	Sanitized hands.
		•	Assembled the equipment.
		•	Completed as much of the cytology request form as possible.
		•	Checked the expiration date and labeled the collection vial.
		•	Greeted the patient and introduced yourself.
		•	Escorted the patient to the examining room.
		•	Identified the patient.
		•	Asked the patient if she has any problems or concerns and documented the information.
		•	Completed the cytology request by asking the necessary questions.
		•	Measured the vital signs and height and weight and documented the results correctly.
			Prepared the patient for the examination:
		•	Asked the patient whether she needs to empty her bladder.
		▷	Explained why the bladder should be empty for the examination.
		•	Instructed the patient to undress and put on the examining gown with the opening in front.
		•	Informed the patient that the physician would be in soon.
		•	Left the room to provide patient privacy.
		•	Made the medical record available for review by the physician (if using a PPR).
		•	Checked to make sure the patient is ready.
		•	Informed the physician that the patient was ready.

347

Trial 1	Trial 2	Point Value	Performance Standards
			Assisted the physician:
		•	Positioned and draped the patient in a supine position for the breast examination.
		•	Positioned and draped the patient in the lithotomy position for the pelvic examination.
		•	Prepared the vaginal speculum and handed it to the physician.
		•	Prepared the light for the physician.
		•	Handed the vaginal speculum to the provider.
		•	Reassured the patient and helped her to relax during the examination.
		▷	Explained why the patient should be relaxed during the examination.
			Assisted with Pap specimen collection:
		•	Applied gloves and removed the cap from the collection vial.
			1a. ThinPrep spatula and brush method
		•	Held the vial to receive the collection device from the provider.
		•	Correctly rinsed each collection device in the liquid preservative.
		▷	Explained why the collection device should be swirled vigorously.
		•	Discarded each collection device in a biohazard waste container.
		•	Tightened the cap on the vial.
			1b. ThinPrep broom method
		•	Held the vial to receive the broom from the provider.
		•	Correctly rinsed the broom in the liquid preservative.
		•	Discarded the broom in a biohazard waste container.
		•	Tightened the cap on the vial.
			2. SurePath spatula and brush method
		•	Held the vial to receive each collection device from the provider.
		•	Broke off or disconnected the tip of each collection device.
		•	Discarded each handle in a regular waste container.
		•	Tightened the cap on the vial.
			Assisted with the remainder of the examination:
		•	Removed the light source.
		•	Discarded the vaginal speculum in a biohazard waste container.
		•	Provided the provider with lubricant for the bimanual and rectal-vaginal examinations.

Trial 1	Trial 2	Point Value	Performance Standards
		•	Assisted as required with the collection of the fecal occult blood specimen.
		•	Assisted the patient into a sitting position and allowed her to rest.
		▷	Explained why the patient should be allowed to rest.
		•	Offered the patient tissues to remove lubricant from the perineum.
		•	Assisted the patient from the examining table.
		•	Instructed the patient to get dressed.
		•	Informed the patient of the method used by the medical office to relay test results.
		•	Tested the fecal occult blood specimen and documented the results.
		•	Prepared the Pap specimen for transport to the laboratory.
		•	Placed the specimen in a biohazard specimen bag and sealed the bag.
		•	Inserted the cytology requisition into the outside pocket of the bag.
		•	Placed the bag in the appropriate location for pickup by the laboratory.
		•	Documented the transport of the Pap specimen to an outside laboratory.
		•	Cleaned the examining room.
			Demonstrated the following affective behavior(s) during this procedure:
		Ⓐ	Incorporated critical thinking skills when performing patient assessment.
		Ⓐ	Showed awareness of a patient's concerns related to the procedure being performed.
		Ⓐ	Protected the integrity of the medical record.
		★	Completed the procedure within 15 minutes.
			Totals
CHART			
Date			

Chapter **8** **The Gynecologic Examination and Prenatal Care**

Evaluation of Student Performance

EVALUATION CRITERIA			COMMENTS
Symbol	**Category**	**Point Value**	
★	Critical Step	16 points	
•	Essential Step	6 points	
Ⓐ	Affective Competency	6 points	
▷	Theory Question	2 points	

Score calculation: 100 points
−_____ points missed
_____ Score
Satisfactory score: 85 or above

CAAHEP Competencies Achieved

Psychomotor (Skills)

☑ I. 3. Perform screening using established protocols.

☑ I. 8. Instruct and prepare a patient for a procedure or a treatment.

☑ I. 9. Assist provider with a patient exam.

☑ V. 1. Use feedback techniques to obtain patient information including: (a) reflection (b) restatement (c) clarification.

☑ V. 4. Coach patients regarding: (a) office policies (b) health maintenance (c) disease prevention (d) treatment plan.

☑ X. 2. Apply HIPAA rules in regard to: (a) privacy (b) release of information.

☑ X. 3. Document patient care accurately in the medical record.

Affective (Behavior)

☑ I. 1. Incorporate critical thinking skills when performing patient assessment.

☑ I. 3. Show awareness of a patient's concerns related to the procedure being performed.

☑ X. 2. Protect the integrity of the medical record.

ABHES Competencies Achieved

☑ 4. a. Follow documentation guidelines.

☑ 7. g. Display professionalism through written and verbal communications.

☑ 9. d. Assist provider with specialty examination including cardiac, respiratory, OB-GYN, neurological, and gastroenterology procedures.

☑ 8. e. Perform specialty procedures including but not limited to minor surgery, cardiac, respiratory, OB-GYN, neurological, and gastroenterology.

☑ 8. h. Teach self-examination, disease management and health promotion.

GYN CYTOLOGY REQUISITION

THOMAS WOODSIDE, MD
501 MAIN ST
ST. LOUIS, MO 63146
(314) 883–0093

PATIENT INFO

Patient's Name (Last)	(First)	(MI)	Date of Birth MO	DAY	YR	Collection Time : AM PM	Collection Date MO	DAY	YR	Patient's ID #

Patient's Address   Phone

City   State   ZIP

RESP. PARTY

Name of Responsible Party (if different from patient)

Address of Responsible Party   APT #

City   State   ZIP

INSURANCE

Patient's Relationship to Responsible Party ☐ 1. Self ☐ 2. Spouse ☐ 3. Child ☐ 4. Other

Insurance Company Name	Plan	Carrier Code

Subscriber/Member #   Location   Group #

Insurance Address   Physician's Provider #

City   State   ZIP

Employer's Name or Number   Insured SSN

Diagnosis/Signs/Symptoms in ICD-9 Format (Highest Specificity)

R E Q U I R E D

ICD-9 codes are the internationally accepted method of describing the clinical picture of the patient. All diagnoses should be provided by the ordering physician or his or her authorized designee. The following is a partial list of common diagnoses in ICD-9 format. Most third party payers require an ICD-9 code to indicate the medical necessity of the test(s) and/or profile(s) ordered. For a complete list of all ICD-9 codes, please refer to a current ICD-9 manual.

V76.2	Routine Cervical Pap Smear	616.0	Cervicitis	626.8	Abnormal Bleeding
V15.89	High Risk Cervical Screening	616.10	Vaginitis	627.1	Postmenopausal Bleeding
V22.2	Pregnancy	617.0	Endometriosis, Uterus	627.3	Atrophic Vaginitis
079.4	Human Papillomavirus	622.1	Dysplasia, Cervix	795.0	Abnormal Cervical Pap Smear
180.0	Malignant Neoplasm, Cervix	623.0	Dysplasia, Vagina		

COLLECTION METHOD

Liquid-Based Prep

192055 ☐ Thin Prep Pap Test

192039 ☐ Thin Prep Pap Test w/reflex to HPV Hybrid Capture when ASC-US or SIL

192047 ☐ Thin Prep Pap Test w/reflex to high-risk only HPV Hybrid Capture when ASC-US

Pap Smear

009100 ☐ 1 Slide   009191 ☐ 2 Slides

Pap Smear and Maturation Index

009209 ☐ 1 Slide   190074 ☐ 2 Slides

SOURCE OF SPECIMEN

☐ Cervical

☐ Endocervical

☐ Vaginal

Date LMP

___ / ___ / ___
Mo   Day   Year

COLLECTION TECHNIQUE

☐ Spatula

☐ Brush

☐ Broom

☐ Other _____

PATIENT HISTORY

☐ Pregnant
☐ Lactating
☐ Oral Contraceptives
☐ Postmenopausal
☐ Hormone Replacement Therapy

☐ PMP Bleeding
☐ Postpartum
☐ IUD
☐ Postcoital Bleeding
☐ DES Exposure
☐ Previous Abnormal Pap Test

☐ Other _____

PREVIOUS TREATMENT   Date/Results

☐ None
☐ Colposcopy and Bx   _____
☐ Cryosurgery   _____
☐ LEEP   _____
☐ Laser Vaporization   _____
☐ Conization   _____
☐ Hysterectomy   _____
☐ Radiation   _____
☐ Chemotherapy   _____

351

Notes

Procedure 8-3: Assisting with a Return Prenatal Examination

Name: _____ Date: _____

Evaluated by: _____ Score: _____

Performance Objective

Outcome:	Prepare the patient and assist with a return prenatal examination.
Conditions:	Using an examining table.
	Given the following: centimeter tape measure, Doppler fetal pulse detector, ultrasound coupling agent, paper towel, disposable vaginal speculum, disposable gloves, lubricant, gauze pads, examining gown and drape, and a biohazard waste container.
Standards:	Time: 15 minutes. Student completed procedure in _____ minutes.
	Accuracy: Satisfactory score on the Performance Evaluation Checklist.

Performance Evaluation Checklist

Trial 1	Trial 2	Point Value	Performance Standards
		•	Sanitized hands.
		•	Set up the tray for the prenatal examination.
		•	Greeted the patient and introduced yourself.
		•	Identified the patient and explained the procedure.
		•	Asked the patient to obtain a urine specimen.
		•	Escorted the patient to the examining room and asked her to be seated.
		•	Asked the patient whether she has experienced any problems since her last visit and documented the information in the prenatal record.
		•	Measured the patient's blood pressure and documented the results correctly.
		•	Weighed the patient and documented the results correctly.
		▷	Stated the importance of weighing the patient.
		•	Instructed and prepared the patient for the examination.
		•	Left the room to provide the patient with privacy.
		•	Made the medical record available for review by the provider (if using a PPR).
		•	Tested the urine specimen for glucose and protein, and documented the results correctly.
		•	Checked to make sure the patient is ready to be seen by the provider.
		•	Informed the provider that the patient was ready.
		▷	Stated how the provider can be informed that the patient is ready.
		•	Assisted the patient into a supine position and properly draped her.

Chapter **8** The Gynecologic Examination and Prenatal Care

Trial 1	Trial 2	Point Value	Performance Standards
			Assisted the provider during the examination:
		•	Handed the provider the tape measure for the determination of fundal height.
		•	Applied coupling gel to the patient's abdomen and handed the provider the Doppler device.
		•	Removed the gel from the patient's abdomen.
		•	Cleaned the probe head of the Doppler device.
		•	Assisted the patient into the lithotomy position if a vaginal specimen is to be obtained or if a vaginal examination is to be performed.
			After completion of the examination:
		•	Assisted the patient into a sitting position and allowed her to rest.
		•	Assisted the patient from the examining table.
		•	Provided patient teaching and explanation of the provider's instructions as required.
		•	Escorted the patient to the reception area.
		•	Cleaned the examining room in preparation for the next patient.
		•	Prepared any specimens collected for transport to an outside laboratory.
			Demonstrated the following affective behavior(s) during this procedure:
		Ⓐ	Incorporated critical thinking skills when performing patient assessment.
		Ⓐ	Showed awareness of a patient's concerns related to the procedure being performed.
		Ⓐ	Protected the integrity of the medical record.
		★	Completed the procedure within 15 minutes.
			Totals

CHART

Date	

Evaluation of Student Performance

EVALUATION CRITERIA			COMMENTS
Symbol	**Category**	**Point Value**	
★	Critical Step	16 points	
•	Essential Step	6 points	
Ⓐ	Affective Competency	6 points	
▷	Theory Question	2 points	

Score calculation: 100 points

− _____ points missed

_____ Score

Satisfactory score: 85 or above

CAAHEP Competencies Achieved

Psychomotor (Skills)

☑ I. 3. Perform screening using established protocols.

☑ I. 8. Instruct and prepare a patient for a procedure or a treatment.

☑ I. 9. Assist provider with a patient exam.

☑ II. 3. Maintain lab test results using flow sheets.

☑ V. 1. Use feedback techniques to obtain patient information including: (a) reflection (b) restatement (c) clarification.

☑ V. 4. Coach patients regarding: (a) office policies (b) health maintenance (c) disease prevention (d) treatment plan.

☑ V. 5. Coach patients appropriately considering: (a) cultural diversity (b) developmental life stage (c) communication barriers.

☑ X. 2. Apply HIPAA rules in regard to: (a) privacy (b) release of information.

☑ X. 3. Document patient care accurately in the medical record.

Affective (Behavior)

☑ I. 1. Incorporate critical thinking skills when performing patient assessment.

☑ I. 3. Show awareness of a patient's concerns related to the procedure being performed.

☑ X. 2. Protect the integrity of the medical record.

ABHES Competencies Achieved

☑ 4. a. Follow documentation guidelines.

☑ 5. d. Adapt care to discuss the developmental stages of life.

☑ 7. g. Display professionalism through written and verbal communications.

☑ 8. b. Obtain vital signs, obtain patient history, and formulate chief complaint.

☑ 8. d. Assist provider with specialty examination including cardiac, respiratory, OB-GYN, neurological, and gastroenterology procedures.

☑ 8. e. Perform specialty procedures including but not limited to minor surgery, cardiac, respiratory, OB-GYN, neurological, and gastroenterology.

☑ 8. h. Teach self-examination, disease management and health promotion.

	PATIENT'S NAME _____

INTERVAL PRENATAL HISTORY

Date 20___	Weeks Gestation	Height of Fundus (cm)	Weight	B/P	Urine Glucose	Urine Protein	FHT	Vaginal Examination	Presentation	Edema	Discharge	Bleeding	Contractions	Fetal Activity	NST	Next Appt.	Initials

9 The Pediatric Examination

√ After Completing	Date Due	Study Guide Pages	STUDY GUIDE ASSIGNMENTS (CTA = Critical Thinking Activity)	Possible Points	Points You Earned
		361	? Pretest	10	
		362	Term Key Term Assessment	12	
		362-365	Evaluation of Learning questions	35	
		366	CTA A: Pediatric Weight	7	
			e Evolve Site: Pounds and Ounces (Record points earned)		
		366	CTA B: Pediatric Length	8	
			e Evolve Site: Inch by Inch (Record points earned)		
		366-367	CTA C: Growth Charts	18	
		368-370	CTA D: Motor and Social Development (5 points each category)	65	
		371	CTA E: Intramuscular Injection	15	
		371-372	CTA F: Vaccine Information Statement	11	
		372	CTA G: Locating and Interpreting a Vaccine Information Statement	20	
		372-373	CTA H: Immunization Administration Record	40	
		374	CTA I: Crossword Puzzle	28	
			e Evolve Site: Apply Your Knowledge questions (Record points earned)	10	
			e Evolve Site: Video Evaluation	31	
		361	? Posttest	10	
			ADDITIONAL ASSIGNMENTS		
			Total points		

357

√ When Assigned by Your Instructor	Study Guide Pages	Practices Required	LABORATORY ASSIGNMENTS (Procedure Number and Name)	Score*
	375	3	**Practice for Competency** 9-A: Carrying an Infant Textbook reference: p. 285-286	
	379-380		**Evaluation of Competency** 9-A: Carrying an Infant	*
	376	5	**Practice for Competency** 9-1: Measuring the Weight and Length of an Infant Textbook reference: pp. 288-289	
	381-383		**Evaluation of Competency** 9-1: Measuring the Weight and Length of an Infant	*
	376	5	**Practice for Competency** 9-2: Measuring Head and Chest Circumference of an Infant Textbook reference: pp. 290-291	
	385-386		**Evaluation of Competency** 9-2: Measuring Head and Chest Circumference of an Infant	*
	376	5	**Practice for Competency** 9-3: Calculating Growth Percentiles Textbook reference: pp. 291-295	
	387-388		**Evaluation of Competency** 9-3: Calculating Growth Percentiles	*
	377	5	**Practice for Competency** 9-4: Applying a Pediatric Urine Collector Textbook reference: pp. 298-300	
	389-391		**Evaluation of Competency** 9-4: Applying a Pediatric Urine Collector	*
	377-378	5	**Practice for Competency** 9-5: Newborn Screening Test Textbook reference: pp. 311-312	
	393-396		**Evaluation of Competency** 9-5: Newborn Screening Test	*
			ADDITIONAL ASSIGNMENTS	

Notes

Name: _____ Date: _____

True or False

_____ 1. A pediatrician is a medical doctor who specializes in the diagnosis and treatment of disease in children.

_____ 2. The first well-child visit is usually scheduled 4 weeks after birth of the infant.

_____ 3. Length is measured with the child standing with his or her back to the measuring device.

_____ 4. Blood pressure should be taken for a child starting at 8 years of age.

_____ 5. It is best not to tell a child that an immunization will hurt.

_____ 6. The vastus lateralis muscle site is recommended for administering an injection to an infant.

_____ 7. An MMR injection includes the following immunizations: measles, meningitis, and rubella.

_____ 8. A Vaccine Information Statement explains the benefits and risks of a vaccine in lay terminology.

_____ 9. The hepatitis B vaccine can be given to a newborn.

_____ 10. The blood specimen for a newborn screening test is obtained from the infant's earlobe.

? POSTTEST

True or False

_____ 1. A well-child visit is also referred to as a health maintenance visit.

_____ 2. A reason for weighing a child is to determine proper medication dosage.

_____ 3. Growth charts can be used to identify children with growth abnormalities.

_____ 4. Measuring pediatric blood pressure helps to identify children at risk for type 1 diabetes.

_____ 5. Using a blood pressure cuff that is too large for the child can result in a falsely low reading.

_____ 6. The length of the needle used for a pediatric IM injection depends on the amount of medication being administered.

_____ 7. The resistance of the body to pathogenic microorganisms or their toxins is known as inflammation.

_____ 8. The recommended route of administration for an MMR vaccine is subcutaneous.

_____ 9. Before administering a pediatric immunization, the National Childhood Vaccine Injury Act (NCVIA) requires that the parent sign a consent form.

_____ 10. If phenylketonuria (PKU) is left untreated, it can lead to malnutrition.

Directions: Match each key term with its definition.

_____ 1. Immunity

_____ 2. Immunization

_____ 3. Infant

_____ 4. Length

_____ 5. Pediatrician

_____ 6. Pediatrics

_____ 7. Preschooler

_____ 8. School-age child

_____ 9. Toddler

_____ 10. Toxoid

_____ 11. Vaccine

_____ 12. Vertex

A. A physician who specializes in the care and development of children and the diagnosis and treatment of children's diseases
B. A child between 1 and 3 years old
C. The top of the head
D. The resistance of the body to the effects of a harmful agent such as a pathogenic microorganism or its toxins
E. The branch of medicine that deals with the care and development of children and the diagnosis and treatment of children's diseases
F. A suspension of attenuated or killed microorganisms administered to an individual to prevent an infectious disease
G. The process of becoming immune or of rendering an individual immune through the use of a vaccine or toxoid
H. The measurement from the vertex of the head to the heel of the foot in a supine position
I. A toxin that has been treated by heat or chemicals to destroy its harmful properties administered to an individual to prevent an infectious disease
J. A child from birth to 12 months old
K. A child from 3 to 6 years old
L. A child from 6 to 12 years old

EVALUATION OF LEARNING

Directions: Fill in each blank with the correct answer.

1. What are the components of the well-child visit?

_____

_____

2. What topics are commonly included in anticipatory guidance?

_____

_____

3. What is the usual schedule for well-child visits?

_____

_____

4. What is the purpose of the sick-child visit?

_____

_____

5. What procedures are often performed by the medical assistant during pediatric office visits?

_____

_____

6. Why is it important for the medical assistant to develop a rapport with the pediatric patient?

_____

_____

_____

7. List the two positions that can be used to safely carry an infant.

_____

8. Why is it important to measure the growth (weight and height or length) of the child during each office visit?

_____

9. What is the difference between height and length?

_____

_____

10. What is the purpose of measuring head circumference?

_____

_____

11. What is the primary use of growth charts?

_____

_____

12. What is the primary cause of childhood obesity?

_____

13. What problems are associated with childhood obesity?

_____

_____

14. List five guidelines for preventing childhood obesity.

_____

_____

_____

15. According to the American Academy of Pediatrics, at what age and how often should blood pressure be measured in children?

_____

_____

16. What is the importance of measuring blood pressure in children?

_____

_____

363

17. What criteria must be followed to determine the correct cuff size for a child?

_____

_____

18. What occurs if the blood pressure cuff is too small or too large?

_____

_____

19. What three factors must be taken into consideration when determining if a child has hypertension?

_____

20. List three reasons for collecting a urine specimen from a child.

_____

_____

_____

21. Why should the child's genitalia be cleansed before applying a pediatric urine collector?

_____

_____

22. What gauge and length (range) of needle are recommended for giving an intramuscular injection to a child?

_____

23. Why is the dorsogluteal site not recommended for use as an intramuscular injection site in infants and young children?

_____

_____

_____

24. Why is the vastus lateralis muscle recommended as a good site for giving an intramuscular injection to an infant or young child? How is this site located?

_____

_____

_____

25. At what age can the deltoid site be used to administer an IM injection to a child? Explain the reason for this.

_____

_____

26. What is the recommended subcutaneous injection site for each of the following?

    a. An infant younger than 12 months of age: _____

    b. A child who is 12 months of age or older: _____

27. What is the difference between a vaccine and a toxoid?

_____

_____

_____

28. What immunizations are included in the following?

   a. DTaP: _____

   b. MMR: _____

29. According to the American Academy of Pediatrics, what immunizations are recommended for each of the following pediatric patients?

   a. 2-month-old infant: _____

   b. 6-month-old infant: _____

   c. 12-month-old infant: _____

   d. 5-year-old child: _____

30. What information must be provided to parents as required by the NCVIA?

_____

_____

31. What information is included in a VIS?

_____

_____

_____

32. According to the NCVIA, what information must be documented in the patient's medical record after a pediatric immunization has been administered?

_____

_____

_____

33. The newborn screening test screens for which metabolic diseases?

_____

_____

34. What are the symptoms of PKU if left untreated?

_____

35. Why can the PKU screening test be performed earlier on infants on formula compared with breast-fed babies?

_____

_____

A. Pediatric Weight

Locate the following weight values on a pediatric balance scale. Place a check mark next to each one after it has been correctly located.

1. 7 lb, 9 oz _____

2. 8 lb, 5 oz _____

3. 12 lb, 10 oz _____

4. 15 lb, 11 oz _____

5. 19 lb, 7 oz _____

6. 23 lb, 6 oz _____

7. 25 lb, 3 oz _____

B. Pediatric Length

Locate the following length values on your pediatric measuring device. Place a check mark next to each after it has been correctly located.

1. 20½ inches _____

2. 22½ inches _____

3. 24 inches _____

4. 25¼ inches _____

5. 28½ inches _____

6. 31 inches _____

7. 33¼ inches _____

8. 36½ inches _____

C. Growth Charts

Matthew Williams, age 2 years (24 months), has had health maintenance visits at the intervals listed below. His length and weight measurements were taken during each visit and are documented here. Plot these on the growth chart provided on the following page. You can also print out a growth chart from your computer by going to the following website: www.cdc.gov/growthcharts. Calculate the percentile for each and document it in the space provided. (*Note:* His birth weight was 7 lb, 8 oz, and his length was 20 inches.)

Well-Child Visit				
Age	Weight	Percentile	Length	Percentile
1 month	9 lb, 10 oz	50	22 in	
2 months	12 lb, 4 oz	50	23½ in	
4 months	16 lb, 5 oz	25	25¼ in	
6 months	18 lb, 8 oz	75	27 in	
9 months	22 lb, 4 oz	75	29¼ in	
12 months	24 lb, 4 oz	75	30½ in	
15 months	26 lb, 8 oz	80	31½ in	
18 months	27 lb	75	32½ in	
24 months	28 lb	50	35¾ in	

Birth to 36 months: Boys
Length-for-age and Weight-for-age percentiles

NAME _____

RECORD # _____

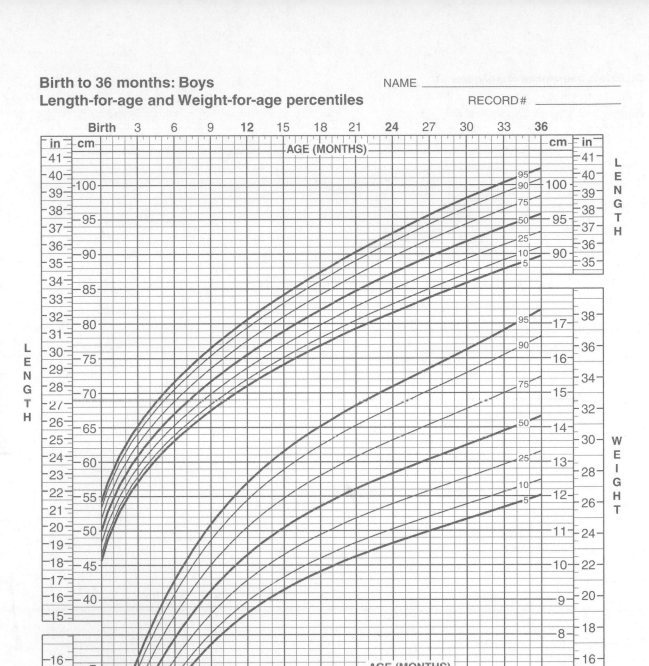

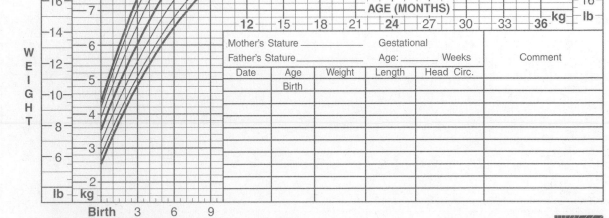

Date	Age	Weight	Length	Head Circ.	Comment
	Birth				

Mother's Stature _____

Father's Stature _____

Gestational Age: _____ Weeks

Published May 30, 2000 (modified 4/20/01).

SOURCE: Developed by the National Center for Health Statistics in collaboration with the National Center for Chronic Disease Prevention and Health Promotion (2000).

http://www.cdc.gov/growthcharts

CDC
SAFER · HEALTHIER · PEOPLE™

D. Motor and Social Development

Using a reference source, describe the motor and social development of the age groups listed here. The first one is done for you.

Age	Motor and Social Development
Birth to 3 months	Raises head but not stable, can turn head from side to side, activities are limited to reflexes, cries when hungry, responsive social smile, coos, eyes can focus on an object and follow a moving object 180 degrees.
4 to 6 months	
7 to 9 months	
10 to 12 months	

Age	Motor and Social Development
1 year	
2 years	
3 years	
4 years	
5 years	

Age	Motor and Social Development
6 years	
7 years	
8 to 10 years	
Preadolescent	
Adolescent	

E. Intramuscular Injection

How would you prepare the following children for an intramuscular injection of penicillin to reduce apprehension and fear? Table 9.2, Techniques for Interacting with Children, on page 285 of your textbook can be used as a reference for this activity.

a. Katie Waugh, age 5

_____

_____

_____

b. Patrick Williams, age 8

_____

_____

_____

c. Julie Anderson, age 15

_____

_____

_____

F. Vaccine Information Statement

Refer to the Diphtheria, Tetanus, and Pertussis Vaccine Information Statement (VIS) in your textbook (pages 306-307), and answer the following questions:

1. How does an individual contract tetanus?

_____

_____

2. What are the symptoms of the following diseases?

   a. Diphtheria _____

   b. Tetanus _____

   c. Pertussis _____

3. Why is DTaP now used instead of DTP?

_____

_____

4. What is the immunization schedule for DTaP?

_____

_____

5. Who should not get a DTaP immunization?

_____

_____

6. What does Td protect against, and what is the recommended immunization schedule for Td?

_____

_____

7. What mild problems may occur from a DTaP vaccine?

_____

_____

8. What moderate problems may occur from a DTaP vaccine?

_____

_____

9. What should be done if the patient develops fever and pain after receiving DTaP?

_____

_____

10. What are the symptoms of a serious reaction to DTaP?

_____

11. What should be done if a moderate or severe reaction occurs after a DTaP immunization?

_____

_____

G. Locating and Interpreting a Vaccine Information Statement

Obtain a VIS for a vaccine that you would like to know more about (other than the DTaP vaccine already included in your textbook). List the information that would be important for a parent to know before this immunization is administered to his or her child. The following Internet sites can be used to obtain a VIS:

www.cdc.gov/vaccines/hcp/vis/index.html

www.immunize.org/vis

Name of Immunization: _____

Publication Date: _____

Information to Relay to a Parent:

_____

_____

_____

_____

_____

_____

_____

_____

_____

_____

H. Immunization Administration Record

Complete the following immunization record form for an infant at his or her 2-month, 4-month, and 6-month visits using Figure 9.11 (immunization schedule) in the textbook to determine which immunizations are administered during these well-child visits. The website (www.immunize.org/catg.d/p2022.pdf) provides an example of a completed immunization administration form to assist you in completing this form.

372

IMMUNIZATION ADMINISTRATION RECORD

Name _____
         (first)   (MI)   (last)

DOB _____

Physician _____

Address _____

_____

SITE ABBREVIATIONS:

RVL: Right vastus lateralis
LVL: Left vastus lateralis
RD: Right deltoid
LD: Left deltoid
PO: By mouth
IN: Intranasal

Vaccine	Type of Vaccine[1] (generic abbreviation)	Date Given (mo/day/yr)	Dose	Site	Vaccine		Vaccine Information Statement		Signature and Title of Vaccinator
					Lot #	Mfr.	Date on VIS	Date Given	
Hepatitis B[2] (e.g., HepB, Hib-HepB, DTaP-HepB-IPV) Give IM.									
Diphtheria, Tetanus, Pertussis[2] (e.g., DTaP, DTaP-Hib, DTaP-HepB-IPV, DT, DTaP-HiB-IPV, Tdap, DTaP-IPV, Td) Give IM.									
Haemophilus influenzae **type b**[2] (e.g., Hib, Hib-HepB, DTaP-HiB-IPV, DTaP-Hib) Give IM.									
Polio[2] (e.g., IPV, DTaP-HepB-IPV, DTaP-HiB-IPV, DTaP-IPV) Give IPV SC or IM. Give all others IM.									
Pneumococcal (e.g., PCV, conjugate; PPV, polysaccharide) Give PCV IM. Give PPV SC or IM.									
Rotovirus Give oral.									
Measles, Mumps, Rubella (e.g., MMR, MMRV) Give SC.									
Varicella (e.g., Var, MMRV) Give SC.									
Hepatitis A (HepA) Give IM									
Meningococcal (e.g., MCV4, MPSV4) Give MCV4 IM and MPSV4 SC.									
Human papillomavirus (e.g., HPV) Give IM									
Influenza (e.g., TIV, inactivated; LAIV, live attenuated) Give TIV IM. Give LAIV IN.									
Other									

1. Record the generic abbreviation for the type of vaccine given (e.g., DTaP-Hib, PCV), *not* the trade name.
2. For combination vaccines, fill in a row for each separate antigen in the combination.

I. Crossword Puzzle: The Pediatric Examination

Directions: Complete the crossword puzzle using the clues provided.

Across

1 Right size for child's BP?
3 Title expires at 1 year
6 Child's vaccine act
9 German measles
10 Not for pregnant women
13 Whooping cough
16 PKU puncture site
17 3-in-1 vaccine
20 Do not weigh infant in this
21 Stand up straight
22 Begin at 3 years
23 First breast milk
24 Baby doctor
25 MMR administration route
26 Can give at birth vaccine
27 Injection site for infants

Down

1 Hold-me position
2 Not a kid reward
4 Common immunization side effect
5 From 1 to 3 years
7 Resistance to microorganisms
8 No phenylalanine enzyme disease
11 Vertex to heel
12 Child's work
14 Childhood obesity can cause this
15 Not caused by chickens
18 Fights with a microorganism
19 Immunization explainer

Procedure 9-A: Carrying an Infant

Practice the procedure for carrying an infant, using a pediatric training mannequin in the following positions: cradle and upright.

Carrying Position	Number of Practices

Procedures 9-1 and 9-3: Weight, Length, and Growth Charts

1. **Weight and Length.** Measure the weight of an infant using a pediatric training mannequin. Document the results in the chart provided.

2. **Growth Charts.** Calculate growth percentiles on a growth chart using the values presented below. Assume these values were taken from the same (female) child over the course of her first year of life.

Age	Weight	Length
2 months	9 pounds	21 inches
4 months	11 pounds, 8 ounces	23½ inches
6 months	14 pounds, 8 ounces	25¼ inches
9 months	18 pounds, 8 ounces	27¼ inches
12 months	21 pounds, 6 ounces	28¾ inches

Procedure 9-2: Head and Chest Circumference

Measure the head and chest circumference of an infant using a pediatric training mannequin. Document the results in the chart provided.

CHART	
Date	

Procedure 9-4: Pediatric Urine Collector

Practice the procedure for applying a pediatric urine collector, using a pediatric training mannequin. Document the procedure in the chart provided.

Procedure 9-5: Newborn Screening Test

1. Complete the information section of the Newborn Screening Test Card provided for you.

2. Practice the procedure for specimen collection for the newborn screening test using a pediatric training mannequin. Document the procedure in the chart provided.

CHART	
Date	

377

Newborn Screening Test

USE BALL-
POINT PEN-
PRESS HARD

ALL
INFORMATION
MUST BE
PRINTED

Birth date: ___ / ___ / ___   Time ___ : ___ (Use 24-hour time only)

Baby's name:
(last, first)

Hospital provider number:

Hospital of birth
or transfer:

Mom's name:
(last, first, initial)

Mom's address:

Mom's city: Ohio   Zip:

Mom's race: Mom's age: Mom's SSN: ___ - ___ - ___

Mom's phone: (___) ___ - ___   Mom's county:

Mom's ID: Baby's ID:

Specimen date ___ ; ___ / ___   Time ___ : ___ (Use 24-hour time only)

Baby's physician:
(last name first)

Physician address:

City: Ohio   Zip

Physician phone: (___) ___ - ___   Physician provider number:

1. SPECIMEN: ☐ FIRST ☐ SECOND
☐ other

2. BIRTH NUMBER/SEX:
☐ SINGLE ☐ MULTIPLE ___ A, B, C, etc.
☐ FEMALE ☐ MALE

3. BIRTH WEIGHT: ___ GRAMS

4. PREMATURE: ☐ YES ☐ NO

5. ANTIBIOTICS: ☐ YES ☐ NO

6. TRANSFUSION: ☐ YES ☐ NO

7. FEEDING: ☐ YES ☐ NO
Type 1. Breast 2. Milk-base
NO. 3. Soy 4. TPN 5. IV-only

8. SUBMITTER:
☐ HOSPITAL/BIRTH CENTER
☐ HEALTH DEPARTMENT
☐ PHYSICIAN
☐ HOME HEALTH CARE AGENCY
☐ CLINICAL LAB
☐ OTHER

☐ SPECIMEN REJECTED _____

Procedure 9-A: Carrying an Infant

Name: _____   Date: _____

Evaluated by: _____   Score: _____

Performance Objective

Outcome:	Carry an infant in the following positions: cradle and upright.
Conditions:	Given a pediatric training mannequin.
Standards:	Time: 5 minutes. Student completed procedure in _____ minutes.
	Accuracy: Satisfactory score on the Performance Evaluation Checklist.

Performance Evaluation Checklist

Trial 1	Trial 2	Point Value	Performance Standards
			Cradle position:
		•	Slid the left hand and arm under the infant's back.
		•	Grasped the infant's upper arm from behind.
		•	Encircled the infant's upper arm with the thumb and fingers.
		•	Supported the infant's head, shoulders, and back on your arm.
		•	Slipped the right arm up and under the infant's buttocks.
		•	Cradled the infant in your arms with the infant's body resting against your chest.
			Upright position:
		•	Slipped the right hand under the infant's head and shoulders.
		•	Spread the fingers apart to support the infant's head and neck.
		•	Slipped the left forearm under the infant's buttocks.
		•	Allowed the infant to rest against your chest.
			Demonstrated the following affective behavior(s) during this procedure:
		Ⓐ	Demonstrated: (a) empathy (b) active listening (c) nonverbal communication.
		★	Completed the procedure within 5 minutes.
			Totals

CHART	
Date	

Evaluation of Student Performance

EVALUATION CRITERIA			COMMENTS
Symbol	**Category**	**Point Value**	
★	Critical Step	16 points	
•	Essential Step	6 points	
Ⓐ	Affective Competency	6 points	
▷	Theory Question	2 points	

Score calculation: 100 points
    − _____ points missed
        _____ Score

Satisfactory score: 85 or above

CAAHEP Competencies Achieved

Psychomotor (Skills)

☑ I. 8. Instruct and prepare a patient for a procedure or a treatment.

Affective (Behavior)

☑ V. 1. Demonstrate: (a) empathy (b) active listening (c) nonverbal communication.

ABHES Competencies Achieved

☑ 8. c. Assist provider with general/physical examination.

Procedure 9-1: Measuring the Weight and Length of an Infant

Name: _____   Date: _____

Evaluated by: _____   Score: _____

Performance Objective

Outcome:	Measure the weight and length of an infant.
Conditions:	Using a pediatric training mannequin and a pediatric balance scale (table model).
	Given a paper protector.
Standards:	Time: 5 minutes. Student completed procedure in _____ minutes.
	Accuracy: Satisfactory score on the Performance Evaluation Checklist.

Performance Evaluation Checklist

Trial 1	Trial 2	Point Value	Performance Standards
			Weight·
		•	Sanitized hands.
		•	Greeted the infant's parent and introduced yourself.
		•	Identified the infant.
		•	Explained the procedure to the child's parent.
		•	Based on the medical office policy, asked the parent to: a. Remove the infant's clothing and put on a dry diaper. b. Remove the infant's clothing, including the diaper.
		▷	Stated why the infant should not be weighed with a wet diaper.
		•	Unlocked the pediatric scale and placed a clean paper protector on it.
		▷	Stated the purpose of the paper protector.
		•	Checked the balance scale for accuracy.
		▷	Stated the purpose for balancing the scale.
		•	Gently placed the infant on his or her back on the scale.
		•	Placed one hand slightly above the infant.
		•	Balanced the scale.
		•	Read the results while the infant was lying still.
		•	Jotted down the value or made a mental note of it.
		★	The reading was identical to the evaluator's reading.
		•	Returned the balance to its resting position and locked the scale.
			Length:
		•	Placed the vertex of the infant's head against the headboard at the zero mark.
		•	Asked the parent to hold the infant's head in position.

381

Trial 1	Trial 2	Point Value	Performance Standards
		•	Straightened the infant's knees and placed the soles of the infant's feet firmly against the upright footboard.
		•	Read the infant's length in inches from the measure.
		•	Jotted down the value or made a mental note of it.
		★	The reading was identical to the evaluator's reading.
		•	Removed the infant from the scale and handed him or her to the parent.
		•	Returned the headboard and footboard to their resting positions.
		•	Sanitized hands.
		•	Documented the results correctly.
			Demonstrated the following affective behavior(s) during this procedure:
		Ⓐ	Incorporated critical thinking skills when performing patient assessment.
		Ⓐ	Demonstrated: (a) empathy (b) active listening (c) nonverbal communication.
		★	Completed the procedure within 5 minutes.
			Totals

CHART

Date	

Evaluation of Student Performance

EVALUATION CRITERIA			COMMENTS
Symbol	**Category**	**Point Value**	
★	Critical Step	16 points	
•	Essential Step	6 points	
Ⓐ	Affective Competency	6 points	
▷	Theory Question	2 points	

Score calculation: 100 points

− _____ points missed

_____ Score

Satisfactory score: 85 or above

CAAHEP Competencies Achieved

Psychomotor (Skills)

☑ I. 1. f. Measure and record weight.

☑ I. 1. g. Measure and record length (infant).

☑ V. 5. Coach patients appropriately considering: (a) cultural diversity (b) developmental life stage (c) communication barriers.

Affective (Behavior)

☑ I. 1. Incorporate critical thinking skills when performing patient assessment.

☑ V. 1. Demonstrate: (a) empathy (b) active listening (c) nonverbal communication.

ABHES Competencies Achieved

☑ 4. a. Follow documentation guidelines.

☑ 5. d. Adapt care to address the developmental stages of life.

☑ 8. c. Assist provider with general/physical examination.

Notes

Procedure 9-2: Measuring Head and Chest Circumference of an Infant

Name: _____   Date: _____

Evaluated by: _____   Score: _____

Performance Objective

Outcome:	Measure the head and chest circumference of an infant.
Conditions:	Given a flexible, nonstretch tape measure (in centimeters).
Standards:	Time: 5 minutes. Student completed procedure in _____ minutes.
	Accuracy: Satisfactory score on the Performance Evaluation Checklist.

Performance Evaluation Checklist

Trial 1	Trial 2	Point Value	Performance Standards
			Measurement of head circumference:
		•	Sanitized hands.
		•	Assembled equipment.
		•	Positioned the infant.
		▷	Stated what positions can be used to measure head circumference.
		•	Positioned the measuring device around the infant's head.
		•	The tape measure was placed slightly above the eyebrows and pinna of the ears and around the occipital prominence at the back of the skull.
		•	Read the results in centimeters (or inches).
		•	Jotted down the value or made a mental note of it.
		★	The reading was identical to the evaluator's reading.
		•	Sanitized hands.
		•	Documented the results correctly.
			Measurement of chest circumference:
		•	Positioned the infant on his or her back on the examining table.
		•	Encircled the measuring device around the infant's chest at the nipple line.
		•	Ensured that the measuring device was snug but not too tight.
		•	Read the results in centimeters (or inches).
		•	Jotted down this value or made a mental note of it.
		★	The reading was identical to the evaluator's reading.
		•	Documented the results correctly.

Trial 1	Trial 2	Point Value	Performance Standards
			Demonstrated the following affective behavior(s) during this procedure:
		Ⓐ	Incorporated critical thinking skills when performing patient assessment.
		★	Completed the procedure within 5 minutes.
			Totals

CHART

Date	

Evaluation of Student Performance

EVALUATION CRITERIA			COMMENTS
Symbol	**Category**	**Point Value**	
★	Critical Step	16 points	
•	Essential Step	6 points	
Ⓐ	Affective Competency	6 points	
▷	Theory Question	2 points	

Score calculation: 100 points
−_____ points missed
_____ Score

Satisfactory score: 85 or above

CAAHEP Competencies Achieved

Psychomotor (Skills)
☑ I. 1. h. Measure and record head circumference (infant).

Affective (Behavior)
☑ I. 1. Incorporate critical thinking skills when performing patient assessment.

ABHES Competencies Achieved

☑ 4. a. Follow documentation guidelines.
☑ 8. c. Assist provider with general/physical examination.

℮ Procedure 9-3: Calculating Growth Percentiles

Name: _____ Date: _____

Evaluated by: _____ Score: _____

Performance Objective

Outcome:	Plot a pediatric growth value on a growth chart.
Conditions:	Given a pediatric growth chart.
Standards:	Time: 5 minutes. Student completed procedure in _____ minutes.
	Accuracy: Satisfactory score on the Performance Evaluation Checklist.

Performance Evaluation Checklist

Trial 1	Trial 2	Point Value	Performance Standards
		•	Selected the proper growth chart.
		•	Located the child's age in the horizontal column at the bottom of the chart.
		•	Located the growth value in the vertical column under the appropriate category.
		•	Drew an (imaginary) vertical line from the child's age mark and an imaginary horizontal line from the growth mark.
		•	Found the site at which the two lines intersected on the graph.
		•	Placed a dot on this site.
		•	Determined the percentile by following the curved percentile line upward.
		•	Read the value located on the right side of the chart.
		•	Estimated the results if the value did not fall exactly on a percentile line.
		•	Documented the results correctly.
		★	The value was within ±2 percentage points of the evaluator's determination.
			Demonstrated the following affective behavior(s) during this procedure:
		Ⓐ	Explained to a patient the rationale for performance of a procedure.
		★	Completed the procedure within 5 minutes.
			Totals

CHART	
Date	

Evaluation of Student Performance

EVALUATION CRITERIA			COMMENTS
Symbol	**Category**	**Point Value**	
★	Critical Step	16 points	
•	Essential Step	6 points	
Ⓐ	Affective Competency	6 points	
▷	Theory Question	2 points	

Score calculation: 100 points

    − _____ points missed

    _____ Score

Satisfactory score: 85 or above

CAAHEP Competencies Achieved

Psychomotor (Skills)

☑ II. 4. Document on a growth chart.

Affective (Behavior)

☑ V. 4. Explain to a patient the rationale for performance of a procedure.

ABHES Competencies Achieved

☑ 4. a. Follow documentation guidelines.

☑ 5. d. Adapt care to address the developmental stages of life.

e **Procedure 9-4: Applying a Pediatric Urine Collector**

Name: _____ Date: _____

Evaluated by: _____ Score: _____

Performance Objective

Outcome:	Apply a pediatric urine collector.
Conditions:	Using a pediatric training mannequin.
	Given the following: disposable gloves, personal antiseptic wipes, pediatric urine collector bag, urine specimen container and label, and a waste container.
Standards:	Time: 10 minutes.　　Student completed procedure in _____ minutes.
	Accuracy: Satisfactory score on the Performance Evaluation Checklist.

Performance Evaluation Checklist

Trial 1	Trial 2	Point Value	Performance Standards
		•	Sanitized hands.
		•	Assembled the equipment.
		•	Greeted the child's parent and introduced yourself.
		•	Identified the child and explained the procedure to the parent.
		•	Applied gloves.
		•	Positioned the child on his or her back with legs spread apart.
			Cleanse the area and apply the bag:
			Females
		•	Cleansed each side of the meatus with a separate wipe using a front-to-back motion.
		•	Cleansed directly down the middle with a third wipe.
		•	Discarded each wipe after cleansing.
		▷	Stated the reason for cleansing the urinary meatus.
		•	Allowed the area to dry completely.
		▷	Explained why the area should be allowed to dry.
		•	Removed the paper backing from the urine collector bag.
		•	Placed the bottom of the adhesive ring on the perineum and worked upward.
		•	Firmly pressed the adhesive surface to the skin surrounding the external genitalia.
		•	Made sure there was no puckering.
		•	The opening of the bag was placed directly over the urinary meatus.
		•	Excess length of the bag was positioned toward the feet.

389

Trial 1	Trial 2	Point Value	Performance Standards
			Males
		•	Retracted the foreskin of the penis if the child is not circumcised.
		•	Cleansed each side of the urethral orifice with a separate wipe.
		•	Cleansed directly over the urethral orifice.
		•	Cleansed the scrotum.
		•	Discarded each wipe after cleansing.
		•	Allowed the area to dry completely.
		•	Removed the paper backing from the urine collector bag.
		•	Positioned the bag so that the child's penis and scrotum are projected through the opening of the bag.
		•	Pressed the adhesive surface firmly to the skin.
		•	Excess length of the bag was positioned toward the feet.
			Completed the procedure:
		•	Loosely diapered the child.
		•	Checked the bag every 15 minutes until the urine specimen was obtained.
		•	Gently removed the collector bag from top to bottom.
		•	Cleansed the genital area with a personal antiseptic wipe and rediapered the child.
		•	Transferred the urine specimen into the specimen container and tightly applied the lid.
		•	Applied a label to the container.
		•	Disposed of the collector bag in a regular waste container.
		•	Tested the specimen or prepared it for transfer to an outside laboratory.
		▷	Explained why the urine specimen should not be allowed to stand at room temperature.
		•	Removed gloves and sanitized hands.
		•	Documented the procedure correctly.
			Demonstrated the following affective behavior(s) during this procedure:
		Ⓐ	Explained to a patient the rationale for performance of a procedure.
		★	Completed the procedure within 10 minutes.
			Totals
CHART			
Date			

390

Evaluation of Student Performance

EVALUATION CRITERIA			COMMENTS
Symbol	**Category**	**Point Value**	
★	Critical Step	16 points	
•	Essential Step	6 points	
Ⓐ	Affective Competency	6 points	
▷	Theory Question	2 points	

Score calculation: 100 points
− _____ points missed
_____ Score

Satisfactory score: 85 or above

CAAHEP Competencies Achieved

Psychomotor (Skills)
☑ I. 11. c. Obtain specimens and perform CLIA waived urinalysis.

Affective (Behavior)
☑ V. 4. Explain to a patient the rationale for performance of a procedure.

ABHES Competencies Achieved

☑ 4. a. Follow documentation guidelines.
☑ 9. d. Collect, label and process specimens.

Chapter **9 The Pediatric Examination**

e **Procedure 9-5: Newborn Screening Test**

Name: _____ Date: _____

Evaluated by: _____ Score: _____

Performance Objective

Outcome:	Collect a capillary blood specimen for a newborn screening test.
Conditions:	Using a pediatric training mannequin.
	Given the following: disposable gloves, sterile lancet, heel warmer or warm compress, antiseptic wipe, newborn testing card, mailing envelope, sterile gauze pad, adhesive bandages, and a biohazard sharps container.
Standards:	Time: 10 minutes. Student completed procedure in _____ minutes.
	Accuracy: Satisfactory score on the Performance Evaluation Checklist.

Performance Evaluation Checklist

Trial 1	Trial 2	Point Value	Performance Standards
		•	Sanitized hands.
		•	Assembled the equipment.
		•	Greeted the infant's parent and introduced yourself.
		•	Identified the infant and explained the procedure to the parent.
		•	Completed the information section of the newborn screening card.
		•	Selected an appropriate puncture site.
		•	Identified the sites that can be used for the heel puncture.
		▷	Explained what could occur if a different site is used.
		•	Warmed the puncture site.
		▷	Stated the purpose of warming the site.
		•	Cleaned the puncture site with an antiseptic wipe and allowed it to air-dry.
		•	Applied gloves and grasped the infant's foot around the puncture site.
		•	Punctured the heel using a sterile lancet, and disposed of the lancet.
		•	Wiped away the first drop of blood with a gauze pad.
		▷	Explained why the first drop of blood should be wiped away.
		•	Encouraged a large drop of blood to form by exerting gentle pressure on the heel.
		•	Did not excessively squeeze the heel.
		▷	Explained why the excessive squeezing should be avoided.
		•	Touched the drop of blood to the center of the first circle on the test card.

393

Trial 1	Trial 2	Point Value	Performance Standards
		•	Completely filled the circle on the test card with blood.
		•	Continued until all the circles are completely filled with blood.
		▷	Explained why each circle must be completely filled with blood.
		•	Did not touch the blood specimen with your gloved hand.
		▷	Stated why the specimen should not be touched.
		•	Held a gauze pad over the puncture site and applied pressure.
		•	Remained with the infant until bleeding stopped. Applied an adhesive bandage if needed.
		•	Removed gloves and sanitized hands.
		•	Allowed the test card to air-dry horizontally for 3 hours at room temperature.
		•	Did not allow the blood specimen to come in contact with any other surface.
		•	Did not place the specimen in a plastic bag.
		▷	Explained what occurs if the specimen is placed in a plastic bag.
		•	Placed the test card in its protective envelope.
		•	Mailed the card to the laboratory within 48 hours.
		▷	Stated why the specimen must be mailed within 48 hours.
		•	Documented the procedure correctly.
			Demonstrated the following affective behavior(s) during this procedure:
		Ⓐ	Applied critical thinking when performing patient assessment.
		Ⓐ	Showed awareness of a patient's concerns related to the procedure being performed.
		Ⓐ	Recognized the implications for failure to comply with Centers for Disease Control and Prevention (CDC) regulations in health care settings.
		★	Completed the procedure within 10 minutes.
			Totals

CHART

Date	

Evaluation of Student Performance

EVALUATION CRITERIA			COMMENTS
Symbol	**Category**	**Point Value**	
★	Critical Step	16 points	
•	Essential Step	6 points	
Ⓐ	Affective Competency	6 points	
▷	Theory Question	2 points	

Score calculation: 100 points
       − _____ points missed
       ____ Score

Satisfactory score: 85 or above

CAAHEP Competencies Achieved

Psychomotor (Skills)

☑ I. 2. c. Perform capillary puncture.

☑ III. 10. Demonstrate proper disposal of biohazardous material (a) sharps (b) regulated waste.

Affective (Behavior)

☑ I. 1. Apply critical thinking when performing patient assessment.

☑ I. 3. Show awareness of a patient's concerns related to the procedure being performed.

☑ III. 1. Recognize the implications for failure to comply with Centers for Disease Control and Prevention (CDC) regulations in health care settings.

ABHES Competencies Achieved

☑ 8. a. Practice standard precautions and perform disinfection/sterilization techniques.

☑ 9. c. Dispose of biohazardous materials.

☑ 9. d. Collect, label, and process specimens: (2) Perform capillary puncture.

Newborn Screening Test

USE BALL-POINT PEN-PRESS HARD

ALL INFORMATION MUST BE PRINTED

Birth date: ☐☐ / ☐☐ / ☐☐

Baby's name: (last, first)

Hospital provider number:

Hospital of birth or transfer:

Mom's name: (last, first, initial)

Mom's address:

Mom's city: Ohio   Zip: ☐☐☐☐☐ - ☐☐☐☐

Mom's race: Mom's age: ☐☐

Mom's phone: (☐☐☐) ☐☐☐ - ☐☐☐☐   Mom's SSN: ☐☐☐ - ☐☐ - ☐☐☐☐

Mom's ID: Mom's county:

                   Baby's ID:

Specimen date ☐☐ / ☐☐ / ☐☐   Time ☐☐ : ☐☐ (Use 24-hour time only)

Baby's physician: (last name first)

Physician address:

City: Ohio   Zip ☐☐☐☐☐ - ☐☐☐☐

Physician phone: (☐☐☐) ☐☐☐ - ☐☐☐☐   Physician provider number:

Time ☐☐ : ☐☐ (Use 24-hour time only)

1. SPECIMEN: ☐ FIRST ☐ SECOND
              ☐ other

2. BIRTH NUMBER/ SEX:
   ☐ SINGLE   ☐ MULTIPLE A, B, C, etc.
   ☐ FEMALE   ☐ MALE

3. BIRTH WEIGHT: ☐☐☐☐ GRAMS

4. PREMATURE: ☐ YES ☐ NO

5. ANTIBIOTICS: ☐ YES ☐ NO

6. TRANSFUSION: ☐ YES ☐ NO

7. FEEDING: ☐ YES ☐ NO
   Type 1. Breast 2. Milk-base
   NO. 3. Soy 4. TPN 5. IV-only

8. SUBMITTER:
   ☐ HOSPITAL/BIRTH CENTER
   ☐ HEALTH DEPARTMENT
   ☐ PHYSICIAN
   ☐ HOME HEALTH CARE AGENCY
   ☐ CLINICAL LAB
   ☐ OTHER

   ☐ SPECIMEN REJECTED _____

10 Minor Office Surgery

√ After Completing	Date Due	Study Guide Pages	STUDY GUIDE ASSIGNMENTS (CTA = Critical Thinking Activity)	Possible Points	Points You Earned
		401	📄 Pretest	10	
		402-403	🔑 Term Key Term Assessment		
		402	A. Definitions	26	
		403	B. Word Parts	9	
			(Add 1 point for each key term)		
		403-408	📝 Evaluation of Learning questions	53	
		408-409	CTA A: Medical and Surgical Asepsis	10	
		410	CTA B: Violation of Surgical Asepsis	10	
		411-412	CTA C: Surgical Instruments (2 points each)	22	
			𝑒 Evolve Site: It's Instrumental (Record points earned)		
			𝑒 Evolve Site: Keep It Sterile (Record points earned)		
		413	CTA D: Pioneers in Surgical Asepsis (5 points each)	15	
		413-415	CTA E: Patient Instruction Sheet	20	
		417	CTA F: Crossword Puzzle	24	
			𝑒 Evolve Site: Apply Your Knowledge questions	10	
			𝑒 Evolve Site: Video Evaluation	69	
		401	📄 Posttest	10	
			ADDITIONAL ASSIGNMENTS		
			Total points		

√ When Assigned by Your Instructor	Study Guide Pages	Practices Required	Laboratory Assignments (Procedure Number and Name)	Score*
	419	5	**Practice for Competency** 10-1: Applying and Removing Sterile Gloves Textbook reference: pp. 325-327	
	421-422		**Evaluation of Competency** 10-1: Applying and Removing Sterile Gloves	*
	419	5	**Practice for Competency** 10-2: Opening a Sterile Package Textbook reference: pp. 328-329	
	423-424		**Evaluation of Competency** 10-2: Opening a Sterile Package	*
	419	5	**Practice for Competency** Using Commercially Prepared Sterile Packages Textbook reference: p. 324-325	
	425-426		**Evaluation of Competency** Using Commercially Prepared Sterile Packages	*
	419	3	**Practice for Competency** 10-3: Pouring a Sterile Solution Textbook reference: p. 329-330	
	427-428		**Evaluation of Competency** 10-3: Pouring a Sterile Solution	*
	419	5	**Practice for Competency** 10-4: Changing a Sterile Dressing Textbook reference: pp. 333-335	
	429-431		**Evaluation of Competency** 10-4: Changing a Sterile Dressing	*
	419	Sutures: 3 Staples: 3	**Practice for Competency** 10-5: Removing Sutures and Staples Textbook reference: pp. 340-343	
	433-435		**Evaluation of Competency** 10-5: Removing Sutures and Staples	*
	419	3	**Practice for Competency** 10-6: Applying and Removing Adhesive Skin Closures Textbook reference: pp. 343-347	
	337-440		**Evaluation of Competency** 10-6: Applying and Removing Adhesive Skin Closures	*
	419	5	**Practice for Competency** 10-7: Assisting with Minor Office Surgery Textbook reference: pp. 352-355	

399

√ When Assigned by Your Instructor	Study Guide Pages	Practices Required	Laboratory Assignments (Procedure Number and Name)	Score*
	441-444		**Evaluation of Competency** 10-7: Assisting with Minor Office Surgery	*
	419	Each bandage turn: 3	**Practice for Competency** 10-A: Bandage Turns Textbook reference: pp. 367-370	
	445-447		**Evaluation of Competency** 10-A: Bandage Turns	*
	420	3	Practice for Competency 10-8: Applying a Tubular Gauze Bandage Textbook reference: pp. 370-372	
	449-451		**Evaluation of Competency** 10-8: Applying a Tubular Gauze Bandage	*
			ADDITIONAL ASSIGNMENTS	

Name: _____ Date: _____

True or False

_____ 1. Surgical asepsis refers to practices that keep objects and areas free from all microorganisms.

_____ 2. Something that is sterile is contaminated if it comes in contact with a pathogen.

_____ 3. Reaching over a sterile field is a violation of sterile technique.

_____ 4. An incision is a jagged tearing of the tissues.

_____ 5. The skin is the first line of defense of the body.

_____ 6. One of the local signs of inflammation is fever.

_____ 7. Sutures approximate the edges of a wound until proper healing occurs.

_____ 8. A biopsy is usually performed to determine if an infection is present.

_____ 9. An ingrown toenail can be caused by shoes that are too tight.

_____ 10. One of the functions of a bandage is to hold a dressing in place.

? POSTTEST

True or False

_____ 1. Measuring a patient's temperature requires the use of surgical asepsis.

_____ 2. Hemostatic forceps are used to clamp off blood vessels.

_____ 3. An instrument with a ratchet should be kept in a closed position when not in use.

_____ 4. The provider would most likely order a tetanus booster for an abrasion.

_____ 5. Inflammation is the protective response of the body to trauma and the entrance of foreign substances.

_____ 6. A serous exudate is red in color.

_____ 7. Size 4-0 sutures have a smaller diameter than size 3 sutures.

_____ 8. Sebaceous cysts are commonly found on the palm of the hand.

_____ 9. Colposcopy is frequently used to evaluate lesions of the cervix.

_____ 10. Cryosurgery is used in the treatment of cervical cancer.

A. Definitions

Directions: Match each key term with its definition.

M ____ 1. Abrasion

E ____ 2. Abscess

T ____ 3. Absorbable suture

U ____ 4. Approximation

V ____ 5. Bandage

L ____ 6. Biopsy

N ____ 7. Capillary action

I ____ 8. Colposcope

S ____ 9. Colposcopy

B ____ 10. Contaminate

K ____ 11. Contusion

R ____ 12. Cryosurgery

Y ____ 13. Fibroblast

O ____ 14. Forceps

J ____ 15. Furuncle

F ____ 16. Hemostasis

W ____ 17. Incision

D ____ 18. Infection

A ____ 19. Inflammation

H ____ 20. Laceration

X ____ 21. Nonabsorbable suture

C ____ 22. Puncture

G ____ 23. Sterile

Z ____ 24. Surgery

P ____ 25. Surgical asepsis

Q ____ 26. Wound

A. A protective response of the body to trauma and the entrance of foreign matter

B. To cause a sterile object or surface to become unsterile

C. A wound made by a sharp pointed object piercing the skin

D. The condition in which the body is invaded by a pathogen

E. A collection of pus in a cavity surrounded by inflamed tissue

F. The arrest of bleeding by natural or artificial means

G. Free of all living microorganisms and bacterial spores

H. A wound in which the tissues are torn apart, leaving ragged and irregular edges

I. A lighted instrument with a binocular magnifying lens used to examine the vagina and cervix

J. A localized staphylococcal infection that originates deep within a hair follicle; also known as a boil

K. An injury to the tissues under the skin that causes blood vessels to rupture, allowing blood to seep into the tissues

L. The surgical removal and examination of tissue from the living body

M. A wound in which the outer layers of the skin are damaged

N. The action that causes liquid to rise along a wick, a tube, or a gauze dressing

O. A two-pronged instrument for grasping and squeezing

P. Practices that keep objects and areas sterile or free from micro-organisms

Q. A break in the continuity of an external or internal surface caused by physical means

R. The therapeutic use of freezing temperatures to destroy abnormal tissue

S. The visual examination of the vagina and cervix using a lighted instrument with a magnifying lens

T. Suture material that is gradually digested and absorbed by the body

U. The process of bringing two parts, such as tissue, together through the use of sutures or other means

V. A strip of woven material used to wrap or cover a part of the body

W. A clean cut caused by a cutting instrument

X. Suture material that is not absorbed by the body

Y. An immature cell from which connective tissue can develop

Z. The branch of medicine that deals with operative and manual procedures for correction of deformities and defects, repair of injuries, and diagnosis and treatment of certain diseases

B. Word Parts

Directions: Indicate the meaning of each word part in the space provided. List as many medical terms as possible that incorporate the word part in the space provided.

Word Part	Meaning of Word Part	Medical Terms That Incorporate Word Part
1. bi/o		
2. -opsy		
3. colp/o		
4. -scope		
5. -scopy		
6. cry/o		
7. fibr/o		
8. hem/o		
9. -stasis		

EVALUATION OF LEARNING

Directions: Fill in each blank with the correct answer.

1. List the characteristics of a minor surgical procedure.

2. List the responsibilities of the medical assistant during a minor surgical operation.

3. What is the purpose of serrations found on some instruments?

4. What is the difference in function between mosquito hemostatic forceps and standard hemostatic forceps?

5. List five guidelines that should be followed in caring for instruments.

_____

_____

_____

_____

6. What is the difference between a closed and an open wound?

_____

_____

7. Why does a puncture wound encourage the growth of tetanus bacteria?

_____

_____

8. What is the purpose of inflammation?

_____

_____

9. List the four local signs that occur during inflammation.

_____

10. What occurs during the inflammatory phase of wound healing?

_____

_____

11. What occurs during the granulation phase of wound healing?

_____

_____

12. What occurs during the maturation phase of wound healing?

_____

13. What is an exudate?

_____

_____

14. Describe the appearance of the following types of exudates:

   a. Serous

   b. Sanguineous

   c. Purulent

   d. Serosanguineous

   e. Purosanguineous

404

15. List two functions of a sterile dressing.

_____

_____

16. The names and sizes of sutures are listed. In each set, circle the suture that has the smaller diameter:
    a. 4-0 silk
       2-0 silk
    b. 0 chromic surgical gut
       3-0 chromic surgical gut
    c. 2-0 polypropylene
       2 polypropylene

17. List five examples of materials used for nonabsorbable sutures.

_____

_____

18. What is a swaged needle? List advantages of using a swaged needle.

_____

_____

19. Why are sutures inserted in the head and neck generally removed sooner than other sutures?

_____

_____

20. List two advantages of using surgical skin staples to approximate a wound.

_____

_____

21. List three advantages of adhesive skin closures.

_____

_____

_____

22. What is the purpose of preparing the patient's skin before minor office surgery?

_____

23. What is the purpose of a fenestrated drape?

_____

_____

24. What are the characteristics of a local anesthetic?

_____

_____

25. What is the purpose of adding epinephrine to a local anesthetic?

_____

405

26. What is the name of the local anesthetic most frequently used in the medical office during minor office surgery?

_____

27. Explain how an instrument should be handed to the provider during minor office surgery.

_____

28. What is a sebaceous cyst, and what causes it to form?

_____

_____

29. What is the purpose of using gauze packing or a rubber Penrose drain after incising a localized infection?

_____

_____

30. What is the difference between congenital nevi and acquired nevi?

_____

_____

31. What are the characteristics of benign moles?

_____

_____

_____

32. What are skin tags? Where are they most frequently found on the body?

_____

_____

_____

33. Describe the appearance of dysplastic nevi. What concern exists with dysplastic nevi?

_____

_____

_____

34. List the characteristics of melanoma.

_____

_____

_____

35. What are the most common methods used to remove moles?

_____

_____

36. What is the purpose of a biopsy?

_____

_____

37. What is an ingrown toenail?

_____

_____

38. List three causes of an ingrown toenail.

_____

_____

_____

39. What are the postoperative instructions for toenail removal?

_____

_____

40. List two reasons for performing a colposcopy.

_____

_____

41. What is the purpose of performing a cervical punch biopsy?

_____

_____

42. List the postoperative instructions that must be relayed to the patient after a cervical punch biopsy.

_____

_____

_____

43. List two uses of cryosurgery.

_____

_____

44. List the postoperative instructions that must be relayed to the patient after cervical cryosurgery.

_____

_____

_____

45. List three functions of a bandage.

_____

_____

_____

46. List four guidelines to follow when applying a bandage.

_____

_____

_____

_____

47. List four signs that may indicate a bandage is too tight.

_____

_____

_____

_____

48. Why should the medical assistant be careful when applying an elastic bandage?

_____

_____

49. What is the purpose of reversing the spiral during a spiral-reverse turn?

_____

_____

50. List two uses of the figure-eight bandage turn.

_____

_____

51. What type of bandage turn is used to anchor a bandage?

_____

_____

52. List four examples of body parts to which a tubular bandage can be applied.

_____

_____

_____

_____

53. List two advantages for using a tubular bandage (compared with a roller bandage).

_____

_____

CRITICAL THINKING ACTIVITIES

A. Medical and Surgical Asepsis
Refer to Chapter 2, and describe the difference between medical asepsis and surgical asepsis.

_____

_____

_____

408

Which technique (medical asepsis or surgical asepsis) would be employed during the following procedures? For procedures requiring surgical asepsis, indicate which of the following reasons necessitates the use of surgical asepsis: caring for broken skin, penetrating a skin surface, or entering a body cavity that is normally sterile.

1. Administering oral medication

_____

_____

2. Inserting sutures

_____

_____

3. Measuring oral temperature

_____

_____

4. Applying a bandage to the forearm

_____

_____

5. Performing a needle biopsy

_____

_____

6. Removing a sebaceous cyst

_____

_____

7. Obtaining a Pap specimen

_____

_____

8. Inserting a urinary catheter

_____

_____

9. Incision and drainage of an abscess

_____

_____

10. Applying a dressing to an open wound

_____

_____

409

B. Violation of Surgical Asepsis

In the situations that follow, the principles of surgical asepsis have been violated. In the space provided, explain why the techniques should not be performed in this manner.

1. Placing a sterile 4 3 4 gauze pad within the 1-inch border around the sterile field

_____

_____

2. Wearing rings during the application of sterile gloves

_____

_____

3. Talking over a sterile field

_____

_____

4. Reaching over a sterile field

_____

_____

5. Holding sterile gauze below waist level

_____

_____

6. Not palming the label when pouring an antiseptic solution

_____

_____

7. Spilling an antiseptic solution on the sterile field

_____

_____

8. Passing a soiled dressing over the sterile field

_____

_____

9. Placing a vial of Xylocaine on the sterile field

_____

_____

10. Using bare hands to arrange articles on the sterile field

_____

_____

C. Surgical Instruments

In the space provided, state the name and use of each of the following types of surgical instruments. Identify any of the following parts present on each instrument by labeling the instrument: box lock, spring handle, ratchets, serrations, cutting edge, and teeth.

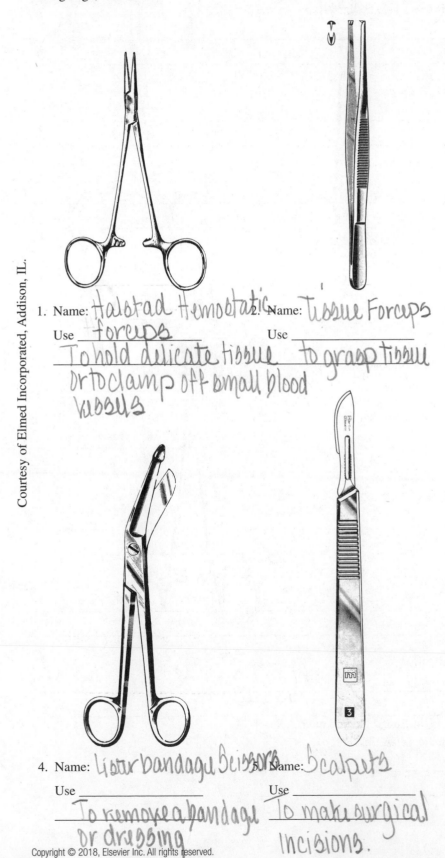
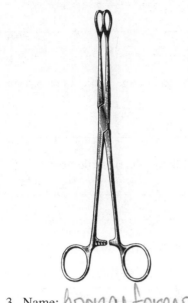
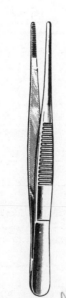

1. Name: _Halstead Hemostatic_
   forceps
   Use _____
   To hold delicate tissue
   or to clamp off small blood
   vessels

2. Name: _Tissue Forceps_
   Use _____
   to grasp tissue

3. Name: _Sponge forceps_
   Use _____
   To hold Sponge

4. Name: _Lister bandage Scissors_
   Use _____
   To remove a bandage
   or dressing

5. Name: _Scalpets_
   Use _____
   To make surgical
   Incisions.

6. Name: _thumb forceps_
   Use _____
   to pick up Tissue

411

7. Name: *Operating Scissors*   blunt blunt
   Use _____
   To cut through tissue

8. Name: *Suture Scissors*
   Use *Cut through tissue*
   _____

9. Name: *Kelly hanson Forceps*
   Use *Straight*
   To clamp off blood
   vessels

10. Name: *Plain Splinter forceps*
    Use _____
    To remove foreign objects
    from Skin.

11. Name: *Crile Needle Holder*
    Use _____
    To grasp a curved Needle.

Courtesy of Elmed Incorporated, Addison, IL.

D. Pioneers in Surgical Asepsis

Using a reference source, describe the contributions the following men made to medicine, especially regarding surgical asepsis:

1. Ignaz Semmelwcis

_____

_____

_____

2. Louis Pasteur

_____

_____

_____

3. Joseph Lister

_____

_____

_____

E. Patient Instruction Sheet

1. You are working for a surgeon who would like you to develop a patient instruction sheet for minor surgery. Select one of the minor operations provided. Using the following instruction sheet, develop a sheet that would be informative and visually appealing to a patient. Be as creative as possible in designing your sheet.

2. Select a partner. Have your partner play the role of a patient who is going to have the minor surgery performed, and explain the information on the sheet. Ask the patient to sign the sheet, and witness the patient's signature.

Minor Office Operations

a. Sebaceous cyst removal
b. Mole removal
c. Needle biopsy
d. Ingrown toenail removal
e. Colposcopy and biopsy
f. Cervical cryosurgery

Notes

PATIENT INSTRUCTION SHEET

NAME OF THE PROCEDURE:

DESCRIPTION OF THE PROCEDURE:

PURPOSE OF THE PROCEDURE:

HOW TO PREPARE FOR THE PROCEDURE:

WHAT TO DO FOLLOWING THE PROCEDURE:

I have received and understand the above instructions:

Patient's Signature _____

Witness: _____ Date: _____

Notes

F. Crossword Puzzle: Minor Office Surgery

Directions: Complete the crossword puzzle using the clues presented below.

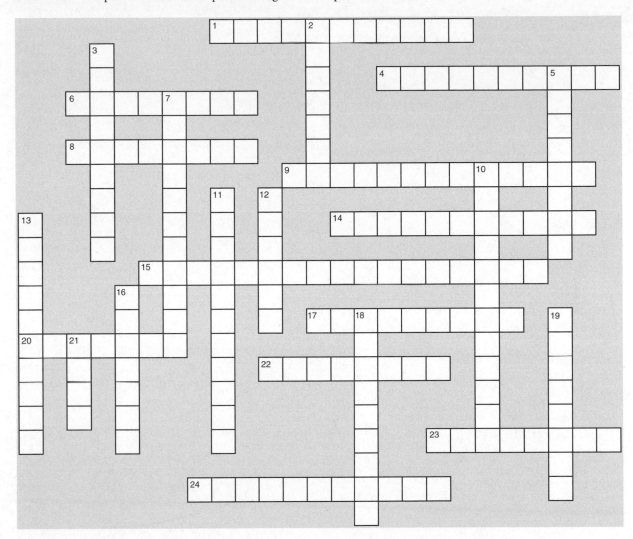

Across

1 Drape with a hole
4 Produces collagen
6 Clean, smooth cut
8 Boil
9 Sac containing oil secretions
14 Pus formation
15 Clamps off blood vessels
17 Local anesthetic brand name
20 Pus in a cavity
22 Tetanus may grow here
23 A local sign of inflammation
24 Bring together

Down

2 Free of all MOs and spores
3 Bruise
5 Scrape
7 Exudate containing blood
10 Suture/needle combination
11 Tx for chronic cervicitis
12 Father of modern surgery
13 Ragged and irregular wound
16 Discovered penicillin
18 Position for colposcopy
19 Antiseptic brand name
21 Nonabsorbable suture material

Sterile Technique

Procedure 10-1: Applying and Removing Sterile Gloves

Apply and remove sterile gloves.

Procedure 10-2: Opening a Sterile Package

Open a sterile package. Add a sterile article to a sterile field using a commercially prepared peel-apart package. Practice each of the methods used to transfer articles to a sterile field as shown in Figure 10-4 of your textbook.

Procedure 10-3: Pouring a Sterile Solution

Pour a sterile solution into a container on a sterile field.

Minor Surgical Procedures

Procedure 10-4: Changing a Sterile Dressing

Change a sterile dressing and document the procedure in the chart provided.

Procedure 10-5: Removing Sutures and Staples

Practice the procedure for removing sutures and staples, and document the procedure in the chart provided.

Procedure 10-6: Applying and Removing Adhesive Skin Closures

Practice the procedure for applying and removing adhesive skin closures, and document the procedure in the chart provided.

Procedure 10-7: Assisting with Minor Office Surgery

Obtain eight index cards. For each of the following minor office surgeries, indicate (on one side of the card) the equipment and supplies required for the side table. On the other side of the card, indicate the equipment and supplies required for the sterile tray setup. Set up a surgical tray for the procedures listed using your index cards. In the chart provided, document the instructions relayed to the patient following the surgery.

a. Suture insertion
b. Sebaceous cyst removal
c. Incision and drainage of a localized infection
d. Mole removal
e. Needle biopsy
f. Ingrown toenail removal
g. Colposcopy
h. Cervical punch biopsy
i. Cervical cryosurgery

Procedure 10-A: Bandage Turns

Practice the following bandage turns:

a. Circular turn
b. Spiral turn
c. Spiral-reverse turn
d. Figure-eight turn
e. Recurrent turn

Procedure 10-8: Tubular Gauze Bandage

Practice the procedure for applying a tubular gauze bandage, and document the procedure in the chart provided.

CHART	
Date	

e Procedure 10-1: Applying and Removing Sterile Gloves

Name: _____ Date: _____

Evaluated by: _____ Score: _____

Performance Objective

Outcome:	Apply and remove sterile gloves.
Conditions:	Given the appropriate-sized sterile gloves.
	Using a clean flat surface.
Standards:	Time: 5 minutes. Student completed procedure in _____ minutes.
	Accuracy: Satisfactory score on the Performance Evaluation Checklist.

Performance Evaluation Checklist

Trial 1	Trial 2	Point Value	Performance Standards
			Application of gloves:
		•	Removed rings and washed hands with an antimicrobial soap.
		▷	Explained why the hands should be washed.
		•	Selected the appropriate-sized gloves.
		▷	Explained what may occur if the gloves are too small or too large.
		•	Placed the glove package on a clean flat surface.
		•	Opened the sterile glove package without touching the inside of the wrapper.
		•	Picked up the first glove on the inside of the cuff without contaminating.
		•	Did not touch the outside of the glove with the bare hand.
		•	Stepped back and pulled on glove and allowed the cuff to remain turned back on itself.
		•	Picked up the second glove by slipping sterile gloved fingers under its cuff and grasping the opposite side with the thumb.
		•	Pulled the glove on and turned back the cuff.
		•	Turned back the cuff of the first glove without contaminating it.
		•	Adjusted the gloves to a comfortable position.
		•	Inspected the gloves for tears.
		▷	Explained what should be done if a glove is torn.
			Removal of gloves:
		•	Grasped the outside of the right glove 1 to 2 inches from the top with the gloved left hand.
		•	Slowly pulled right glove off the hand.

421

Trial 1	Trial 2	Point Value	Performance Standards
		•	Pulled the right glove free and scrunched it into a ball with the gloved left hand.
		•	Placed the index and middle fingers of the right hand on the inside of left glove.
		•	Did not allow the clean hand to touch the outside of the glove.
		•	Pulled the glove off the left hand, enclosing the balled-up right glove.
		•	Discarded both gloves in an appropriate waste container.
		▷	Stated how to discard gloves if they are visibly contaminated with blood.
		•	Sanitized hands.
			Demonstrated the following affective behavior(s) during this procedure:
		Ⓐ	Recognized the implications for failure to comply with Centers for Disease Control and Prevention (CDC) regulations in health care settings.
		★	Completed the procedure within 5 minutes.
			Totals

Evaluation of Student Performance

EVALUATION CRITERIA			COMMENTS
Symbol	**Category**	**Point Value**	
★	Critical Step	16 points	
•	Essential Step	6 points	
Ⓐ	Affective Competency	6 points	
▷	Theory Question	2 points	

Score calculation: 100 points
− _____ points missed
_____ Score

Satisfactory score: 85 or above

CAAHEP Competencies Achieved

Psychomotor (Skills)

☑ III. 2. Select appropriate barrier/personal protective equipment (PPE).

Affective (Behavior)

☑ III. 1. Recognize the implications for failure to comply with Centers for Disease Control and Prevention (CDC) regulations in health care settings.

ABHES Competencies Achieved

☑ 4. f. Comply with federal, state and local health laws as they relate to health care settings.
☑ 8. a. Practice standard precautions and perform disinfection/sterilization techniques.

e **Procedure 10-2: Opening a Sterile Package**

Name: _____ Date: _____

Evaluated by: _____ Score: _____

Performance Objective

Outcome:	Open a sterile package.
Conditions:	Given a sterile package.
	Using a clean flat surface.
Standards:	Time: 5 minutes. Student completed procedure in _____ minutes.
	Accuracy: Satisfactory score on the Performance Evaluation Checklist.

Performance Evaluation Checklist

Trial 1	Trial 2	Point Value	Performance Standards
		•	Sanitized hands.
		•	Assembled the equipment.
		•	Checked the pack to make sure it is not wet, torn, or opened.
		•	Checked the autoclave tape on the pack.
		▷	Stated the purpose of the autoclave tape.
		•	Positioned the pack on the table so that the top flap of wrapper will open away from the body.
		•	Removed the fastener on the wrapped package and discarded it.
		•	Opened the first flap away from the body.
		•	Opened the left and right flaps without contaminating the contents.
		•	Opened the flap closest to the body.
		•	In all cases, touched only the outside of the wrapper.
		•	In all cases, did not reach over the sterile contents of the package.
		▷	Stated why the medical assistant should not reach over the contents of the package.
		•	Adjusted the sterile wrapper by the corners as needed.
		•	Checked the sterilization indicator on the inside of the pack.
		▷	Stated the reason for checking the sterilization indicator.
		★	Completed the procedure within 5 minutes.
			Totals

Evaluation of Student Performance

EVALUATION CRITERIA			COMMENTS
Symbol	**Category**	**Point Value**	
★	Critical Step	16 points	
•	Essential Step	6 points	
Ⓐ	Affective Competency	6 points	
▷	Theory Question	2 points	

Score calculation: 100 points
− _____ points missed
_____ Score

Satisfactory score: 85 or above

CAAHEP Competencies Achieved

Psychomotor (Skills)
☑ III. 6. Prepare a sterile field.
☑ III. 7. Perform within a sterile field.

ABHES Competencies Achieved

☑ 8. e. Perform specialty procedures including but not limited to minor surgery, cardiac, respiratory, OB-GYN, neurological, and gastroenterology.

EVALUATION OF COMPETENCY

Using Commercially Prepared Sterile Packages

Name: _____   Date: _____

Evaluated by: _____   Score: _____

Performance Objective

Outcome:	Add a sterile article to a sterile field from a peel-apart package by ejecting its contents onto the field.
Conditions:	Given the following: peel-apart package and a sterile field.
Standards:	Time: 3 minutes. Student completed procedure in _____ minutes.
	Accuracy: Satisfactory score on the Performance Evaluation Checklist.

Performance Evaluation Checklist

Trial 1	Trial 2	Point Value	Performance Standards
		•	Sanitized hands.
		•	Grasped the two unsterile flaps of the peel-pack between the thumbs.
		•	Pulled the package apart using a rolling-outward motion.
		▷	Stated what parts of the peel-pack must remain sterile.
		•	Stepped back slightly from the sterile field.
		▷	Explained the reason for stepping back.
		•	Gently ejected the contents of the peel-pack onto the center of the sterile field.
		★	Completed the procedure within 3 minutes.
			Totals

Evaluation of Student Performance

EVALUATION CRITERIA			COMMENTS
Symbol	**Category**	**Point Value**	
★	Critical Step	16 points	
•	Essential Step	6 points	
Ⓐ	Affective Competency	6 points	
▷	Theory Question	2 points	

Score calculation: 100 points
  − _____ points missed
     _____ Score

Satisfactory score: 85 or above

CAAHEP Competencies Achieved

Psychomotor (Skills)

☑ III. 7. Perform within a sterile field.

ABHES Competencies Achieved

☑ 8. e. Perform specialty procedures including but not limited to minor surgery, cardiac, respiratory, OB-GYN, neurological, and gastroenterology.

Procedure 10-3: Pouring a Sterile Solution

Name: _____   Date: _____

Evaluated by: _____   Score: _____

Performance Objective

Outcome:	Pour a sterile solution.
Conditions:	Given the following: sterile solution, sterile container, and a sterile towel.
Standards:	Time: 5 minutes. Student completed procedure in _____ minutes.
	Accuracy: Satisfactory score on the Performance Evaluation Checklist.

Performance Evaluation Checklist

Trial 1	Trial 2	Point Value	Performance Standards
		•	Checked the label of the solution.
		•	Checked the expiration date on the solution.
		▷	Explained why an outdated solution should not be used.
		•	Checked the solution label a second time.
		•	Palmed the label of the bottle.
		▷	Explained why the label should be palmed.
		•	Removed the cap and placed it on a flat surface with the open end up.
		▷	Stated why the cap should be placed with the open end up.
		•	Rinsed the lip of the bottle.
		▷	Explained why the lip of the bottle should be rinsed.
		•	Poured the proper amount of solution into a sterile container at a height of 6 inches.
		•	Did not allow the neck of the bottle to come in contact with the container.
		•	Did not allow any of the solution to splash onto the sterile field.
		▷	Explained why the sterile solution should not be allowed to splash onto the sterile field.
		•	Replaced the cap on the container without contaminating.
		•	Checked the label a third time.
		★	Completed the procedure within 5 minutes.
			Totals

Evaluation of Student Performance

EVALUATION CRITERIA			COMMENTS
Symbol	**Category**	**Point Value**	
★	Critical Step	16 points	
•	Essential Step	6 points	
Ⓐ	Affective Competency	6 points	
▷	Theory Question	2 points	

Score calculation: 100 points

      −   _____ points missed

           _____ Score

Satisfactory score: 85 or above

CAAHEP Competencies Achieved

Psychomotor (Skills)

☑ III. 7. Perform within a sterile field.

ABHES Competencies Achieved

☑ 8. e. Perform specialty procedures including but not limited to minor surgery, cardiac, respiratory, OB-GYN, neurological, and gastroenterology.

Procedure 10-4: Changing a Sterile Dressing

Name: _____ Date: _____

Evaluated by: _____ Score: _____

Performance Objective

Outcome:	Change a sterile dressing.
Conditions:	Given the following: Mayo stand, biohazard waste container, clean and disposable gloves, antiseptic swabs, sterile gloves, plastic waste bag, adhesive tape and scissors, sterile dressing, and thumb forceps.
Standards:	Time: 10 minutes. Student completed procedure in _____ minutes.
	Accuracy: Satisfactory score on the Performance Evaluation Checklist.

Performance Evaluation Checklist

Trial 1	Trial 2	Point Value	Performance Standards
		•	Washed hands with an antimicrobial soap.
		•	Assembled the equipment.
		•	Set up nonsterile items on a side table or counter.
		•	Positioned the plastic waste bag in a convenient location.
		•	Greeted the patient and introduced yourself.
		•	Identified the patient and explained the procedure.
		•	Instructed the patient not to move during the procedure.
		•	Adjusted the light.
		•	Applied clean gloves.
		•	Loosened the tape and carefully removed soiled dressing by pulling it upward.
		•	Did not touch the inside of the dressing next to the wound.
		▷	Explained why the inside of the dressing should not be touched.
		▷	Described what should be done if the dressing is stuck to the wound.
		•	Placed the soiled dressing in the waste bag without touching the outside of the bag.
		•	Inspected the wound.
		▷	Stated what type of inspection should be performed.
		•	Opened the antiseptic swabs and placed the pouch in a convenient location or held the pouch in your hand.
		•	Applied the antiseptic to the wound.
		•	Used a new swab for each motion.
		•	Discarded each contaminated swab in the waste bag after use.

429

Trial 1	Trial 2	Point Value	Performance Standards
		•	Removed gloves and discarded them without contaminating.
		•	Sanitized hands and prepared the sterile field.
		•	Instructed the patient not to talk, laugh, sneeze, or cough over the sterile field.
		•	Opened a sterile glove package and applied sterile gloves.
		•	Picked up a sterile dressing from the tray using sterile gloves or sterile forceps.
		•	Placed the sterile dressing over the wound by lightly dropping it in place.
		•	Did not move the dressing after dropping it in place.
		▷	Explained why the dressing should be dropped onto the wound and then not moved.
		•	Discarded the gloves (and forceps) in the waste bag.
		•	Applied hypoallergenic tape to hold the sterile dressing in place.
		•	Provided the patient with written wound care instructions.
		•	Instructed the patient in wound care.
		▷	Described the wound care that should be relayed to the patient.
		•	Asked the patient to sign the instruction sheet.
		•	Witnessed the patient's signature.
		•	Gave a signed copy to the patient.
		•	Filed the original in the patient's medical record.
		▷	Stated the purpose of filing the original in the patient's medical record.
		•	Returned the equipment.
		•	Disposed of the plastic bag in a biohazard waste container.
		•	Sanitized hands.
		•	Documented the procedure correctly.
			Demonstrated the following affective behavior(s) during this procedure:
		Ⓐ	Incorporated critical thinking skills when performing patient care.
		Ⓐ	Showed awareness of a patient's concerns related to the procedure being performed.
		Ⓐ	Explained to a patient the rationale for performance of a procedure.
		★	Completed the procedure within 10 minutes.
			Totals

CHART

Date	

Evaluation of Student Performance

EVALUATION CRITERIA			COMMENTS
Symbol	**Category**	**Point Value**	
★	Critical Step	16 points	
•	Essential Step	6 points	
Ⓐ	Affective Competency	6 points	
▷	Theory Question	2 points	

Score calculation: 100 points
− _____ points missed
_____ Score

Satisfactory score: 85 or above

CAAHEP Competencies Achieved

Psychomotor (Skills)

☑ I. 8. Instruct and prepare a patient for a procedure or a treatment.

☑ III. 6. Prepare a sterile field.

☑ III. 7. Perform within a sterile field.

☑ III. 8. Perform wound care.

☑ III. 9. Perform dressing change.

☑ III. 10. Demonstrate proper disposal of biohazardous material: (a) sharps (b) regulated wastes.

☑ V. 4. Coach patient regarding: (a) office policies (b) health maintenance (c) disease prevention (d) treatment plan.

☑ X. 3. Document patient care accurately in the medical record.

Affective (Behavior)

☑ I. 2. Incorporate critical thinking skills when performing patient care.

☑ I. 3. Show awareness of a patient's concerns related to the procedure being performed.

☑ V. 4. Explain to a patient the rationale for performance of a procedure.

ABHES Competencies Achieved

☑ 4. a. Follow documentation guidelines.

☑ 7. g. Display professionalism through written and verbal communications.

☑ 8. e. Perform specialty procedures including but not limited to minor surgery, cardiac, respiratory, OB-GYN, neurological, and gastroenterology.

☑ 8. h. Teach self-examination, disease management and health promotion.

☑ 9. c. Dispose of biohazardous materials.

Notes

e Procedure 10-5: Removing Sutures and Staples

Name: _____ Date: _____

Evaluated by: _____ Score: _____

Performance Objective

Outcome:	Apply and remove sterile gloves.
Conditions:	Given the following: Mayo stand, antiseptic swabs, clean and disposable gloves, sterile 4 × 4 gauze, surgical tape, biohazard waste container, suture removal kit, and staple removal kit.
Standards:	Time: 10 minutes. Student completed procedure in _____ minutes.
	Accuracy: Satisfactory score on the Performance Evaluation Checklist.

Performance Evaluation Checklist

Trial 1	Trial 2	Point Value	Performance Standards
		•	Washed hands with an antimicrobial soap.
		•	Assembled the equipment.
		•	Greeted the patient and introduced yourself.
		•	Identified the patient and explained the procedure.
		•	Positioned the patient as required.
		•	Adjusted the light.
		•	Checked to make sure the sutures (or staples) were intact.
		•	Checked to make sure the incision line was approximated and free from infection.
		▷	Explained what to do if the incision line is not approximated.
		•	Opened the suture or staple removal kit.
		•	Applied clean gloves.
		•	Cleaned the incision line with antiseptic swabs using a new swab for each motion.
		•	Allowed the skin to dry.
		•	Informed the patient that he or she would feel a pulling sensation as each suture (or staple) is removed.
		Removed sutures as follows:	
		•	Picked up the knot of suture with thumb forceps.
		•	Placed the curved tip of suture scissors under the suture.
		•	Cut suture below the knot on the side of the suture closest to the skin.
		•	Gently pulled the suture out of the skin, using a smooth, continuous motion.
		•	Did not allow any portion of the suture previously on the outside to be pulled through the tissue lying beneath the incision line.

433

Trial 1	Trial 2	Point Value	Performance Standards
		•	Placed the suture on the gauze.
		•	Repeated the above sequence until all sutures were removed.
			Removed staples as follows:
		•	Gently placed the jaws of the staple remover under the staple.
		•	Squeezed the staple handles until they were fully closed.
		•	Lifted the staple remover upward to remove the staple.
		•	Placed the staple on gauze.
		•	Continued until all the staples were removed.
		•	Counted the number of sutures or staples and checked the number with the medical record.
		•	Cleansed the site with an antiseptic swab.
		•	Applied adhesive skin closures if directed by the provider.
		•	Applied DSD, if directed to do so by the provider.
		•	Disposed of the sutures or staples and gauze in a biohazard waste container.
		•	Removed gloves and sanitized hands.
		•	Documented the procedure correctly.
			Demonstrated the following affective behavior(s) during this procedure:
		Ⓐ	Incorporated critical thinking skills when performing patient care.
		Ⓐ	Showed awareness of a patient's concerns related to the procedure being performed.
		Ⓐ	Demonstrated: (a) empathy (b) active listening (c) nonverbal communication.
		★	Completed the procedure within 10 minutes.
			Totals

CHART	
Date	

Evaluation of Student Performance

EVALUATION CRITERIA			COMMENTS
Symbol	**Category**	**Point Value**	
★	Critical Step	16 points	
•	Essential Step	6 points	
Ⓐ	Affective Competency	6 points	
▷	Theory Question	2 points	

Score calculation: 100 points

− _____ points missed

_____ Score

Satisfactory score: 85 or above

CAAHEP Competencies Achieved

Psychomotor (Skills)

☑ I. 8. Instruct and prepare a patient for a procedure or a treatment.

☑ III. 8. Perform wound care.

☑ III. 10. Demonstrate proper disposal of biohazardous material: (a) sharps (b) regulated wastes.

☑ V. 4. Coach patient regarding: (a) office policies (b) health maintenance (c) disease prevention (d) treatment plan.

☑ X. 3. Document patient care accurately in the medical record.

Affective (Behavior)

☑ I. 2. Incorporate critical thinking skills when performing patient care.

☑ I. 3. Show awareness of a patient's concerns related to the procedure being performed.

☑ V. 1. Demonstrate: (a) empathy (b) active listening (c) nonverbal communication.

ABHES Competencies Achieved

☑ 4. a. Follow documentation guidelines.

☑ 7. g. Display professionalism through written and verbal communications.

☑ 8. e. Perform specialty procedures including but not limited to minor surgery, cardiac, respiratory, OB-GYN, neurological, and gastroenterology.

☑ 8. h. Teach self-examination, disease management and health promotion.

☑ 9. c. Dispose of biohazardous materials.

Notes

EVALUATION OF COMPETENCY

Procedure 10-6: Applying and Removing Adhesive Skin Closures

Name: _____   Date: _____

Evaluated by: _____   Score: _____

Performance Objective

Outcome:	Apply and remove adhesive skin closures.
Conditions:	Given the following: clean and disposable gloves, sterile gloves, antiseptic solution, surgical scrub brush, antiseptic swabs, tincture of benzoin, sterile cotton-tipped applicator, adhesive skin closure strips, sterile 4 × 4 gauze pads, surgical tape, and a biohazard waste container.
Standards:	Time: 10 minutes. Student completed procedure in _____ minutes.
	Accuracy: Satisfactory score on the Performance Evaluation Checklist.

Performance Evaluation Checklist

Trial 1	Trial 2	Point Value	Performance Standards
			Application of adhesive skin closures:
		•	Washed hands with an antimicrobial soap.
		•	Assembled the equipment.
		•	Checked the expiration date on the adhesive skin closures.
		•	Greeted the patient and introduced yourself.
		•	Identified the patient and explained the procedure.
		•	Positioned the patient as required.
		•	Adjusted the light.
		•	Applied clean gloves.
		•	Inspected the wound for redness, swelling, and drainage.
		•	Scrubbed the wound with an antiseptic solution.
		•	Allowed the skin to dry or patted dry with gauze pads.
		•	Applied antiseptic, using a new swab for each motion.
		•	Allowed the skin to dry.
		▷	Explained why the skin must be completely dry.
		•	Applied tincture of benzoin without letting it touch the wound.
		▷	Stated the purpose of tincture of benzoin.
		•	Allowed the skin to dry.
		•	Removed gloves and washed hands.
		•	Opened the package of adhesive strips and laid them on a flat surface.

Trial 1	Trial 2	Point Value	Performance Standards
		•	Applied sterile gloves and tore the tab off the card of strips.
		•	Peeled a strip of tape off the card.
		•	Checked to make sure the skin surface was dry.
		•	Positioned the first strip over the center of the wound.
		•	Secured one end of the strip to the skin by pressing down firmly on the tape.
		•	Stretched the strip across the incision until the edges of the wound were approximated.
		•	Secured the strip to the skin on the other side of the wound.
		•	Applied the second strip on one side of the center strip at a $^1/_8$-inch interval.
		•	Applied a third strip at a $^1/_8$-inch interval on the other side of the center strip.
		•	Continued to apply the strips at $^1/_8$-inch intervals until the edges of the wound were approximated.
		▷	Explained why the strips should be spaced at $^1/_8$-inch intervals.
		•	Applied two closures approximately $^1/_2$ inch from the ends of the strips.
		▷	Stated the purpose of applying a strip along each edge.
		•	Applied a sterile dressing over the strips if indicated by the provider.
		•	Removed gloves and sanitized hands.
		•	Provided the patient with written wound care instructions.
		•	Explained the wound care instructions to the patient.
		•	Asked the patient to sign the instruction sheet and witnessed the patient's signature.
		•	Gave a signed copy to the patient and filed the original in the patient's medical record.
		•	Documented the procedure correctly.
			Removal of adhesive skin closures:
		•	Sanitized hands.
		•	Greeted patient and introduced yourself.
		•	Identified the patient and explained the procedure.
		•	Positioned the patient as required.
		•	Adjusted the light.
		•	Checked to make sure the incision line was approximated and free from infection.
		•	Positioned a 4 × 4 gauze pad in a convenient location.
		•	Applied clean gloves.
		•	Peeled off each half of the strip from the outside toward the wound margin.

Trial 1	Trial 2	Point Value	Performance Standards
		•	Stabilized the skin with one finger.
		•	Gently lifted the strip up and away from the wound and placed it on the gauze.
		•	Continued until all closures were removed.
		•	Cleansed the site with an antiseptic swab.
		•	Applied a sterile dressing if indicated by the provider.
		•	Disposed of the strips and gauze in a biohazard waste container.
		•	Removed gloves and sanitized hands.
		•	Documented the procedure correctly.
			Demonstrated the following affective behavior(s) during this procedure:
		Ⓐ	Incorporated critical thinking skills when performing patient care.
		Ⓐ	Showed awareness of a patient's concerns related to the procedure being performed.
		Ⓐ	Explained to a patient the rationale for performance of a procedure.
		★	Completed the procedure within 10 minutes.
			Totals

CHART

Date	

Evaluation of Student Performance

EVALUATION CRITERIA			COMMENTS
Symbol	**Category**	**Point Value**	
★	Critical Step	16 points	
•	Essential Step	6 points	
Ⓐ	Affective Competency	6 points	
▷	Theory Question	2 points	

Score calculation: 100 points
　　　　　　　　−_____ points missed
　　　　　　　　_____ Score

Satisfactory score: 85 or above

CAAHEP Competencies Achieved

Psychomotor (Skills)

☑ I. 8. Instruct and prepare a patient for a procedure or a treatment.

☑ III. 8. Perform wound care.

☑ V. 4. Coach patient regarding: (a) office policies (b) health maintenance (c) disease prevention (d) treatment plan.

☑ X. 3. Document patient care accurately in the medical record.

Affective (Behavior)

☑ I. 2. Incorporate critical thinking skills when performing patient care.

☑ I. 3. Show awareness of a patient's concerns related to the procedure being performed.

☑ V. 4. Explained to a patient the rationale for performance of a procedure.

ABHES Competencies Achieved

☑ 4. a. Follow documentation guidelines.

☑ 7. g. Display professionalism through written and verbal communications.

☑ 8. e. Perform specialty procedures including but not limited to minor surgery, cardiac, respiratory, OB-GYN, neurological, and gastroenterology.

☑ 8. h. Teach self-examination, disease management and health promotion.

☑ 9. c. Dispose of biohazardous materials.

Procedure 10-7: Assisting with Minor Office Surgery

Name: _____ Date: _____

Evaluated by: _____ Score: _____

Performance Objective

Outcome:	Apply and remove sterile gloves.
Conditions:	Given a Mayo stand, biohazard waste container, and the instruments and supplies required for a specific minor office surgery as designed by the instructor.
Standards:	Time: 15 minutes. Student completed procedure in _____ minutes.
	Accuracy: Satisfactory score on the Performance Evaluation Checklist.

Performance Evaluation Checklist

Trial 1	Trial 2	Point Value	Performance Standards
		•	Determined the type of minor office surgery to be performed.
		•	Prepared the examining room.
		•	Sanitized hands.
		•	Set up the articles required that are not sterile on a side table or counter.
		•	Labeled the specimen container (if included in the setup).
		•	Washed hands with an antimicrobial soap.
		•	Set up the minor office surgery tray on a clean, dry, flat surface, using the principles of surgical asepsis.
		Prepackaged sterile setup:	
		•	Selected the appropriate package from the supply shelf and placed it on a flat surface.
		•	Opened the setup using the inside of the wrapper as the sterile field.
		•	Checked the sterilization indicator on the inside of the pack.
		•	Added any additional articles required for the surgery and covered the tray setup with a sterile towel.
		Transferring articles to a sterile field:	
		•	Placed a sterile towel on a flat surface by two corner ends, making sure not to contaminate it.
		•	Transferred sterile articles to the field from wrapped or peel-apart packages.
		•	Applied a sterile glove.
		•	Arranged articles neatly on the sterile field with the sterile glove.
		•	Checked to make sure all articles were available on the sterile field.
		•	Covered the tray setup with a sterile towel without allowing arms to pass over the sterile field.

Trial 1	Trial 2	Point Value	Performance Standards
			Prepared the patient:
		•	Greeted the patient and introduced yourself.
		•	Identified the patient, explained the procedure, and reassured the patient.
		•	Asked the patient whether he or she needs to void before the surgery.
		•	Instructed the patient on clothing removal.
		•	Instructed the patient not to move during the procedure or to talk, laugh, sneeze, or cough over the sterile field.
		•	Positioned the patient as required for the type of surgery to be performed.
		•	Adjusted the light so that it was focused on the operative site.
			Prepared the patient's skin:
		•	Applied clean disposable gloves.
		•	Shaved the skin (if required).
		•	Cleansed the skin with an antiseptic solution.
		•	Rinsed and dried the area.
		•	Applied antiseptic using antiseptic swabs.
		•	Allowed the skin to dry.
		•	Removed gloves and sanitized hands.
		•	Checked to make sure that everything was ready and informed the provider.
			Assisted the provider:
		•	Uncovered the tray setup.
		•	Opened the outer glove wrapper for the provider.
		•	Held the vial while the provider withdrew the local anesthetic.
		•	Adjusted the light as required.
		•	Restrained the patient (e.g., a child).
		•	Relaxed and reassured the patient.
		•	Handed instruments and supplies to the provider. Sterile gloves are required.
		•	Kept the sterile field neat and orderly. Sterile gloves are required.
		•	Held a basin for the provider to deposit soiled instruments and supplies. Clean gloves are required.
		•	Retracted the tissue. Sterile gloves are required.
		•	Sponged blood from the operative site. Sterile gloves are required.
		•	Added instruments and supplies as necessary to the sterile field.

Trial 1	Trial 2	Point Value	Performance Standards
		•	Held the specimen container to accept the specimen. Clean gloves are required.
		•	Cut the ends of suture material after insertion by the provider. Sterile gloves are required.
			After surgery:
		•	Applied a sterile dressing to the surgical wound if ordered by the provider.
		•	Stayed with the patient as a safety precaution.
		•	Assisted and instructed the patient as required.
		•	Verified that the patient understood postoperative instructions.
		•	Provided the patient with verbal and written wound care instructions.
		▷	Stated the patient instructions that should be relayed for wound and suture care.
		•	Asked the patient to sign the instruction sheet and witnessed the patient's signature.
		•	Gave a signed copy to the patient and filed the original in the patient's medical record.
		•	Relayed information regarding the return visit.
		•	Assisted the patient off the table.
		•	Instructed the patient to get dressed.
		•	Prepared any specimens collected for transfer to the laboratory with a completed biopsy request.
		•	Documented correctly.
		•	Cleaned the examining room.
		•	Discarded disposable contaminated articles in a biohazard waste container.
		•	Sanitized and sterilized instruments.
			Demonstrated the following affective behavior(s) during this procedure:
		Ⓐ	Showed awareness of a patient's concerns related to the procedure being performed.
		Ⓐ	Demonstrated: (a) empathy (b) active listening (c) nonverbal communication.
		Ⓐ	Explained to a patient the rationale for performance of a procedure.
		★	Completed the procedure within 15 minutes.
			Totals

CHART	
Date	

Evaluation of Student Performance

<table>
<tr><th colspan="3">EVALUATION CRITERIA</th><th>COMMENTS</th></tr>
<tr><th>Symbol</th><th>Category</th><th>Point Value</th><td rowspan="9"></td></tr>
<tr><td>★</td><td>Critical Step</td><td>16 points</td></tr>
<tr><td>•</td><td>Essential Step</td><td>6 points</td></tr>
<tr><td>Ⓐ</td><td>Affective Competency</td><td>6 points</td></tr>
<tr><td>▷</td><td>Theory Question</td><td>2 points</td></tr>
<tr><td colspan="3">Score calculation: 100 points
    − _____ points missed
      _____ Score</td></tr>
<tr><td colspan="3">Satisfactory score: 85 or above</td></tr>
</table>

CAAHEP Competencies Achieved

Psychomotor (Skills)

☑ I. 8. Instruct and prepare a patient for a procedure or a treatment.

☑ III. 6. Prepare a sterile field.

☑ III. 7. Perform within a sterile field.

☑ III. 10. Demonstrate proper disposal of biohazardous material: (a) sharps (b) regulated wastes.

☑ V. 4. Coach patient regarding: (a) office policies (b) health maintenance (c) disease prevention (d) treatment plan.

☑ X. 3. Document patient care accurately in the medical record.

☑ X. 4. Apply the Patient's Bill of Rights as it relates to: (a) choice of treatment (b) consent for treatment (c) refusal of treatment.

Affective (Behavior)

☑ I. 3. Show awareness of a patient's concerns related to the procedure being performed.

☑ V. 1. Demonstrate: (a) empathy (b) active listening (c) nonverbal communication.

☑ V. 4. Explain to a patient the rationale for performance of a procedure.

ABHES Competencies Achieved

☑ 4. a. Follow documentation guidelines.

☑ 7.g. Display professionalism through written and verbal communications.

☑ 8. d. Assist provider with specialty examination including cardiac, respiratory, OB-GYN, neurological, and gastroenterology procedures.

☑ 8. e. Perform specialty procedures including but not limited to minor surgery, cardiac, respiratory, OB-GYN, neurological, and gastroenterology.

☑ 8. g. Recognize and respond to medical office emergencies.

☑ 8. h. Teach self-examination, disease management and health promotion.

☑ 8. j. Make adaptations for patients with special needs (psychological or physical limitations)

☑ 9. c. Dispose of biohazardous materials.

Procedure 10-A: Bandage Turns

Name: _____ Date: _____

Evaluated by: _____ Score: _____

Performance Objective

Outcome:	Apply the following bandage turns: circular, spiral, spiral-reverse, figure-eight, and recurrent.
Conditions:	Given the following: a roller bandage and an elastic bandage.
Standards:	Time: 15 minutes. Student completed procedure in _____ minutes.
	Accuracy: Satisfactory score on the Performance Evaluation Checklist.

Performance Evaluation Checklist

Trial 1	Trial 2	Point Value	Performance Standards
			Circular turn:
		•	Placed the end of a bandage on a slant.
		•	Encircled the body part while allowing the corner of the bandage to extend.
		•	Turned down the corner of the bandage.
		•	Made another circular turn around the body part.
		▷	Stated a use of the circular turn.
			Spiral turn:
		•	Anchored the bandage by using a circular turn.
		•	Encircled the body part while keeping the bandage at a slant.
		•	Carried each spiral turn upward at a slight angle.
		•	Overlapped each previous turn by one half to two thirds of the width of the bandage.
		▷	Stated a use of the spiral turn.
			Spiral-reverse turn:
		•	Anchored the bandage by using a circular turn.
		•	Encircled the body part while keeping the bandage at a slant.
		•	Reversed the spiral turn by using the thumb or index finger.
		•	Directed the bandage downward and folded it on itself.
		•	Kept the bandage parallel to the lower edge of the previous turn.
		•	Overlapped each previous turn by two thirds the width of the bandage.
		▷	Stated a use of the spiral-reverse turn.

Trial 1	Trial 2	Point Value	Performance Standards
			Figure-eight turn:
		•	Anchored the bandage by using a circular turn.
		•	Slanted bandage turns to alternately ascend and descend around the body part.
		•	Crossed the turns over one another in the middle to resemble a figure eight.
		•	Overlapped each previous turn by two thirds of the width of the bandage.
		▷	Stated a use of the figure-eight turn.
			Recurrent turn:
		•	Anchored the bandage by using two circular turns.
		•	Passed the bandage back and forth over the tip of the body part being bandaged.
		•	Overlapped each previous turn by two thirds of the width of the bandage.
		▷	Stated a use of the recurrent turn.
			Demonstrated the following affective behavior(s) during this procedure:
		Ⓐ	Incorporated critical thinking skills when performing patient care.
		★	Completed the procedure within 15 minutes.
			Totals

CHART	
Date	

Evaluation of Student Performance

EVALUATION CRITERIA			COMMENTS
Symbol	**Category**	**Point Value**	
★	Critical Step	16 points	
•	Essential Step	6 points	
Ⓐ	Affective Competency	6 points	
▷	Theory Question	2 points	

Score calculation: 100 points
    − _____ points missed
     _____ Score

Satisfactory score: 85 or above

CAAHEP Competencies Achieved

Psychomotor (Skills)

☑ I. 8. Instruct and prepare a patient for a procedure or a treatment.

☑ V. 4. Coach patient regarding: (a) office policies (b) health maintenance (c) disease prevention (d) treatment plan.

Affective (Behavior)

☑ I. 2. Incorporate critical thinking skills when performing patient care.

ABHES Competencies Achieved

☑ 87. h. Teach self-examination, disease management and health promotion.

☑ 8. j. Make adaptations for patients with special needs (psychological or physical limitations).

Notes

EVALUATION OF COMPETENCY

Procedure 10-8: Applying a Tubular Gauze Bandage

Name: _____   Date: _____

Evaluated by: _____   Score: _____

Performance Objective

Outcome:	Apply a tubular gauze bandage.
Conditions:	Given the following: applicator, tubular gauze, adhesive tape and bandage scissors.
Standards:	Time: 5 minutes. Student completed procedure in _____ minutes.
	Accuracy: Satisfactory score on the Performance Evaluation Checklist.

Performance Evaluation Checklist

Trial 1	Trial 2	Point Value	Performance Standards
		•	Sanitized hands.
		•	Greeted the patient and introduced yourself
		•	Identified the patient and explained the procedure.
		•	Assembled the equipment.
		•	Selected the proper applicator.
		•	Pulled a sufficient length of gauze from the dispensing box roll.
		•	Spread apart the open end of the gauze.
		•	Slid the gauze over one end of the applicator.
		•	Continued loading the applicator by gathering enough gauze on it to complete the bandage.
		•	Cut the roll of gauze near the opening of the box.
		•	Placed the applicator over the proximal end of the patient's finger.
		•	Moved the applicator from the proximal to the distal end of the patient's finger.
		•	Held the bandage in place with the fingers.
		▷	Explained why the bandage should be held in place.
		•	Pulled the applicator 1 to 2 inches past the end of the patient's finger.
		•	Rotated the applicator one full turn to anchor the bandage.
		•	Moved the applicator forward toward the proximal end of the patient's finger.
		•	Moved the applicator forward approximately 1 inch past the original starting point of the bandage.
		•	Rotated the applicator one full turn.
		▷	Stated the reason for rotating the applicator.

Chapter **10 Minor Office Surgery**

Trial 1	Trial 2	Point Value	Performance Standards
		•	Repeated the procedure for the number of layers desired.
		•	Finished the last layer at the proximal end.
		•	Cut the gauze from the applicator.
		•	Removed the applicator.
		•	Applied adhesive tape at the base of the patient's finger.
		•	Sanitized hands.
		•	Documented the procedure correctly.
			Demonstrated the following affective behavior(s) during this procedure:
		Ⓐ	Incorporated critical thinking skills when performing patient care.
		★	Completed the procedure within 5 minutes.
			Totals

CHART	
Date	

Evaluation of Student Performance

EVALUATION CRITERIA			COMMENTS
Symbol	**Category**	**Point Value**	
★	Critical Step	16 points	
•	Essential Step	6 points	
Ⓐ	Affective Competency	6 points	
▷	Theory Question	2 points	

Score calculation: 100 points
−_____ points missed
_____ Score

Satisfactory score: 85 or above

CAAHEP Competencies Achieved

Psychomotor (Skills)

☑ I. 8. Instruct and prepare a patient for a procedure or a treatment.

☑ V. 4. Coach patient regarding: (a) office policies (b) health maintenance (c) disease prevention (d) treatment plan.

Affective (Behavior)

☑ I. 2. Incorporate critical thinking skills when performing patient care.

ABHES Competencies Achieved

☑ 87. h. Teach self-examination, disease management and health promotion.

☑ 8. j. Make adaptations for patients with special needs (psychological or physical limitations).

11 Administration of Medication and Intravenous Therapy

√ After Completing	Date Due	Study Guide Pages	STUDY GUIDE ASSIGNMENTS (CTA = Critical Thinking Activity)	Possible Points	Points You Earned
		459	?≡ Pretest	10	
		460-461	Term Key Term Assessment		
		460	A. Definitions	26	
		461	B. Word Parts	13	
			(Add 1 point for each key term)		
		461-168	Evaluation of Learning questions	65	
		468-470	CTA A: Using the PDR	38	
		470-472	CTA B: Locating Information in a Drug Insert	15	
		472	CTA C: Drug Classifications (3 points each)	30	
			e Evolve Site: Road to Recovery: Drug Classifications		
		473	CTA D: Medication Record	20	
		474	CTA E: Seven Rights of Medication Administration	35	
			e Evolve Site: Script It! (Record points earned)		
		475	CTA F: Liquid Measurement	11	
		475	CTA G: Parts of a Needle and Syringe	11	
			e Evolve Site: Take the Plunge (Record points earned)		
		475-476	CTA H: Hypodermic Syringe Calibrations	10	
			e Evolve Site: Which Needle? (Record points earned)		
		476	CTA I: Insulin Syringe Calibrations	20	
		476-477	CTA J: Tuberculin Syringe Calibrations	14	

√ After Completing	Date Due	Study Guide Pages	STUDY GUIDE ASSIGNMENTS (CTA = Critical Thinking Activity)	Possible Points	Points You Earned
			Evolve Site: Draw It Up! (Record points earned)		
		477	CTA K: Syringe and Needle Labels (3 points each)	12	
		477	CTA L: Angle of Insertion for Injections	3	
		478-479	CTA M: Preparing and Administering Parenteral Medication	18	
		479	CTA N: Measuring Mantoux Test Reactions	5	
		480	CTA O: Interpreting Mantoux Skin Test Reactions	11	
		480-481	CTA P: Anaphylactic Reaction	20	
		482-497	CTA Q: Researching Drugs (5 points per drug researched)	325	
		498	CTA R: Crossword Puzzle	37	
			Evolve Site: Math Review (Record points earned)		
			Evolve Site: Apply Your Knowledge questions	10	
			Evolve Site: Video Evaluation	60	
		459	Posttest	10	
			ADDITIONAL ASSIGNMENTS		
			Total points		

√ After Completing	Date Due	Study Guide Pages	STUDY GUIDE ASSIGNMENTS Drug Dosage Calculation: Supplemental Education for Chapter 11	Possible Points	Points You Earned
		535	Unit 1: The Metric System A. Units of Measurement	10	
		535	Unit 1: The Metric System B. Metric Abbreviations	6	
		536	Unit 1: The Metric System C. Metric Notation	15	
		536	Unit 2: The Household System A. Units of Measurements	4	
		536-537	Unit 3: Medication Orders A. Medical Abbreviations	25	
		537-538	Unit 3: Medication Orders B. Interpreting Medication Orders (3 points each)	30	
		539	Unit 4: Converting Units of Measurement A. Using Conversion Tables (2 points each)	40	
		540-541	Unit 4: Converting Units of Measurement B. Converting Units Within the Metric System (2 points each)	40	
		542-543	Unit 4: Converting Units of Measurement C. Converting Units Within the Household System (2 points each)	20	
		544-546	Unit 5: Ratio and Proportion A. Ratio and Proportion Guidelines (6 points each)	48	
		546-547	Unit 5: Ratio and Proportion B. Converting Units Using Ratio and Proportion (2 points each)	20	
		547-553	Unit 6: Determining Drug Dosage A. Oral Administration (2 points each)	30	
		553-556	Unit 6: Determining Drug Dosage B. Parenteral Administration (2 points each)	20	

Chapter **11 Administration of Medication and Intravenous Therapy**

√ After Completing	Date Due	Study Guide Pages	STUDY GUIDE ASSIGNMENTS Drug Dosage Calculation: Supplemental Education for Chapter 11	Possible Points	Points You Earned
			ADDITIONAL ASSIGNMENTS		
			Total points		

√ When Assigned by Your Instructor	Study Guide Pages	Practices Required	LABORATORY ASSIGNMENTS (Procedure Number and Name)	Score*
	499	5	**Practice for Competency** 11-1: Administering Oral Medication Textbook reference: pp. 412-413	
	501-507		**Evaluation of Competency** 11-1: Administering Oral Medication	*
	499	Vial: 5 Ampule: 5	**Practice for Competency** 11-2: Preparing an Injection Textbook reference: pp. 423-426	
	509-511		**Evaluation of Competency** 11-2: Preparing an Injection	*
	499	3	**Practice for Competency** 11-3: Reconstituting Powdered Drugs Textbook reference: p. 427	
	513-514		**Evaluation of Competency** 11-3: Reconstituting Powdered Drugs	*
	499	5	**Practice for Competency** 11-4: Administering a Subcutaneous Injection Textbook reference: pp. 428-429	
	515-517		**Evaluation of Competency** 11-4: Administering a Subcutaneous Injection	*
	501	5	**Practice for Competency** 11-A: Locating Intramuscular Injection Sites Textbook reference: pp. 420-421	
	519-521		**Evaluation of Competency** 11-A: Locating Intramuscular Injection Sites	*
	501	5	**Practice for Competency** 11-5: Administering an Intramuscular Injection Textbook reference: pp. 430-432	
	523-525		**Evaluation of Competency** 11-5: Administering an Intramuscular Injection	*
	501	5	**Practice for Competency** 11-6: Z-Track Intramuscular Injection Technique Textbook reference: p. 432-433	
	527-529		**Evaluation of Competency** 11-6: Z-Track Intramuscular Injection Technique	*

Chapter **11 Administration of Medication and Intravenous Therapy**

	501	5	*e* **Practice for Competency** 11-7: Administering an Intradermal Injection Textbook reference: pp. 446-449	
	531-534		**Evaluation of Competency** 11-7: Administering an Intradermal Injection	*
			ADDITIONAL ASSIGNMENTS	

Name: _____ Date: _____

True or False

_____T_____ 1. A drug is a chemical that is used for treatment, prevention, or diagnosis of disease.

_____T_____ 2. The generic name of a drug is assigned by the pharmaceutical manufacturer that develops the drug.

_____T_____ 3. The Rx symbol comes from the Latin word recipe and means "take."

_____T_____ 4. An anaphylactic reaction can be life threatening.

_____F_____ 5. The dorsogluteal site is the most common site for administering injections in infants.

_____F_____ 6. A subcutaneous injection is given into muscle tissue.

_____T_____ 7. The purpose of aspirating when administering an injection is to make sure the needle is not in a blood vessel.

_____F_____ 8. The Mantoux tuberculin skin test is administered through a subcutaneous injection.

_____T_____ 9. The peripheral veins of the arm and hand are used most often for administering IV therapy.

_____T_____ 10. Chemotherapy is the use of chemicals to treat disease.

True or False

_____F_____ 1. OSHA is responsible for determining whether drugs are safe before release for human use.

_____T_____ 2. An enteric-coated tablet does not dissolve until it reaches the intestines.

_____F_____ 3. The apothecary system is most often used to administer medication in the medical office.

_____F_____ 4. The parenteral route of administering medications is used when the patient is allergic to the oral form of the drug.

_____T_____ 5. Hypodermic syringes are calibrated in milliliters.

_____F_____ 6. The maximum amount of medication that can be administered through the subcutaneous route is 2 mL.

_____T_____ 7. A patient with latent tuberculosis infection has a negative reaction to a TB test.

_____F_____ 8. A tuberculin skin test result should be read 15 to 20 minutes after administration.

_____T_____ 9. The administration of fluids, medications, or nutrients through the IV route is known as an infusion.

_____F_____ 10. The administration of blood through the IV route is known as an IV push.

A. Definitions

Directions: Match each key term with its definition.

_____ 1. Adverse reaction

_____ 2. Allergen

_____ 3. Allergy

_____ 4. Ampule

_____ 5. Anaphylactic reaction

_____ 6. Chemotherapy

_____ 7. Controlled drug

_____ 8. Dose

_____ 9. Drug

_____ 10. Gauge

_____ 11. Induration

_____ 12. Infusion

_____ 13. Inhalation administration

_____ 14. Intradermal injection

_____ 15. Intramuscular injection

_____ 16. Intravenous therapy

_____ 17. Oral administration

_____ 18. Parenteral

_____ 19. Pharmacology

_____ 20. Prescription

_____ 21. Subcutaneous injection

_____ 22. Sublingual administration

_____ 23. Topical administration

_____ 24. Transfusion

_____ 25. Vial

_____ 26. Wheal

A. Application of a drug to a particular spot, usually for a local action
B. Introduction of medication into the dermal layer of the skin
C. A small, sealed glass container that holds a single dose of medication
D. A provider's order authorizing the dispensing of a drug by a pharmacist
E. An unintended and undesirable effect produced by a drug
F. An abnormal hypersensitivity of the body to substances that are ordinarily harmless
G. The administration of a liquid agent directly into a patient's vein, where it is distributed throughout the body by way of the circulatory system
H. A tense, pale raised area of the skin
I. Introduction of medication beneath the skin, into the subcutaneous or fatty layer of the body
J. An abnormally raised hardened area of the skin with clearly defined margins
K. A closed glass container with a rubber stopper that holds medication
L. The administration of medication by way of air or other vapor being drawn into the lungs
M. A serious allergic reaction that requires immediate treatment
N. Administration of medication by mouth
O. A drug that has restrictions placed on it by the federal government because of its potential for abuse
P. Introduction of medication into the muscular layer of the body
Q. Administration of medication by placing it under the tongue
R. The quantity of a drug to be administered at one time
S. A substance that is capable of causing an allergic reaction
T. A chemical used for the treatment, prevention, or diagnosis of disease
U. The diameter of the lumen of a needle used to administer medication
V. Administration of medication by injection
W. The study of drugs
X. The use of chemicals to treat disease; most often refers to the treatment of cancer using antineoplastic medications
Y. The administration of fluids, medications, or nutrients into a vein
Z. The administration of whole blood or blood products through the intravenous route

B. Word Parts

Directions: Indicate the meaning of each word part in the space provided. List as many medical terms as possible that incorporate the word part in the space provided.

Word Part	Meaning of Word Part	Medical Terms That Incorporate Word Part
1. chem/o		
2. -therapy		
3. intra-		
4. derm/o		
5. muscul/o		
6. -ar		
7. ven/o		
8. -ous		
9. pharmac/o		
10. sub-		
11. cutane/o		
12. lingu/o		
13. trans-		

EVALUATION OF LEARNING

Directions: Fill in each blank with the correct answer.

Administration of Medication

1. What is the difference between administering, prescribing, and dispensing medication at the medical office?

_____

_____

_____

_____

2. What is the difference between the generic name and the brand name of a drug?

_____

_____

_____

_____

3. What is a liniment?

_____

_____

_____

4. What is a spray?

_____

_____

5. What is a syrup?

_____

_____

6. What is a tablet?

_____

7. What is the purpose of scoring a tablet?

_____

8. List two drugs that come in the form of chewable tablets.

_____

9. List two reasons for enterically coating a tablet.

_____

_____

10. What is a capsule?

_____

11. Why must a suppository have a cylindrical or conical shape?

_____

_____

12. What is a transdermal patch?

_____

_____

13. Why is the metric system used most often to administer medication?

_____

_____

14. Define the term volume.

_____

15. Describe the use of the household system of measurement.

_____

_____

16. When is conversion required?

_____

_____

17. What is a controlled drug?

_____

18. In what forms can a prescription be authorized?

_____

_____

_____

19. What requirements must be followed when issuing a prescription for a schedule II drug?

_____

_____

_____

20. List five brand names of schedule II analgesics.

_____

_____

21. What requirements must be followed when issuing a prescription for a schedule III drug?

_____

_____

_____

22. What is a schedule IV drug?

_____

_____

23. List two brand names of schedule IV analgesics.

_____

_____

24. List three brand names of schedule IV antianxiety agents.

_____

_____

25. What is included in each of the following parts of a prescription?

    a. Superscription: _____

    b. Inscription: _____

    c. Subscription: _____

    d. Signatura: _____

26. Why is it important for the patient's age to be indicated on a prescription?

    _____

    _____

27. What functions can be performed by an EMR prescription program?

    _____

    _____

    _____

28. What types of medications should be documented on a medication record form?

    _____

29. List and describe three factors that affect the action of drugs in the body.

    _____

    _____

    _____

30. What are the symptoms and treatment of an anaphylactic reaction?

    _____

    _____

31. What are the advantages and disadvantages of using the parenteral route of administration?

    _____

    _____

    _____

    _____

32. How do safety-engineered syringes reduce the risk of a needlestick injury?

    _____

33. What is the purpose of using a filter needle when withdrawing medication from an ampule?

    _____

34. What sites are used most frequently to administer a subcutaneous injection?

    _____

    _____

35. List three medications commonly administered through a subcutaneous injection.

_____

_____

_____

36. Why is medication absorbed faster through the intramuscular route than through the subcutaneous route?

_____

_____

37. List the four intramuscular (IM) injection sites, and explain why these sites must be used to administer an IM injection.

_____

_____

_____

_____

_____

38. What types of medications are given using the Z-track technique?

_____

_____

39. What sites are used most frequently to administer an intradermal injection?

_____

40. What is the most frequent use of an intradermal injection?

_____

41. What are the symptoms of active pulmonary tuberculosis?

_____

42. What is latent tuberculosis infection?

_____

43. What are examples of categories of individuals who should have a tuberculin test?

_____

_____

44. Why might a person who was recently infected with tuberculosis have a negative tuberculin skin test result?

_____

_____

Chapter **11 Administration of Medication and Intravenous Therapy**

45. What is induration, and what causes it?

_____

_____

46. What procedures are performed if a patient has a positive reaction to a tuberculin skin test?

_____

_____

47. Who should have a two-step tuberculin skin test?

_____

_____

48. What does it mean if the first test of a two-step tuberculin skin test is negative and the second test is positive? What does it mean if both tests are negative?

_____

_____

_____

49. What is the name of the blood test for tuberculosis?

_____

50. What are 10 examples of common allergens?

_____

_____

_____

_____

51. What is the general treatment for allergies?

_____

52. What is the purpose of patch testing?

_____

_____

53. How long does it take for a reaction to occur with a skin-prick test?

_____

54. Explain what is meant by each of the following intradermal skin test reactions.

a. ±1 _____

b. +2 _____

c. +3 _____

55. What are the advantages of in vitro blood testing over direct skin testing?

_____

_____

_____

Intravenous Therapy

1. What is intravenous therapy?

_____

2. Which veins are most often used for IV therapy?

_____

3. What types of liquid agents are administered through IV therapy?

_____

4. List examples of outpatient sites in which IV therapy may be administered.

_____

_____

5. List five reasons for administering IV therapy in an outpatient setting.

_____

_____

_____

6. What are the advantages of outpatient IV therapy?

_____

_____

7. What requirements must be met before an entry-level medical assistant (MA) can perform IV therapy at a medical office?

_____

_____

8. What must be determined by the provider before prescribing IV therapy?

_____

_____

9. What are the responsibilities of the provider in prescribing IV therapy?

_____

_____

Chapter **11** **Administration of Medication and Intravenous Therapy**

10. What instructions should the MA relay to a patient scheduled for outpatient IV therapy?

_____

_____

CRITICAL THINKING ACTIVITIES

A. Using the PDR

This activity assists you in learning how to use the *Physicians' Desk Reference* (PDR). Refer to Figure 11-1 in your textbook to answer the following questions.

Manufacturer's Index

1. What information is included in the Manufacturer's Index?

_____

_____

2. What company manufactures the drugs listed in the Manufacturer's Index?

_____

3. What number would you call if you had an emergency on the weekend regarding one of these drugs?

_____

4. What page would you turn to in the PDR for product information on Nitrostat tablets?

_____

5. Is a photograph included in the PDR for Accupril tablets?

_____

6. What page would you turn to in the PDR to find a color photograph of Nardil tablets?

_____

Brand and Generic Name Index

1. What information is included in the Brand and Generic Name Index?

_____

2. To what page in the current PDR edition would you turn to find product information on Lipitor tablets manufactured by Parke-Davis?

_____

3. What is the generic name of Prinivil tablets?

_____

4. What company manufactures Prinivil tablets?

_____

5. What page would you turn to in the PDR to find product information on Prinivil tablets?

_____

6. What page would you turn to in the PDR to find product identification information on Prinivil tablets?

_____

7. Who manufactures lisinopril tablets?

_____

8. Does the PDR contain full product information on lisinopril tablets?

_____

Product Category Index

1. What information is included in the Product Category Index?

_____

2. What is the drug category for Flexeril tablets?

_____

3. Who manufactures Soma tablets?

_____

4. What page would you turn to in the current PDR edition to find product information on Skelaxin tablets?

_____

5. Who manufactures Valium tablets?

_____

Product Identification Guide

1. What is included in the Product Identification Guide?

_____

_____

2. How can this section assist the user?

_____

_____

Product Information

Under which heading would you look in this section to find information on the following subjects?

1. Conditions the drug is approved by the FDA to treat

_____

2. Information to relay to the patient to ensure safe and effective use of the drug

_____

3. Route of administration

_____

4. Symptoms associated with an overdose of the drug

_____

5. Diseased states or situations that require special consideration when the drug is being taken

_____

6. Generic name of the drug

_____

7. How the drug functions in the body to produce its therapeutic effect

_____

8. Situations in which the drug should not be used

_____

9. Recommended adult dosage and duration of treatment

_____

10. How to pronounce the brand name of the drug

_____

11. Handling and storage conditions

_____

12. Serious adverse reactions that may occur with the drug

_____

13. The dosage forms in which the drug is available

_____

14. Unintended and undesirable effects that may occur with the use of the drug

_____

15. Modification of dosage needed for children

_____

16. Laboratory tests that may be affected when taking the drug

_____

17. Interactions of the drug that may occur with other drugs

_____

B. Locating Information in a Drug Insert

Obtain a drug insert for a prescription drug, and answer the following questions:

1. What is the brand name of the drug?

_____

470

2. What is the generic name of the drug?

_____

3. What is the drug category of this drug?

_____

4. What are the dosage forms for this drug?

_____

5. What is the route of administration of this drug?

_____

6. What are the indications and usage for this drug?

_____

_____

_____

7. What are the contraindications for this drug?

_____

_____

_____

8. List the warnings for this drug.

_____

_____

_____

9. What are the general precautions for this drug?

_____

_____

_____

10. What information should be relayed to patients regarding this drug?

_____

_____

_____

11. What laboratory tests may be affected when taking this drug?

_____

12. What are the adverse reactions for this drug?

_____

_____

_____

13. What are the symptoms associated with an overdose of this drug?

_____

14. What is the dosage and administration for this medication?

_____

_____

15. How should this drug be stored?

_____

_____

C. Drug Classifications

Inspect the package labels of 10 drugs (or use other means) to assess the classification of each drug based on preparation and action. List the name of each drug along with its appropriate category in the spaces provided. Compare results. Example: drug: Tylenol elixir; classification based on preparation: elixir; classification based on action: analgesic, antipyretic.

	Classification Based On	
Drug	Preparation	Action
1. _____	_____	_____
2. _____	_____	_____
3. _____	_____	_____
4. _____	_____	_____
5. _____	_____	_____
6. _____	_____	_____
7. _____	_____	_____
8. _____	_____	_____
9. _____	_____	_____
10. _____	_____	_____

D. Medication Record

Complete the following medication record form using yourself as the patient. Make sure to include all prescription medications and OTC medications, including vitamin supplements and herbal products. Use Figure 11-5 in your textbook as a guide in completing this form.

MEDICATION RECORD

Patient _____

Birth date _____

ALLERGY

DATE	MEDICATION AND DOSAGE	FREQUENCY	RX	OTC	REFILLS			STOP

E. Seven Rights of Medication Administration

You are the office manager at a large clinic. Six new MAs were just hired. Your provider asks you to design an illustrated poster portraying the seven rights of medication administration to remind the new employees of the importance of following these guidelines. Use the diagram below to design your poster.

Follow the Seven Rights	
Right Drug	Right Dose
Right Time	Right Patient
Right Route	Right Technique
Right Documentation	

F. Liquid Measurement

Obtain a medicine cup that is graduated into the metric (milliliters), apothecary (drams and ounces), and household (teaspoons and tablespoons) systems. Complete the following:

1. What is its capacity?

_____ ounces

_____ milliliters

_____ tablespoons

_____ drams

2. Practice pouring oral liquid medication by pouring the following amounts of water into the medicine cup. Place a check mark by each amount after it has been properly poured.

20 mL _____

4 drams _____

1 ounce _____

10 mL _____

½ ounce _____

1 tablespoon _____

2 drams _____

G. Parts of a Needle and Syringe

Obtain a needle and syringe. Locate the following parts of each and explain their function.

Needle   **Function**

1. Hub _____

2. Shaft _____

3. Lumen _____

4. Point _____

5. Bevel _____

6. What is the gauge of the needle? _____

7. What is the length of the needle? _____

Syringe   **Function**

8. Barrel _____

9. Flange _____

10. Plunger _____

11. What is the capacity of the syringe? _____

H. Hypodermic Syringe Calibrations

1. Obtain a 3-mL syringe that is divided into tenths of a milliliter. Locate the following calibrations on the syringe. Place a check mark in the blank next to each calibration after it has been correctly located.

Calibration (mL)

0.5 mL _____

1.0 mL _____

1.2 mL _____

2.5 mL _____

2.7 mL _____

475

2. Locate each calibration (listed in the previous question) on the illustration of the hypodermic syringe by placing an arrow on the correct calibration line and labeling it with the calibration.

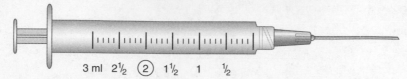

3 ml 2½ ② 1½ 1 ½

I. Insulin Syringe Calibrations

1. Obtain a U-100 insulin syringe. Locate the following calibrations (units) on the syringe, and place a check mark in the blank next to each calibration after it has been correctly located.

Calibration (units)

10 _____

16 _____

20 _____

44 _____

60 _____

68 _____

70 _____

86 _____

90 _____

100 _____

2. Locate each calibration (listed in the previous question) on the illustration of the insulin syringe by placing an arrow on the correct calibration line and labeling it with the calibration.

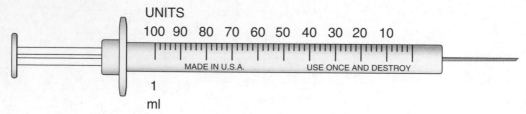

UNITS
100 90 80 70 60 50 40 30 20 10
MADE IN U.S.A. USE ONCE AND DESTROY
1
ml

J. Tuberculin Syringe Calibrations

1. Obtain a 1-mL tuberculin syringe that is divided into tenths and hundredths of a milliliter. Locate the following calibrations on the syringe. Place a check mark in the blank next to each calibration after it has been correctly located.

Calibration (mL)

0.05 mL _____

0.10 mL _____

0.15 mL _____

0.34 mL _____

0.52 mL _____

0.75 mL _____

0.92 mL _____

2. Locate each calibration (listed in the previous question) on the illustration of the tuberculin syringe by placing an arrow on the correct calibration line and labeling it with the calibration.

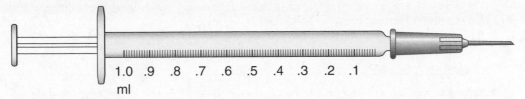

1.0 .9 .8 .7 .6 .5 .4 .3 .2 .1
ml

K. Syringe and Needle Labels

Refer to Figure 11-8 in your textbook, and indicate the following information for each syringe and needle: the syringe capacity and the gauge and length of the needle.

a. _____

b. _____

c. _____

d. _____

L. Angle of Insertion for Injections

In the diagram that follows, draw three lines indicating the angle of insertion into the correct body tissue for an intradermal, a subcutaneous, and an intramuscular injection. Label the lines.

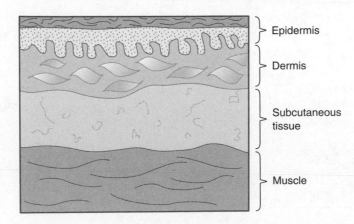

Epidermis

Dermis

Subcutaneous tissue

Muscle

M. Preparing and Administering Parenteral Medication

For each of the following situations involving the preparation and administration of medication, write **C** if the technique is correct and **I** if it is incorrect. If the technique is correct, state the principle underlying the technique. If the technique is incorrect, explain what might happen if it were performed.

_____ 1. The expiration date of the medication is checked before administering the medication.

_____

_____ 2. The MA is unfamiliar with the drug to be administered, so he or she looks it up in a drug reference.

_____

_____ 3. The MA compares the medication label with the provider's instructions three times: as it is taken from the shelf, before preparing the medication, and after preparing the medication.

_____

_____ 4. The rubber stopper of the multidose vial is cleansed with an antiseptic wipe before withdrawing the medication.

_____

_____ 5. Air is not injected into the multidose vial before withdrawing the medication.

_____

_____ 6. Air bubbles are present in the medication in the syringe that has been withdrawn from an ampule.

_____

_____ 7. The injection sites are not rotated when repeated injections are given.

_____

_____ 8. The antiseptic is not allowed to dry before administering an injection.

_____

_____ 9. The skin is stretched taut before an intramuscular injection is given.

_____

_____10. The needle is inserted slowly and steadily for an IM injection.

_____

_____11. An IM injection is given in the deltoid site to a patient who has a tight sleeve.

_____

_____12. An IM injection is given into the dorsogluteal site when the site is not fully exposed.

_____

_____13. The MA does not aspirate when giving an intramuscular injection.

_____

_____14. The medication is injected quickly for an IM injection.

_____

_____15. The needle is withdrawn at the same angle as for insertion.

_____

_____16. The intradermal needle is inserted with the bevel facing downward.

_____

_____17. The MA does not aspirate when giving an intradermal injection.

_____

_____18. Pressure is applied to the injection site after an intradermal injection is given.

_____

N. Measuring Mantoux Test Reactions

Measure the diameter of the following circles, which represent induration from a Mantoux tuberculin skin test. A millimeter ruler is provided below. Cut it out and use it to measure the tuberculin reactions. Document results in the chart provided.

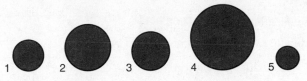

1   2   3   4   5

TB Skin Testing
(mm ruler)
0   10   20

CHART	
Date	

O. Interpreting Mantoux Skin Test Reactions

Tuberculin skin test reactions are listed for various individuals. Using Table 11-7 in your textbook as a reference, determine if the individual's test results are positive or negative, and indicate your answer in the space provided.

_____ a. 2 mm of induration; an individual who is caring for a parent with active TB

_____ b. 7 mm of induration; a student attending college

_____ c. 12 mm of induration; an individual who is 12% below ideal body weight

_____ d. 8 mm of induration; an HIV-infected individual

_____ e. Erythema that is 6 mm wide (no induration); an individual with rheumatoid arthritis on Enbrel

_____ f. 16 mm of induration; a dietitian working in a nursing home

_____ g. 12 mm of induration; an individual who recently traveled to Canada

_____ h. 5 mm of induration; a child living with a parent who has active TB

_____ i. 6 mm of induration; an individual with diabetes mellitus

_____ j. 11 mm of induration; a recent immigrant from Africa

_____ k. 9 mm of induration; an individual working in a home and garden center

P. Anaphylactic Reaction

Create a profile of an individual who is experiencing an anaphylactic reaction following these guidelines:

1. Using a blank piece of paper and colored pencils, crayons, or markers, draw a figure of an individual exhibiting the symptoms of an anaphylactic reaction. Be as creative as possible.

2. Do not use any text on your drawing other than to label items you have drawn in your picture. (A picture is worth a thousand words!)

3. Try to include as many of the symptoms of an anaphylactic reaction as possible.

4. In the classroom, find a partner, and trade drawings. Identify the symptoms in your partner's drawing. With your partner, discuss what causes an anaphylactic reaction and how to prevent it. Also discuss the method of treatment for an anaphylactic reaction.

Chapter **11** **Administration of Medication and Intravenous Therapy**

Q. Researching Drugs

Obtain a drug reference book, and look up the following information for each of the drugs listed on the Pharmacology Drug Sheets: generic name and drug classification, indications, and patient teaching. Document this information in the appropriate space on the Pharmacology Drug Sheets.

Pharmacology Drug Sheet

Name: _____

Generic Name and Drug Classification	Indications	Patient Teaching
Abilify		
Accupril		
Adderall		
Adrenalin		

Pharmacology Drug Sheet

Name: _____

Advair Diskus		
Ambien		
Amoxil		
Aricept		

Chapter **11** **Administration of Medication and Intravenous Therapy**

Pharmacology Drug Sheet

Name: _____

Ativan		
Bentyl		
Cardizem		
Catapres		

Pharmacology Drug Sheet

Name: _____

Celebrex		
Cipro		
Coumadin		
Cozaar		

Pharmacology Drug Sheet

Name: _____

Crestor		
Cymbalta		
Depo-Medrol		
Depo-Provera		

Chapter **11** **Administration of Medication and Intravenous Therapy**

Pharmacology Drug Sheet

Name: _____

Detrol		
Diflucan		
Dilantin		
Flagyl		

Chapter **11** **Administration of Medication and Intravenous Therapy**

Pharmacology Drug Sheet

Name: _____

Flexeril		
Flonase		
Fosamax		
Glucotrol XL		

Pharmacology Drug Sheet

Name: _____

Humulin		
Imitrex		
InFeD		
Keflex		

Pharmacology Drug Sheet

Name: _____

Lamisil		
Lanoxin		
Lasix		
Lipitor		

Pharmacology Drug Sheet

Name: _____

Loestrin Fe		
Lomotil		
Lyrica		
Macrobid		

Pharmacology Drug Sheet

Name: _____

Mexate		
Nitro-Bid		
Norvasc		
Percocet		

Pharmacology Drug Sheet

Name: _____

Phenergan		
Plavix		
Premarin		
Prevacid		

Prinivil		
Prozac		
Requip		
Rocephin		

Pharmacology Drug Sheet

Name: _____

Singulair		
Synthroid		
Tessalon		
Toprol XL		

Pharmacology Drug Sheet

Name: _____

Valium		
Valtrex		
Viagra		
Vicodin		

Pharmacology Drug Sheet

Name: _____

Xanax		
Zithromax		
Zyban		
Zyloprim		
Zyrtec		

Chapter **11** **Administration of Medication and Intravenous Therapy**

R. Crossword Puzzle: Administration of Medication

Directions: Complete the crossword puzzle using the clues provided.

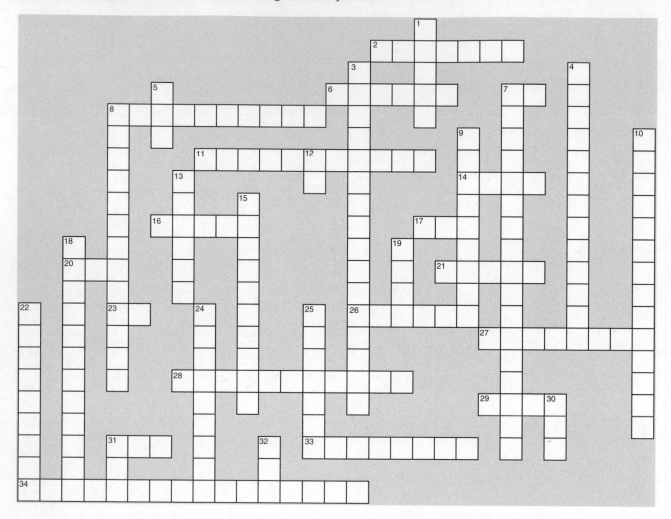

Across

- **2** Discovered penicillin
- **6** Most aggressive Hymenoptera
- **7** 1 mL = 1 _____
- **8** Present with a + Mantoux
- **11** Used to treat anaphylactic reaction
- **14** Metric weight unit
- **16** Ranges between 18 and 27
- **17** Aspirin
- **20** Available w/o a Rx
- **21** Needle opening
- **23** Before meals
- **26** Sym: wheezing and dyspnea
- **27** Allergy to molds and pollen
- **28** Conditions a drug is approved to treat
- **29** Immediately!
- **31** Tuberculin is made of this
- **33** Causes house dust allergy
- **34** Runny and inflamed allergic nose

Down

- **1** Slant of the needle
- **3** Do not use this drug!
- **4** Drug to d/c before allergy testing
- **5** Approves drugs
- **7** Symptoms include itching, erythema, vesiculation
- **8** Abnormal or peculiar reaction
- **9** Medication label info
- **10** Calibrated in units
- **12** By mouth
- **13** Prevents syringe from rolling
- **15** This drug may cause an allergic reaction
- **18** Do not use this IM site for children
- **19** Blood test for allergies
- **22** Hives
- **24** Rx requirement for controlled drug
- **25** Max of 1 mL at this site
- **30** Three times per day
- **31** Drug reference (ex)
- **32** As needed

Prerequisite. Complete the Drug Dosage Calculation: Supplemental Education for Chapter 11 (pp. 535-556 in this manual).

Procedure 11-1: Oral Medication

Administer oral solid and liquid medication, and document the procedure in the chart provided.

Procedure 11-2: Preparing the Injection

Prepare an injection from an ampule and a vial.

Procedure 11-3: Reconstituting Powdered Drugs

Reconstitute a powdered drug for parenteral administration.

Procedure 11-4: Subcutaneous Injection

Administer an allergy injection, and document the procedure in the allergy injection form provided on the following page.

ALLERGY INJECTION (IMMUNOTHERAPY) RECORD

Name _____

Date of Birth _____

ADMINISTRATION GUIDELINES:

Allergy injections are administered weekly. The allergy extract should be increased by 0.05 mL per week until symptomatic improvement is achieved or until a maximum dosage of 0.5 mL is reached.

The patient should remain in the office for 20 minutes following the injection, and the reaction should be noted. If no reaction occurs, the abbreviation NR should be recorded. If a reaction occurs, it should be recorded in mm.

Do not administer the allergy injection in the following situations:
  a. The patient is ill with a temperature that is greater than 101° F
  b. The patient is having an acute asthma attack
  c. The patient is experiencing shortness of breath

Vial Number: **Vial Expiration Date:** _____
  ____ 1
  ____ 2
  ____ 3
  ____ 4

DATE	DOSAGE (mL)	Left Arm	Right Arm	REACTION (mm)	ADMINISTERED BY:

Procedure 11-A: Intramuscular Injection Sites

Locate the following intramuscular injection sites: dorsogluteal, deltoid, vastus lateralis, and ventrogluteal.

Procedure 11-5: Intramuscular Injection

Administer an intramuscular injection, and document the procedure in the chart provided.

Procedure 11-6: Z-Track Method

Administer an intramuscular injection using the Z-track method. Document the procedure in the chart provided.

Procedure 11-7: Intradermal Injection

Administer an intradermal injection, and document the procedure in the chart provided. Read and interpret the test results, and document them in the chart. Complete three TB test record cards located on the following page.

CHART	
Date	

Notes

CHART	
Date	

TUBERCULOSIS TEST RECORD

Name	Date Admin: / /
	Date Read: / /

MANTOUX TEST	RESULT
	____ mm

Logan Family Practice
401 St. George St.
St. Augustine, FL 32084
(904) 555-3933

Performed by _____

TUBERCULOSIS TEST RECORD

Name	Date Admin: / /
	Date Read: / /

MANTOUX TEST	RESULT
	____ mm

Logan Family Practice
401 St. George St.
St. Augustine, FL 32084
(904) 555-3933

Performed by _____

TUBERCULOSIS TEST RECORD

Name	Date Admin: / /
	Date Read: / /

MANTOUX TEST	RESULT
	____ mm

Logan Family Practice
401 St. George St.
St. Augustine, FL 32084
(904) 555-3933

Performed by _____

Notes

Procedure 11-1: Administering Oral Medication

Name: _____ Date: _____

Evaluated by: _____ Score: _____

Performance Objective

Outcome:	Administer oral solid and liquid medication.
Conditions:	Given the following: appropriate medication, medicine cup, and a medication tray.
Standards:	Time: 5 minutes. Student completed procedure in _____ minutes.
	Accuracy: Satisfactory score on the Performance Evaluation Checklist.

Performance Evaluation Checklist

Trial 1	Trial 2	Point Value	Performance Standards
		•	Sanitized hands.
		•	Assembled the equipment.
		•	Worked in a quiet, well-lit atmosphere.
		•	Selected the correct medication from the shelf.
		•	Compared the medication with the provider's instructions.
		•	Checked the drug label.
		•	Checked the expiration date.
		•	Calculated the correct dose to be given, if needed.
		•	Removed the bottle cap.
		•	Checked the drug label and poured the medication.
			Solid medication
		★	Poured the correct number of capsules or tablets into the bottle cap.
		▷	Explained why the medication is poured into the bottle cap.
		•	Transferred the medication to a medicine cup.
			Liquid medication
		•	Placed lid of bottle on a flat surface with the open end facing up.
		•	Palmed the surface of the drug label.
		▷	Explained why the surface of the drug label should be palmed.
		•	Placed thumbnail at the proper calibration on the medicine cup.
		•	Held the medicine cup at eye level.
		★	Poured the correct amount of medication and read the dose at the lowest level of the meniscus.

505

Trial 1	Trial 2	Point Value	Performance Standards
		•	Replaced the bottle cap.
		•	Checked the drug label and returned the medication to its storage location.
		•	Greeted the patient and introduced yourself.
		•	Identified the patient and explained the procedure.
		•	Handed the medicine cup to the patient.
		•	Offered water to the patient.
		▷	Stated one instance when water should not be offered.
		•	Remained with the patient until the medication was swallowed.
		•	Sanitized hands.
		•	Documented the procedure correctly.
			Demonstrated the following affective behavior(s) during this procedure:
		Ⓐ	Incorporated critical thinking skills when performing patient care.
		Ⓐ	Showed awareness of a patient's concerns related to the procedure being performed.
		★	Completed the procedure within 10 minutes.
			Totals

CHART

Date	

Evaluation of Student Performance

EVALUATION CRITERIA			COMMENTS
Symbol	**Category**	**Point Value**	
★	Critical Step	16 points	
•	Essential Step	6 points	
Ⓐ	Affective Competency	6 points	
▷	Theory Question	2 points	

Score calculation: 100 points
−   _____ points missed
  _____ Score

Satisfactory score: 85 or above

CAAHEP Competencies Achieved

Psychomotor (Skills)

☑ I. 4. Verify the rules of medication administration: (a) right patient (b) right medication (c) right dose (d) right route (e) right time (f) right documentation.

☑ I. 6. Administer oral medication.

☑ II. 1. Calculate proper dosages of medication for administration.

☑ X. 3. Document patient care accurately in the medical record.

Affective (Behavior)

☑ I. 2. Incorporate critical thinking skills when performing patient care.

☑ I. 3. Show awareness of a patient's concerns related to the procedure being performed.

ABHES Competencies Achieved

☑ 4. a. Follow documentation guidelines.

☑ 6. b. Demonstrate accurate occupational math and metric conversion for proper medication administration.

☑ 8. f. Prepare and administer oral and parenteral medications and monitor intravenous (IV) infusions.

Notes

Procedure 11-2: Preparing an Injection

Name: _____ Date: _____

Evaluated by: _____ Score: _____

Performance Objective

Outcome:	Prepare an injection from an ampule and a vial.
Conditions:	Given the following: medication ordered by the provider, needle and syringe, antiseptic wipe, and medication tray.
Standards:	Time: 10 minutes. Student completed procedure in _____ minutes.
	Accuracy: Satisfactory score on the Performance Evaluation Checklist.

Performance Evaluation Checklist

Trial 1	Trial 2	Point Value	Performance Standards
		•	Sanitized hands.
		•	Assembled the equipment.
		•	Worked in a quiet, well-lit atmosphere.
		★	Selected the proper medication from its storage location.
		•	Checked the drug label.
		•	Compared the medication with the provider's instructions.
		•	Checked the expiration date.
		★	Calculated the correct dose to be given, if needed.
		•	Opened syringe and needle packages.
		•	Assembled the needle and syringe, if necessary.
		•	Made sure that the needle is attached firmly to the syringe and moved the plunger back and forth.
		•	Checked the drug label a second time.
		•	If required, mixed the medication.
			Withdrew medication from a vial
		•	Removed the metal or plastic cap if vial is new.
		•	Cleansed the rubber stopper of the vial with an antiseptic wipe and allowed it to dry.
		•	Placed the vial in an upright position on a flat surface.
		•	Removed the needle guard.
		•	Drew air into the syringe equal to the amount of medication to be withdrawn.
		•	Inserted the needle through the rubber stopper until it reached the empty space between the stopper and the fluid level.

Chapter **11 Administration of Medication and Intravenous Therapy**

Trial 1	Trial 2	Point Value	Performance Standards
		•	Pushed down on the plunger to inject air into the vial.
		•	Kept the needle above the fluid level.
		▷	Explained why air must be injected into the vial.
		•	Inverted the vial while holding onto the syringe and plunger.
		★	Held the syringe at eye level and withdrew the proper amount of medication.
		•	Kept the needle opening below the fluid level.
		▷	Explained why the needle opening must be kept below the fluid level.
		•	Removed any air bubbles in the syringe by tapping the barrel with the fingertips.
		▷	Explained why air bubbles should be removed from the syringe.
		•	Removed any air remaining at the top of the syringe by pushing the plunger forward.
		•	Held the syringe at eye level and checked to make sure the proper amount of medication had been drawn up.
		•	Removed the needle from the rubber stopper and replaced the needle guard.
		•	If required, removed the needle and replaced it with a new needle.
		•	Checked the drug label for a third time and returned the medication to its storage location.
			Withdrew medication from an ampule
		•	Removed the regular needle from the syringe and attached a filter needle.
		▷	Stated the purpose of a filter needle.
		•	Cleansed the neck of the vial with an antiseptic wipe.
		•	Tapped the stem of the ampule lightly to remove any medication in the neck of the ampule.
		•	Checked the medication label a second time.
		•	Placed a piece of gauze around the neck of the ampule.
		•	Broke off the stem by snapping it quickly and firmly away from the body.
		•	Discarded the stem and gauze in a biohazard sharps container.
		•	Placed the ampule on a flat surface.
		•	Removed the needle guard.
		•	Inserted the needle opening below the fluid level.
		★	Withdrew the proper amount of medication.
		•	Kept the needle opening below the fluid level.
		▷	Explained why the needle opening must be kept below the fluid level.
		•	Held the syringe at eye level and checked to make sure the proper amount of medication had been drawn up.

Trial 1	Trial 2	Point Value	Performance Standards
		•	Removed the needle from the ampule and replaced the needle guard.
		•	Checked the drug label for a third time.
		•	Discarded the ampule in a biohazard sharps container.
		•	Removed the filter needle and reapplied the regular needle (and guard) to the syringe.
		•	Tapped the syringe to remove air bubbles.
		•	Removed the needle guard and expelled air remaining at the top of the syringe.
		•	Replaced the needle guard.
			Demonstrated the following affective behavior(s) during this procedure:
		Ⓐ	Incorporated critical thinking skills when performing patient care.
		★	Completed the procedure within 10 minutes.
			Totals

Evaluation of Student Performance

EVALUATION CRITERIA			COMMENTS
Symbol	**Category**	**Point Value**	
★	Critical Step	16 points	
•	Essential Step	6 points	
Ⓐ	Affective Competency	6 points	
▷	Theory Question	2 points	

Score calculation: 100 points
−_____ points missed
_____ Score

Satisfactory score: 85 or above

CAAHEP Competencies Achieved

Psychomotor (Skills)

☑ I. 4. Verify the rules of medication administration: (a) right patient (b) right medication (c) right dose (d) right route (e) right time (f) right documentation.

☑ II. 1. Calculate proper dosages of medication for administration.

Affective (Behavior)

☑ I. 2. Incorporate critical thinking skills when performing patient care.

ABHES Competencies Achieved

☑ 6. b. Demonstrate accurate occupational math and metric conversion for proper medication administration.

☑ 8. f. Prepare and administer oral and parenteral medications and monitor intravenous (IV) infusions.

Notes

Procedure 11-3: Reconstituting Powdered Drugs

Name: _____ Date: _____

Evaluated by: _____ Score: _____

Performance Objective

Outcome:	Reconstitute a powdered drug for parenteral administration.
Conditions:	Given the following: vial containing the powdered drug, reconstituting liquid, and a needle and syringe.
Standards:	Time: 5 minutes. Student completed procedure in _____ minutes.
	Accuracy: Satisfactory score on the Performance Evaluation Checklist.

Performance Evaluation Checklist

Trial 1	Trial 2	Point Value	Performance Standards
		•	Sanitized hands.
		•	Assembled the equipment.
		★	Selected the proper medication from its storage location.
		•	Checked the drug label.
		•	Compared the medication with the provider's instructions.
		•	Checked the expiration date.
		★	Calculated the correct dose to be given, if needed.
		•	Opened the syringe and needle packages.
		•	Assembled the needle and syringe, if necessary.
		•	Made sure that the needle is attached firmly to the syringe and moved the plunger back and forth.
		•	Checked the drug label a second time.
		•	Withdrew an amount of air equal to the amount of liquid to be injected into the vial from the vial containing the powdered drug.
		•	Injected the air into the vial of diluent.
		★	Inverted the diluent vial and withdrew the proper amount of liquid into the syringe.
		•	Removed air bubbles from the syringe.
		•	Held the syringe at eye level and checked to make sure the proper amount of diluent had been drawn up.
		•	Removed the needle from the vial.
		•	Inserted the needle into the powdered drug vial.
		•	Injected the diluent into the vial.

Trial 1	Trial 2	Point Value	Performance Standards
		•	Removed the needle from the vial and discarded the syringe and needle in a biohazard sharps container.
		•	Rolled the vial between the hands to mix it.
		•	Labeled multiple-dose vials with the date of preparation and your initials.
		•	Prepared the injection and administered the medication.
		•	Stored multiple-dose vials as indicated in the manufacturer's instructions.
		▷	Explained the importance of checking the date of preparation of a reconstituted multiple-dose vial before administering it.
			Demonstrated the following affective behavior(s) during this procedure:
		Ⓐ	Incorporated critical thinking skills when performing patient care.
		★	Completed the procedure within 5 minutes.
			Totals

Evaluation of Student Performance

EVALUATION CRITERIA			COMMENTS
Symbol	**Category**	**Point Value**	
★	Critical Step	16 points	
•	Essential Step	6 points	
Ⓐ	Affective Competency	6 points	
▷	Theory Question	2 points	

Score calculation: 100 points
     − _____ points missed
        _____ Score

Satisfactory score: 85 or above

CAAHEP Competencies Achieved

Psychomotor (Skills)

☑ I. 4. Verify the rules of medication administration: (a) right patient (b) right medication (c) right dose (d) right route (e) right time (f) right documentation.

☑ II. 1. Calculate proper dosages of medication for administration.

Affective (Behavior)

☑ I. 2. Incorporate critical thinking skills when performing patient care.

ABHES Competencies Achieved

☑ 6. b. Demonstrate accurate occupational math and metric conversion for proper medication administration.

☑ 8. f. Prepare and administer oral and parenteral medications and monitor intravenous (IV) infusions.

Procedure 11-4: Administering a Subcutaneous Injection

Name: _____ Date: _____

Evaluated by: _____ Score: _____

Performance Objective

Outcome:	Administer a subcutaneous injection.
Conditions:	Given the following: appropriate medication, appropriate needle and syringe, antiseptic wipe, 2 × 2 gauze pad, disposable gloves, and a biohazard sharps container.
Standards:	Time: 5 minutes. Student completed procedure in _____ minutes.
	Accuracy: Satisfactory score on the Performance Evaluation Checklist.

Performance Evaluation Checklist

Trial 1	Trial 2	Point Value	Performance Standards
		•	Sanitized hands.
		•	Prepared the injection.
		•	Greeted the patient and introduced yourself.
		•	Identified the patient and explained the procedure and purpose of the injection.
		•	Selected an appropriate subcutaneous injection site.
		▷	Stated the sites that can be used to administer a subcutaneous injection.
		•	Cleansed the area with an antiseptic wipe and allowed it to dry completely.
		▷	Explained why the site should be allowed to dry.
		•	Applied gloves.
		•	Removed the needle guard.
		•	Properly positioned the hand on the area surrounding the injection site.
		▷	Explained when the area should be grasped and when it should be held taut.
		•	Inserted needle to the hub at a 45-degree or 90-degree angle (depending on the length of the needle) with a quick, smooth motion.
		▷	Explained how needle length determines the angle of insertion for a subcutaneous injection.
		•	Removed the hand from the skin.
		▷	Explained why the hand should be removed from the skin.
		▷	Explained why aspiration of a subcutaneous injection is not necessary.
		•	Injected the medication slowly and steadily while holding the syringe steady.
		▷	Described what would happen if the medication were injected rapidly.

515

Trial 1	Trial 2	Point Value	Performance Standards
		•	Placed a gauze pad gently over the injection site and removed needle quickly at the same angle as insertion.
		▷	Explained why the needle should be removed at the angle of insertion.
		•	Applied gentle pressure to the injection site.
		▷	Stated why the site should not be vigorously massaged.
		•	Activated the safety shield on the needle.
		•	Properly disposed of needle and syringe.
		•	Removed gloves and sanitized hands.
		•	Documented the procedure correctly.
		•	Remained with the patient to make sure there were no unusual reactions.
		▷	Stated the steps to follow if the patient has been given an allergy injection.
			Demonstrated the following affective behavior(s) during this procedure:
		Ⓐ	Incorporated critical thinking skills when performing patient care.
		Ⓐ	Showed awareness of a patient's concerns related to the procedure being performed.
		Ⓐ	Explained to a patient the rationale for performance of a procedure.
		★	Completed the procedure within 5 minutes.
			Totals
CHART			
Date			

Evaluation of Student Performance

EVALUATION CRITERIA			COMMENTS
Symbol	**Category**	**Point Value**	
★	Critical Step	16 points	
•	Essential Step	6 points	
Ⓐ	Affective Competency	6 points	
▷	Theory Question	2 points	

Score calculation: 100 points
   −_____ points missed
   _____ Score

Satisfactory score: 85 or above

CAAHEP Competencies Achieved

Psychomotor (Skills)

☑ I. 4. Verify the rules of medication administration: (a) right patient (b) right medication (c) right dose (d) right route (e) right time (f) right documentation.

☑ I. 5. Select proper sites for administering parenteral medication.

☑ I. 7. Administer parenteral (excluding IV) medications.

☑ III. 10. Demonstrate proper disposal of biohazardous material: (a) sharps (b) regulated waste.

☑ V. 2. Respond to nonverbal communication.

☑ X. 3. Document patient care accurately in the medical record.

☑ XII. 2. c. Demonstrate proper use of sharps disposal containers.

Affective (Behavior)

☑ I. 2. Incorporate critical thinking skills when performing patient care.

☑ I. 3. Show awareness of a patient's concerns related to the procedure being performed.

☑ V. 4. Explain to a patient the rationale for performance of a procedure.

ABHES Competencies Achieved

☑ 4. a. Follow documentation guidelines.

☑ 8. f. Prepare and administer oral and parenteral medications and monitor intravenous (IV) infusions.

☑ 9. c. Dispose of biohazardous materials.

Notes

Procedure 11-A: Locating Intramuscular Injection Sites

Name: _____ Date: _____

Evaluated by: _____ Score: _____

Performance Objective

Outcome:	Locate intramuscular injection sites.
Conditions:	None required.
Standards:	Time: 5 minutes. Student completed procedure in _____ minutes.
	Accuracy: Satisfactory score on the Performance Evaluation Checklist.

Performance Evaluation Checklist

Trial 1	Trial 2	Point Value	Performance Standards
			DORSOGLUTEAL SITE
			Method 1:
		•	Asked the patient to lie on the abdomen with the toes pointed inward.
		•	Made sure the injection site was fully exposed.
		▷	Stated why the injection site should be fully exposed.
		•	Located the greater trochanter through palpation.
		•	Located the posterior superior iliac spine through palpation.
		•	Drew an imaginary line between these two points.
		•	Stated that the injection is administered above and outside this area.
			Method 2:
		•	Asked the patient to lie on the abdomen with the toes pointed inward.
		•	Made sure the injection area was fully exposed.
		•	Divided the buttocks into quadrants.
		•	Stated that the injection is administered into the upper outer quadrant approximately 2 to 3 inches below the iliac crest.
		▷	Explained why it is important to maintain proper boundary lines.
			DELTOID SITE
		•	Placed the patient in a sitting position.
		•	Pulled up the patient's sleeve or removed the sleeve from the arm.
		▷	Explained why a tight sleeve should be avoided.
		•	Ensured that the entire arm was exposed.
		•	Palpated the lower edge of the acromion process.

Trial 1	Trial 2	Point Value	Performance Standards
		•	Placed 4 fingers horizontally across the deltoid muscle with the top finger along the acromion process.
		•	Explained that the injection site is located 2 to 3 finger-widths below the acromion process (approximately 1 to 2 inches below the acromion process).
		▷	Identified the maximum amount of medication that can be administered into this site.
			VASTUS LATERALIS SITE
			Adult:
		•	Placed the patient in a supine or sitting position.
		•	Located the midanterior thigh (on the front of the leg).
		•	Located the midlateral thigh (on the side of the leg).
		•	Located the proximal boundary by coming down a hand's breadth from the greater trochanter.
		•	Located the distal boundary by coming up a hand's breadth from the knee.
		•	Stated that the injection is administered within the boundaries identified above.
			Infants and Children:
		•	Placed the infant or child in a supine position or asked the parent to hold the infant in a sitting position on his or her lap.
		•	Located the midanterior thigh (on the front of the leg).
		•	Located the midlateral thigh (on the side of the leg).
		•	Located the greater trochanter through palpation.
		•	Located the knee joint through palpation.
		•	Divided the area between the greater trochanter and knee joint into thirds and made a mental note of the middle third of the divided area.
		•	Stated that the injection is administered within the boundaries identified above.
		▷	Explained why this site is commonly used with children younger than 3 years of age.
			VENTROGLUTEAL SITE
		•	Placed the patient in a prone position or lying on one side.
		•	Located the greater trochanter through palpation.
		•	Located the anterior superior iliac spine and the iliac crest through palpation.
			For an injection being administered into the left side:
		•	Placed the palm of the right hand on the greater trochanter.
		•	Placed the index finger on the anterior superior iliac spine.
		•	Spread the middle finger posteriorly as far as possible away from the index finger to touch the iliac crest.

520

Trial 1	Trial 2	Point Value	Performance Standards
		•	Stated that the injection is administered into the triangle formed by the fingers.
			For an injection being administered into the right side:
		•	Placed the palm of the left hand on the greater trochanter.
		•	Placed the index finger on the anterior superior iliac spine.
		•	Spread the middle finger posteriorly as far as possible away from the index finger to touch the iliac crest.
		•	Stated that the injection is administered into the triangle formed by the fingers.
			Demonstrated the following affective behavior(s) during this procedure:
		Ⓐ	Incorporated critical thinking skills when performing patient care.
		★	Completed the procedure within 5 minutes.
			Totals

Evaluation of Student Performance

EVALUATION CRITERIA			COMMENTS
Symbol	**Category**	**Point Value**	
★	Critical Step	16 points	
•	Essential Step	6 points	
Ⓐ	Affective Competency	6 points	
▷	Theory Question	2 points	

Score calculation: 100 points
− _____ points missed
_____ Score

Satisfactory score: 85 or above

CAAHEP Competencies Achieved

Psychomotor (Skills)
☑ I. 4. Verify the rules of medication administration: (a) right patient (b) right medication (c) right dose (d) right route (e) right time (f) right documentation.
☑ I. 5. Select proper sites for administering parenteral medication.

Affective (Behavior)
☑ I. 2. Incorporate critical thinking skills when performing patient care.

ABHES Competencies Achieved

☑ 8. f. Prepare and administer oral and parenteral medications and monitor intravenous (IV) infusions.

Chapter **11** **Administration of Medication and Intravenous Therapy**

Notes

Procedure 11-5: Administering an Intramuscular Injection

Name: _____   Date: _____

Evaluated by: _____   Score: _____

Performance Objective

Outcome:	Administer an intramuscular injection.
Conditions:	Given the following: appropriate medication, appropriate needle and syringe, antiseptic wipe, 2 × 2 gauze pad, disposable gloves, and a biohazard sharps container.
Standards:	Time: 5 minutes. Student completed procedure in _____ minutes.
	Accuracy: Satisfactory score on the Performance Evaluation Checklist.

Performance Evaluation Checklist

Trial 1	Trial 2	Point Value	Performance Standards
		•	Sanitized hands.
		•	Prepared the injection.
		•	Greeted the patient and introduced yourself.
		•	Identified the patient and explained the procedure and purpose of the injection.
		★	Located the appropriate intramuscular injection site.
		▷	Stated what tissue layer of the body the medication will be injected into.
		•	Cleansed area with an antiseptic wipe and allowed it to dry completely.
		•	Applied gloves.
		•	Removed the needle guard.
		•	Stretched the skin taut over the injection site.
		▷	Explained why the skin should be stretched taut.
		•	Held the barrel of the syringe like a dart and inserted the needle quickly at a 90-degree angle to the patient's skin with a firm motion.
		•	Inserted the needle to the hub.
		▷	Explained why the needle should be inserted at a 90-degree angle and to the hub.
		★	Aspirated to make sure that the needle was not in a blood vessel.
		▷	Described what would happen if the medication was injected into a blood vessel.
		•	Injected the medication slowly and steadily.
		▷	Described what would happen if the medication was injected rapidly.
		•	Placed a gauze pad gently over the injection site and removed the needle quickly at the same angle as insertion.
		•	Applied gentle pressure to the injection site.

Trial 1	Trial 2	Point Value	Performance Standards
		▷	Stated the reason for applying pressure to the injection site.
		•	Activated the safety shield on the needle.
		•	Properly disposed of the needle and syringe.
		•	Removed gloves and sanitized hands.
		•	Documented the procedure correctly.
		▷	Stated the purpose of the lot number on the medication vial.
		•	Remained with the patient to make sure there were no unusual reactions.
			Demonstrated the following affective behavior(s) during this procedure:
		Ⓐ	Incorporated critical thinking skills when performing patient care.
		Ⓐ	Showed awareness of a patient's concerns related to the procedure being performed.
		Ⓐ	Explained to a patient the rationale for performance of a procedure.
		★	Completed the procedure within 5 minutes.
			Totals

CHART	
Date	

Evaluation of Student Performance

EVALUATION CRITERIA			COMMENTS
Symbol	**Category**	**Point Value**	
★	Critical Step	16 points	
•	Essential Step	6 points	
Ⓐ	Affective Competency	6 points	
▷	Theory Question	2 points	

Score calculation: 100 points
     − _____ points missed
         _____ Score

Satisfactory score: 85 or above

CAAHEP Competencies Achieved

Psychomotor (Skills)

☑ I. 4. Verify the rules of medication administration: (a) right patient (b) right medication (c) right dose (d) right route (e) right time (f) right documentation.

☑ I. 5. Select proper sites for administering parenteral medication.

☑ I. 7. Administer parenteral (excluding IV) medications.

☑ III. 10. Demonstrate proper disposal of biohazardous material: (a) sharps (b) regulated waste.

☑ V. 2. Respond to nonverbal communication.

☑ X. 3. Document patient care accurately in the medical record.

☑ XII. 2. c. Demonstrate proper use of sharps disposal containers.

Affective (Behavior)

☑ I. 2. Incorporate critical thinking skills when performing patient care.

☑ I. 3. Show awareness of a patient's concerns related to the procedure being performed.

☑ V. 4. Explain to a patient the rationale for performance of a procedure.

ABHES Competencies Achieved

☑ 4. a. Follow documentation guidelines.

☑ 8. f. Prepare and administer oral and parenteral medications and monitor intravenous (IV) infusions.

☑ 9. c. Dispose of biohazardous materials.

Notes

Procedure 11-6: Z-Track Intramuscular Injection Technique

Name: _____   Date: _____

Evaluated by: _____   Score: _____

Performance Objective

Outcome:	Administer an intramuscular injection using the Z-track method.
Conditions:	Given the following: appropriate medication, appropriate needle and syringe, antiseptic wipe, disposable gloves, and a biohazard sharps container.
Standards:	Time: 5 minutes. Student completed procedure in _____ minutes.
	Accuracy: Satisfactory score on the Performance Evaluation Checklist.

Performance Evaluation Checklist

Trial 1	Trial 2	Point Value	Performance Standards
		•	Sanitized hands.
		•	Prepared the injection.
		•	Greeted the patient and introduced yourself.
		•	Identified the patient and explained the procedure and purpose of the injection.
		•	Selected and properly located the intramuscular injection site.
		•	Cleansed the area with an antiseptic wipe and allowed it to dry completely.
		•	Applied gloves.
		•	Removed the needle guard.
		•	Pulled the skin away laterally from the injection site with the nondominant hand approximately 1 to 1 ½ inches.
		•	Inserted the needle quickly and smoothly at a 90-degree angle.
		★	Aspirated to make sure that the needle was not in a blood vessel.
		•	Injected the medication slowly and steadily.
		•	Waited 10 seconds before withdrawing the needle.
		▷	Explained why there should be a 10-second waiting period.
		•	Withdrew the needle quickly at the same angle as that of insertion.
		•	Released the traction on the skin.
		▷	Described what occurs when the skin traction is released.
		•	Did not apply pressure to the injection site.
		▷	Stated why pressure should not be applied to the injection site.
		•	Activated the safety shield on the needle.

527

Trial 1	Trial 2	Point Value	Performance Standards
		•	Properly disposed of the needle and syringe.
		•	Removed gloves and sanitized hands.
		•	Documented the procedure correctly.
		•	Remained with the patient to make sure there were no unusual reactions.
			Demonstrated the following affective behavior(s) during this procedure:
		Ⓐ	Incorporated critical thinking skills when performing patient care.
		Ⓐ	Showed awareness of a patient's concerns related to the procedure being performed.
		Ⓐ	Explained to a patient the rationale for performance of a procedure.
		★	Completed the procedure within 5 minutes.
			Totals

CHART

Date	

Evaluation of Student Performance

EVALUATION CRITERIA			COMMENTS
Symbol	**Category**	**Point Value**	
★	Critical Step	16 points	
•	Essential Step	6 points	
Ⓐ	Affective Competency	6 points	
▷	Theory Question	2 points	

Score calculation: 100 points
− _____ points missed
_____ Score

Satisfactory score: 85 or above

CAAHEP Competencies Achieved

Psychomotor (Skills)

☑ I. 4. Verify the rules of medication administration: (a) right patient (b) right medication (c) right dose (d) right route (e) right time (f) right documentation.

☑ I. 5. Select proper sites for administering parenteral medication.

☑ I. 7. Administer parenteral (excluding IV) medications.

☑ III. 10. Demonstrate proper disposal of biohazardous material: (a) sharps (b) regulated waste.

☑ V. 2. Respond to nonverbal communication.

☑ X. 3. Document patient care accurately in the medical record.

☑ XII. 2. c. Demonstrate proper use of sharps disposal containers.

Affective (Behavior)

☑ I. 2. Incorporate critical thinking skills when performing patient care.

☑ I. 3. Show awareness of a patient's concerns related to the procedure being performed.

☑ V. 4. Explain to a patient the rationale for performance of a procedure.

ABHES Competencies Achieved

☑ 4. a. Follow documentation guidelines.

☑ 8. f. Prepare and administer oral and parenteral medications and monitor intravenous (IV) infusions.

☑ 9. c. Dispose of biohazardous materials.

Notes

Chapter **11** **Administration of Medication and Intravenous Therapy**

Procedure 11-7: Administering an Intradermal Injection

Name: _____   Date: _____

Evaluated by: _____   Score: _____

Performance Objective

Outcome:	Administer an intradermal injection and read the test results.
Conditions:	Given the following: skin testing solution, appropriate needle and syringe, antiseptic wipe, 2 × 2 gauze pad, disposable gloves, millimeter ruler, TB skin test record card, and a biohazard sharps container.
Standards:	Time: 5 minutes. Student completed procedure in _____ minutes.
	Accuracy: Satisfactory score on the Performance Evaluation Checklist.

Performance Evaluation Checklist

Trial 1	Trial 2	Point Value	Performance Standards
		•	Sanitized hands.
		•	Prepared the injection.
		•	Greeted the patient and introduced yourself.
		•	Identified the patient and explained the procedure and purpose of the injection.
		•	Selected an appropriate intradermal injection site.
		▷	Stated the recommended sites for an intradermal injection.
		•	Cleansed the area with an antiseptic wipe and allowed it to dry completely.
		•	Applied gloves.
		•	Removed needle guard.
		•	Stretched the skin taut at the site of administration.
		▷	Explained why the skin is held taut.
		•	Inserted the needle at an angle of 10 to 15 degrees and with the bevel upward.
		•	The bevel of the needle just penetrated the skin.
		▷	Stated why the bevel should face upward.
		•	Injected the medication slowly and steadily, ensuring that a wheal formed (approximately 6 to 10 mm in diameter).
		▷	Explained what to do if a wheal does not form.
		•	Placed a gauze pad gently over the injection site and removed the needle quickly at the same angle as that of insertion.
		•	Did not apply pressure to the injection site.
		▷	Explained why pressure should not be applied to the site.

531

Trial 1	Trial 2	Point Value	Performance Standards
		•	Activated the safety shield on the needle.
		•	Properly disposed of the needle and syringe.
		•	Removed gloves and sanitized hands.
		•	Remained with the patient to make sure that there were no unusual reactions.
			Allergy skin tests
		•	Read the test results within 20 to 30 minutes.
		•	Inspected and palpated the site of the skin tests.
		•	Interpreted the skin test results.
		•	Documented the procedure correctly.
			Mantoux tuberculin test
		•	Informed the patient to return in 48 to 72 hours to have the results read.
		▷	Stated what must be done if the patient does not return to have the results read.
		•	Instructed the patient in the care of the test site.
		▷	Stated the instructions that must be relayed to the patient.
		•	Documented the procedure correctly.
			Reading Mantoux test results
		•	Greeted the patient and introduced yourself.
		•	Identified the patient and explained the procedure.
		•	Worked in a quiet, well-lit atmosphere.
		•	Checked the patient's medical record to determine the site of administration of the test.
		•	Sanitized hands and applied gloves.
		•	Positioned the patient's arm on a firm surface with the arm flexed at the elbow.
		•	Located the application site.
		•	Gently rubbed the fingertip over the test site.
		•	If induration is present, rubbed the area lightly, going from the area of normal skin to the indurated area to assess the size of the indurated area.
		•	Measured the diameter of the induration with a millimeter ruler.
		★	The measurement was documented in millimeters and was identical to the evaluator's measurement.
		•	Removed gloves and sanitized hands.
		•	Documented the results correctly.
		•	Completed a TB test record card and gave it to the patient.

Trial 1	Trial 2	Point Value	Performance Standards
			Demonstrated the following affective behavior(s) during this procedure:
		Ⓐ	Incorporated critical thinking skills when performing patient care.
		Ⓐ	Showed awareness of a patient's concerns related to the procedure being performed.
		Ⓐ	Explained to a patient the rationale for performance of a procedure.
		★	Completed the procedure within 10 minutes.
			Totals

CHART

Date	

Evaluation of Student Performance

EVALUATION CRITERIA			COMMENTS
Symbol	**Category**	**Point Value**	
★	Critical Step	16 points	
•	Essential Step	6 points	
Ⓐ	Affective Competency	6 points	
▷	Theory Question	2 points	

Score calculation: 100 points
−_____ points missed
_____ Score

Satisfactory score: 85 or above

CAAHEP Competencies Achieved

Psychomotor (Skills)

☑ I. 4. Verify the rules of medication administration: (a) right patient (b) right medication (c) right dose (d) right route (e) right time (f) right documentation.

☑ I. 5. Select proper sites for administering parenteral medication.

☑ I. 7. Administer parenteral (excluding IV) medications.

☑ III. 10. Demonstrate proper disposal of biohazardous material: (a) sharps (b) regulated waste.

☑ V. 2. Respond to nonverbal communication.

☑ X. 3. Document patient care accurately in the medical record.

☑ XII. 2. c. Demonstrate proper use of sharps disposal containers.

Affective (Behavior)

☑ I. 2. Incorporate critical thinking skills when performing patient care.

☑ I. 3. Show awareness of a patient's concerns related to the procedure being performed.

☑ V. 4. Explain to a patient the rationale for performance of a procedure.

ABHES Competencies Achieved

☑ 4. a. Follow documentation guidelines.

☑ 8. f. Prepare and administer oral and parenteral medications and monitor intravenous (IV) infusions.

☑ 9. c. Dispose of biohazardous materials.

DRUG DOSAGE CALCULATION: SUPPLEMENTAL EDUCATION FOR CHAPTER 11

This section is designed as supplemental education for Chapter 11 (Administration of Medication) in your textbook. Completion of these exercises will enable you to calculate drug dosage effectively and accurately, which is essential for administering the proper amount of medication to patients and preventing medication errors. Because each unit builds on the next one, you should become completely familiar with each step before proceeding to the next.

LEARNING OBJECTIVES

After completing this chapter, you should be able to:
1. Identify metric abbreviations.
2. Indicate dose quantity using metric notation guidelines.
3. Identify common medical abbreviations used in writing medication orders.
4. Interpret medication orders.
5. Convert units of measurement within the following systems: metric and household.
6. Convert units of measurement using ratio and proportion.
7. Convert units of measurement between the metric and household systems.
8. Determine oral drug dosage.
9. Determine parenteral drug dosage.

UNIT 1: THE METRIC SYSTEM

A. Units of Measurement: Practice Problems

The basic units of measurement in the metric system are the gram, liter, and meter. The gram is a unit of weight used to measure solids, the liter is a unit volume used to measure liquids, and the meter is a unit of length used to measure distance. In the space provided, indicate whether each of the following metric units of measurement is a unit of weight (W), volume (V), or length (L).

_____ 1. milligram

_____ 2. cubic centimeter

_____ 3. meter

_____ 4. kilogram

_____ 5. liter

_____ 6. milliliter

_____ 7. kiloliter

_____ 8. millimeter

_____ 9. microgram

_____10. gram

B. Metric Abbreviations: Practice Problems

Review the metric abbreviations in your textbook before completing these problems. In the space provided, indicate the correct abbreviation for each of the metric units of measurement.

_____ 1. milligram

_____ 2. gram

_____ 3. kilogram

_____ 4. liter

_____ 5. microgram

_____ 6. milliliter

C. Metric Notation: Practice Problems

To read prescriptions and medication orders, to record medication administration, and to avoid medication errors, the MA must be able to use metric notation guidelines. Review the Metric Notation Guidelines on page 399 of your textbook before completing the following practice problems. In the space provided, use metric notation guidelines to indicate the dose quantities.

_____ 1. 25 milligrams

_____ 2. 5 grams

_____ 3. 1½ liters

_____ 4. 10 milliliters

_____ 5. ½ gram

_____ 6. 50 milligrams

_____ 7. 4 milliliters

_____ 8. 2 kilograms

_____ 9. 120 milliliters

_____10. ¼ gram

_____11. 250 milligrams

_____12. ½ liter

_____13. 500 milliliters

_____14. 5 kilograms

_____15. 2½ grams

UNIT 2: THE HOUSEHOLD SYSTEM

The household system is a more complicated and less accurate method for administering medication than the metric system. However, most individuals are familiar with this system because of its frequent use in the United States. This system of measurement may be the only one the patient can fully relate to and therefore may safely use to administer liquid medication at home.

A. Units of Measurement: Practice Problems

Volume is the only household unit of measurement used to administer medication. The basic unit of liquid volume is the drop. The remaining units, in order of increasing volume, are the teaspoon, tablespoon, ounce, cup, and glass. In the space provided, indicate the correct abbreviation for each of the household units of measurement listed.

_____ 1. drop

_____ 2. teaspoon

_____ 3. tablespoon

_____ 4. ounce

UNIT 3: MEDICATION ORDERS

A. Medical Abbreviations: Practice Problems

To safely administer medication, the MA must be completely familiar with common medical abbreviations. Review Table 11-5 in your textbook before completing the following practice problems. In the space provided, write the meaning of the following medical abbreviations.

_____ 1. NPO

_____ 2. prn

_____ 3. tab

_____ 4. ac

_____ 5. DAW

_____ 6. pc

_____ 7. qid

_____ 8. $\bar{c}$

_____ 9. $\bar{s}$

_____ 10. bid

_____ 11. tid

_____ 12. qh

_____ 13. gtts

_____ 14. q4h

_____ 15. qs

_____ 16. IM

_____ 17. caps

_____ 18. po

_____ 19. ad lib

_____ 20. $\overline{aa}$

_____ 21. OTC

_____ 22. subcut

_____ 23. per

_____ 24. SL

_____ 25. STAT

B. Interpreting Medication Orders: Practice Problems

To safely administer medication and instruct patients on administering medication at home, the medical assistant must be able to interpret medication orders. Interpret the following medication orders, and using a drug reference, indicate the drug category based on action and a brand name for each medication.

1. Tetracycline 250 mg po qid × 10 days

   _____

   Drug category: _____

   Brand name: _____

2. Lansoprazole 30 mg po every day ac

   _____

   Drug category: _____

   Brand name: _____

3. Alprazolam 0.25 mg po tid

   _____

   Drug category: _____

   Brand name: _____

4. Diltiazem 50 mg po q4h

   _____

   Drug category: _____

   Brand name: _____

5. Ciprofloxacin 500 mg q12h

   _____

   Drug category: _____

   Brand name: _____

6. Hydrocodone/acetaminophen 5 mg q4h prn

   _____

   Drug category: _____

   Brand name: _____

7. Furosemide 40 mg po q AM

   _____

   Drug category: _____

   Brand name: _____

8. Paroxetine 20 mg po every day in AM

   _____

   Drug category: _____

   Brand name: _____

9. Cetirizine 5 mg po every day

   _____

   Drug category: _____

   Brand name: _____

10. Cyclobenzaprine 10 mg po tid × 1 wk

   _____

   Drug category: _____

   Brand name: _____

UNIT 4: CONVERTING UNITS OF MEASUREMENT

A. Using Conversion Tables

Changing from one unit of measurement to another is known as *conversion*. Conversion is required when medication is ordered in one unit of measurement and the medication label expresses the drug strength in a different unit. The dose quantity must be mathematically translated or converted to the unit of measurement of the medication on hand. For example, if the provider orders 5 grams of an oral solid medication and the medication label expresses the drug strength in milligrams, the medical assistant must convert the grams into milligrams to know how much medication to administer. Converting units of measurement can be classified as follows:

1. Conversion of units within a measurement system
2. Conversion of units from one measurement system to another

Converting units within a measurement system allows a quantity to be expressed in a different but equal unit of measurement within the same system. An example of converting between units of weight within the metric system is as follows: 1 gram is equal to 1000 milligrams.

Converting from one measurement system to another allows a quantity to be expressed in a unit of measurement of another system. An example of a conversion between the household and metric systems is as follows: 1 ounce (household system) is equivalent to 30 milliliters (metric system). Methods used to convert units of measurement are presented in this unit and in Unit 5.

Conversion requires the use of a conversion table to indicate the equivalent values between units of measurement. The practice problems that follow can assist you in attaining competency in using conversion tables.

Conversion Tables: Practice Problems

Refer to the conversion tables at the end of this chapter. Locate and document the equivalent value for each of the units of measurement listed.

                                          ANSWER

1 g	=	_____ mg
1 ounce	=	_____ mL
1 tablespoon	=	_____ teaspoons
1 mg	=	_____ mcg
1 liter	=	_____ mL
1 kiloliter	=	_____ liters
1 teacup	=	_____ ounces
1 teaspoon	=	_____ drops
1 mL	=	_____ cc
1 cup	=	_____ ounces
1 drop	=	_____ mL
1 kg	=	_____ g
1 mL	=	_____ drops
1 teaspoon	=	_____ mL
1 ounce	=	_____ tablespoons
1 tablespoon	=	_____ mL
1 ounce	=	_____ teaspoons
1 glass	=	_____ mL
1 glass	=	_____ ounces

B. Converting Units Within the Metric System

Drug administration often requires conversion within the metric system to prepare the correct dose. Metric conversion involves converting a larger unit to a smaller unit (e.g., grams to milligrams) or converting a smaller unit to a larger unit (e.g., milliliters to liters). Methods used to convert one metric unit to another are described in the next sections.

Converting a Larger Unit to a Smaller Unit

Converting a larger unit to a smaller unit within the metric system can be accomplished using one of three methods. The method chosen is based on personal preference and the level of difficulty of the conversion problem. For example, more difficult problems require the use of ratio and proportion as the method of conversion. Examples of converting a larger unit to a smaller unit are as follows:

1. Grams to milligrams
2. Liters to milliliters
3. Kilograms to grams

> **Methods of Conversion:** To convert a larger unit to a smaller unit within the metric system, use one of the following:
> *Method 1:* Multiply the unit to be changed by 1000.
> *Method 2:* Move the decimal point of the unit to be changed three places to the right.
> *Method 3:* Ratio and proportion (see Unit 5).
> **Guideline:** When converting a larger unit to a smaller unit, expect the quantity to become larger. Use this guideline to assist in making accurate conversions. The problems illustrate this guideline.

EXAMPLES

PROBLEM   2 L = _____ mL
Method 1:   Multiply the unit to be changed by 1000.
                     $2 \times 1000 = 2000$ mL
Method 2:   Move the decimal point of the unit to be changed three places to the right.
                     2.0 0 0. = 2000 mL

Answer	2 L = 2000 mL

PROBLEM   4 g = _____ mg
Method 1:   Multiply the unit to be changed by 1000.
                     $4 \times 1000 = 4000$ mg
Method 2:   Move the decimal point of the unit to be changed three places to the right.
                     4.0 0 0. = 4000 mL

Answer	4 g = 4000 mg

Converting a Smaller Unit to a Larger Unit

Converting a smaller unit to a larger unit within the metric system can be accomplished using one of three methods of conversion as outlined below. Examples of converting a smaller unit to a larger unit are as follows:

1. Milligrams to grams
2. Milliliters to liters
3. Grams to kilograms

> **Methods of Conversion:** To convert a smaller unit to a larger unit within the metric system, use one of the following:
> *Method 1:* Divide the unit to be changed by 1000.
> *Method 2:* Move the decimal point of the unit to be changed three places to the left.
> *Method 3:* Ratio and proportion (see Unit 5).
> **Guideline:** When converting a smaller unit to a larger unit, expect the quantity to become smaller. The problems illustrate this guideline.

PROBLEM   250 mg = _____ g
Method 1:   Divide the unit to be changed by 1000.
                 250 ÷ 1000 = 0.25 g
Method 2:   Move the decimal point of the unit to be changed three places to the left.
                 .2 5 0. = 0.25 g

Answer	250 mg = 0.25 g

PROBLEM   1500 mL = _____ L
Method 1:   Divide the unit to be changed by 1000.
                 1500 ÷ 1000 = 1.5 L
Method 2:   Move the decimal point of the unit to be changed three places to the left.
                 1.5 0 0. = 1.5 L

Answer	1500 mL = 1.5 L

Converting Units Within the Metric System: Practice Problems

Directions: Convert the following metric units of measurement using Method 1 or Method 2. In the space provided, indicate if the conversion is going from a larger to smaller unit (L→S) or smaller to larger unit (S→L).

		ANSWER		CONVERSION
1. 1 g	=	_____ mg		_____
2. 750 mg	=	_____ g		_____
3. 2 kg	=	_____ g		_____
4. 1000 g	=	_____ kg		_____
5. 1.5 L	=	_____ mL		_____
6. 250 mL	=	_____ L		_____
7. 5 g	=	_____ mg		_____
8. 0.25 kg	=	_____ g		_____
9. 1000 mg	=	_____ g		_____
10. 2.5 g	=	_____ mg		_____
11. 475 mL	=	_____ L		_____
12. 0.05 g	=	_____ mg		_____
13. 0.5 L	=	_____ mL		_____
14. 1000 mL	=	_____ L		_____
15. 500 g	=	_____ kg		_____
16. 50 mg	=	_____ g		_____
17. 1 L	=	_____ mL		_____
18. 40 g	=	_____ mg		_____
19. 50 mL	=	_____ L		_____
20. 1 kg	=	_____ g		_____

Chapter **11** **Administration of Medication and Intravenous Therapy**

C. Converting Units Within the Household System

Household system conversion involves converting a larger unit to a smaller unit (e.g., tablespoons to teaspoons) or converting a smaller unit to a larger unit (e.g., tablespoons to ounces). Methods used to convert one unit to another are described.

Converting a Larger Unit to a Smaller Unit

Converting a larger unit to a smaller unit within the household system is accomplished using the equivalent value method or the ratio and proportion method. The method chosen is based on personal preference and on the level of difficulty of the conversion problem. Examples of converting a larger unit to a smaller unit follow:

Volume:
teaspoons to drops
tablespoons to teaspoons
ounces to teaspoons
ounces to tablespoons
teacup to ounces
glass to ounces

Method of Conversion: To convert a larger unit to a smaller unit within the household system, use one of the following:
    Method 1:
    a. Look at Table 11-2 (Household Conversion) at the end of this chapter to determine the equivalent value between the two units of measurement.
    b. Multiply the equivalent value by the number next to the larger unit of measurement.
    Method 2: Ratio and proportion (see Unit 5).

EXAMPLES

PROBLEM   2 tablespoons = _____ teaspoons
    Method 1:
    a. Look at the conversion table to determine the equivalent value:
       1 tablespoon = 3 teaspoons
       3 = the equivalent value
    b. Multiply the equivalent value by the number next to the larger unit of measurement:
       $2 \times 3 = 6$

Answer	2 tablespoons = 6 teaspoons

PROBLEM   ½ teaspoon = _____ drops
    Method 1:
    a. Look at the conversion table to determine the equivalent value:
       1 teaspoon = 60 drops
       60 = the equivalent value
    b. Multiply the equivalent value by the number next to the larger unit of measurement:
       $½ \times 60 = 30$ drops

Answer	½ tablespoon = 30 drops

Converting a Smaller Unit to a Larger Unit

Converting a smaller unit to a larger unit within the household system is accomplished using the equivalent value method or the ratio and proportion method. Examples of converting from a smaller unit to a larger unit follow:

Volume
drops to teaspoons
teaspoons to tablespoons
teaspoons to ounces
tablespoons to ounces

542

ounces to teacups
ounces to glasses

> **Method of Conversion:** To convert a smaller unit to a larger unit within the household system, use one of the following:
> *Method 1:*
>   a. Look at Table 11-2 (Household Conversion) at the end of this chapter to determine the equivalent value between the two units of measurement.
>   b. Divide the equivalent value into the number next to the smaller unit of measurement.
> *Method 2:* Ratio and proportion (see Unit 5).

EXAMPLES

PROBLEM   4 tablespoons = _____ ounces
   Method 1:
   a. Look at the conversion table to determine the equivalent value:
     1 ounce = 2 tablespoons
     2 = the equivalent value
   b. Divide the equivalent value into the number next to the smaller unit of measurement:
     4 ÷ 2 = 2

Answer	4 tablespoons = 2 ounces

PROBLEM   24 ounces = _____ glasses
   Method 1:
   a. Look at the conversion table to determine the equivalent value:
     1 glass = 8 ounces
     8 = the equivalent value
   b. Divide the equivalent value into the number next to the smaller unit of measurement:
     24 ÷ 8 = 3 glasses

Answer	24 ounces = 3 glasses

Converting Units Within the Household System: Practice Problems

Directions: Convert the following household units of measurement using the equivalent value method of conversion. In the space provided, indicate the equivalent value for each problem.

		ANSWER	EQUIVALENT VALUE
1. 12 teaspoons	=	_____ ounces	_____
2. 4 ounces	=	_____ glasses	_____
3. 90 drops	=	_____ teaspoons	_____
4. ½ ounce	=	_____ tablespoons	_____
5. 6 teaspoons	=	_____ tablespoons	_____
6. 3 tablespoons	=	_____ ounces	_____
7. 18 ounces	=	_____ teacups	_____
8. ½ ounce	=	_____ teaspoons	_____
9. 3 tablespoons	=	_____ teaspoons	_____
10. ½ teaspoon	=	_____ drops	_____

Ratio and proportion are used to convert units of measurement. This method of conversion has the advantage of clarifying the mathematical rationale for the methods of conversion previously presented. It is also useful in converting units of measurement that are more difficult to calculate, such as converting between systems—for example, when converting a metric unit of measurement to a household unit of measurement.

A. Ratio and Proportion Guidelines

Some guidelines must be followed when using ratio and proportion:

1. A **ratio** is composed of two related numbers separated by a colon. It indicates the relationship between two quantities or numbers. The ratio example shows a relationship between milligrams and grams (i.e., 1000 mg = 1 g).

    EXAMPLE   1000 mg : 1 g

2. A proportion shows the relationship between two equal ratios. The proportion consists of two ratios separated by an equal sign (=), which indicates that the two ratios are equal. This proportion example shows the relationship between two equal ratios of milligrams and grams.

    EXAMPLE   1000 mg : 1 g = 2000 mg : 2 g

3. The units of measurement in the two ratios of a proportion must be expressed in the same sequence. The correct sequencing in the proportion example is mg : g = mg : g, not mg : g = g : mg.

    EXAMPLE   *Correct:*   1000 mg : 1 g = 2000 mg : 2 g
                   Incorrect: 1000 mg : 1 g = 2g : 2000 mg

4. The numbers on the ends of a proportion are called the extremes, and the numbers in the middle of the proportion are known as the means. In this example, the means consist of 1 g and 2000 mg, and the extremes are 1000 mg and 2 g.

    EXAMPLE   1000 mg : 1 g = 2000 mg : 2g
                                └── means ──┘
                   └────────── extremes ──────────┘

5. The product of the means equals the product of the extremes. The calculation of the product of the means in the example is $1 \times 2000 = 2000$. The calculation of the product of the extremes is $1000 \times 2 = 2000$. The product of the means equals the product of the extremes, or 2000 = 2000.

    EXAMPLE   1000 mg : 1 g = 2000 mg : 2 g
                   $1 \times 2000 = 1000 \times 2$
                   $2000 = 2000$

6. In setting up a proportion, one side of the equation consists of the known quantities, and the other side of the equation consists of the unknown quantity. The letter x is commonly used to express the unknown quantity. To be consistent, the known quantities are indicated on the left side of the equation, and the unknown quantity is indicated on the right side of the equation. Using the previous proportion example, but inserting an unknown quantity, or x, the equation is set up as follows:

    EXAMPLE   1000 mg : 1 g   = x mg : 2 g
                          (known quantities)   (unknown quantity)

Ratio and Proportion: Practice Problems

Answer the following questions.

1. What is a ratio?

   _____

2. In the space provided, place a check mark next to each correct example of a ratio.

   _____ a. 1000 mg × 10 grams

   _____ b. 1000 mL = 1 L

   _____ c. 1 mg : 1000 mcg

   _____ d. 1000 mg/1 gram

   _____ e. 1 tablespoon : 1 ounce

   _____ f. 1 mL : 1 cc

3. What is a proportion?

   _____

   _____

   _____

4. In the space provided, place a check mark next to each correct example of a proportion.

   _____ a. 1 mL : 1 cc

   _____ b. 2 tablespoons : 1 ounce = 4 tablespoons : 2 ounces

   _____ c. $2x$ = 60 mg

   _____ d. 1000 mL : 1 L = 500 mL : 0.5 L

   _____ e. 1000 mg : 1 gram = 1000 mL : 1 L

5. In the space provided, place a check mark next to each proportion that has correct sequencing for the units of measurement.

   _____ a. 1000 g : 1 kg = 1500 g : 1.5 kg

   _____ b. 3 teaspoons : 1 tablespoon = 2 tablespoons : 6 teaspoons

   _____ c. 1000 mg : 1 g = 2000 mg : x g

6. Circle the means and underline the extremes in each of the following proportions:
   a. 1000 mg : 1 g = 500 mg : 0.5 g
   b. 8 ounces : 1 glass = 16 ounces : 2 glasses
   c. 1 mL : 1 cc = 2 mL : 2cc

7. In each of the following proportions, what is the product of the means, and what is the product of the extremes?
   a. 1000 g : 1 kg = 1500 g : 1.5 kg

   _____ product of the means

   _____ product of the extremes

   b. 60 drops : 1 teaspoon = 120 drops : 2 teaspoons

   _____ product of the means

   _____ product of the extremes

545

c. 1 ounce : 30 mL = 4 ounces : 120 mL

_____ product of the means

_____ product of the extremes

8. In each of the following proportions, circle the known quantities and underline the unknown quantity.
   a. 1000 mg : 1 g = 500 mg : x g
   b. 2 tablespoons : 1 ounce = 6 tablespoons : x ounces
   c. 1000 mL : 1 L = x mL : 2 L

B. Converting Units Using Ratio and Proportion

Units can be converted using ratio and proportion.

Method of Conversion:
To convert a unit of measurement using ratio and proportion, use the following steps:
  a. Look at the appropriate conversion table at the end of this chapter to determine what is known about the two units of measurement (equivalent value).
  b. State the known quantities as a ratio.
  c. Determine the unknown quantity.
  d. State the unknown quantity as a ratio.
  e. Set up the proportion with the known quantities on the left side and the unknown quantity on the right side of the equation.
  f. To solve the equation, multiply the product of the means and the product of the extremes. Divide the equation by the number before the x.
  g. Include the unit of measure corresponding to x in the original equation with the answer.

EXAMPLES
PROBLEM   2 g = _____ mg
  a. Look at Table 11-1 (Metric Conversion) to determine what is known about the two units of measurement:
     1000 mg = 1 g
  b. State the known quantities as a ratio:
     1000 mg : 1 g
  c. Determine the unknown quantity:
     2 g = x mg
  d. State the unknown quantity as a ratio using the correct unit of measurement sequencing:
     x mg : 2 g
  e. Set up the proportion with the known quantities on the left side and the unknown quantity on the right side of the equation:
     1000 mg : 1 g = x mg : 2 g
  f. Solve the equation by multiplying the product of the means and the product of the extremes and dividing the equation by the number before the x:
     1000 mg : 1 g = x mg : 2 g
     $1 \times x = 1000 \times 2$
     $1x = 2000$
     $x = 2000$
  g. Include the unit of measure corresponding to x in the original equation with the answer:
     $x = 2000$ mg

Answer	2 g = 2000 mg

PROBLEM   4 ounces = _____ mL
The steps previously outlined are followed here. However, they are combined as they would be in working an actual conversion problem.
   1 ounce : 30 mL = 4 ounces : x mL
   $30 \times 4 = 1 \times x$
   $120 = 1x$
   $x = 120$ mL

Answer	4 ounces = 120 mL

Converting Units Using Ratio and Proportion: Practice Problems

Directions: Use ratio and proportion to convert between the metric and household systems by completing the problems below. In the space at the right, indicate what is known regarding the two units of measurement.

	ANSWER		KNOWN QUANTITIES
1. 30 drops	=	_____ mL	_____
2. 2 ounces	=	_____ mL	_____
3. 90 mL	=	_____ ounces	_____
4. 2 glasses	=	_____ mL	_____
5. 360 mL	=	_____ teacups	_____
6. 10 mL	=	_____ teaspoons	_____
7. 60 drops	=	_____ mL	_____
8. 60 mL	=	_____ tablespoons	_____
9. 3 teaspoons	=	_____ mL	_____
10. 5 mL	=	_____ drops	_____

UNIT 6: DETERMINING DRUG DOSAGE

A. Oral Administration

Dosage refers to the amount of medication to be administered to the patient. Each medication has a certain dosage range, or range of quantities that produce therapeutic effects. It is important to administer the exact drug dosage. If a dose is too small, it will not produce a therapeutic effect, whereas too large a dose could harm or even kill the patient. The steps to follow in determining drug dosage depend on the unit of measurement in which the drug is ordered and the unit of measurement of the drug you have available, or the dose on hand.

1. If the dose on hand is the same as that ordered, no calculation is required. In this example, the dose ordered and the dose on hand are in the same unit of measurement, and one tablet is administered to the patient.

    EXAMPLE   The provider orders 50 mg of a medication po.
    The drug label reads 50 mg/tablet.

2. If the dosage ordered is in the same unit of measurement as that indicated on the medication label, only one calculation step is required. In this example, the dose ordered and the dose on hand are in the same unit of measurement, or milligrams. The calculation determines the number of tablets to administer to the patient.

    EXAMPLE   The provider orders 500 mg of a medication po.
    The drug label reads 250 mg/tablet.

3. If the dosage ordered is in a different unit of measurement than indicated on the drug label, two calculation steps are required to determine the amount of medication to administer to the patient. In this example, the dose ordered and the dose on hand are stated in different units of measurement, or in grams and milligrams. The first step requires conversion of the dose ordered to the unit of measurement of the dose on hand; in this example, grams must be converted to milligrams. The second step is to determine the number of tablets to administer to the patient.

    EXAMPLE   The provider orders 1 g of a medication po.
    The drug label reads 500 mg/tablet.

A detailed discussion of determining drug dosage for administration of oral medication follows. The method used to calculate drug dosage when the units of measurement are the same is presented first, followed by the method used when the units of measurement are different.

Determining Drug Dosage with the Same Units of Measurement

Determining the correct drug dosage to be administered when the units of measurement are the same requires the use of a drug dosage formula.

Drug Dosage Formula

$$\frac{D\,(\textit{dose ordered})}{H\,(\textit{on hand})} \times V\,(\textit{vehicle}) = x\,(\text{amount of medication to be administered})$$

D (*dose ordered*): This is the amount of medication ordered by the provider.

H (*drug strength on hand*): This is the dosage strength available as indicated on the medication label or the dose on hand.

V (*vehicle*): The vehicle refers to the type of preparation containing the dose on hand (e.g., tablet, capsule, liquid).

x: The letter *x* is used to express the unknown quantity or the amount of medication to be administered.

Guidelines

1. The units of measurement must be included when setting up the problem.
2. The values for D and H must be in the same unit of measurement.
3. The value of *x* is expressed in the same unit as V.
4. When determining the drug dosage for oral liquid medication, the vehicle must also include the amount of liquid in which the available drug is contained. For example, if the medication label reads 250 mg/5 mL, the value of V is 5 mL.

The method to follow to determine drug dosage using this formula is outlined in the following examples. The first problem illustrates determining the dosage for solid medication taken orally.

EXAMPLES

PROBLEM   *Oral solid medication:*
           The provider orders 50 mg of a medication po.
           The medication label reads 25 mg/tablet.
           How much medication should be administered to the patient?

Drug dosage formula:

$$\frac{D}{H} \times V = x$$

a. Identify the dose ordered.
   D = 50 mg

b. Identify the strength of the drug on hand.
   H = 25 mg

c. Determine the vehicle containing the dose on hand.
   V = 1 tablet

d. Calculate the amount of medication to administer to the patient. The units of measurement must be included when setting up the problem, and the values for D and H must be in the same unit of measurement. The value of *x* is expressed in the same unit as V; in this problem V = 1 tablet.

$$\frac{50\text{ mg}}{25\text{ mg}} \times 1\text{ tablet} = x$$
$$(50 \div 25 = 2) \times 1\text{ tablet} = x$$
$$2 \times 1\text{ tablet} = x$$
$$x = 2\text{ tablets}$$

Answer	2 tablets administered to the patient

The next problem illustrates the determination of drug dosage for liquid medication taken orally. The steps previously outlined are followed; however, they are combined as should be done when working out drug dosage problems. Remember, with oral liquid medication, the vehicle must also include the amount of liquid in which the available drug is contained; in the following problem, V = 5 mL.

PROBLEM   *Oral liquid medication:*
           The provider orders 500 mg of a medication.
           The medication label reads 250 mg/5 mL.
           How much medication should be administered to the patient?

$$\frac{D}{H} \times 1 \text{ tablet} = x$$

$$\frac{500 \text{ mg}}{250 \text{ mg}} \times 1 \text{ tablet} = x$$

$(500 \div 250 = 2) \times 5 \text{ mL} = x$

$2 \times 5 \text{ mL} = x$

$x = 10 \text{ mL}$

Answer	A dose of 10 mL of medication is administered to the patient.

Determining Drug Dosage with Different Units of Measurement

Sometimes, the medication ordered is in a different unit of measurement than indicated on the drug label. In this case, the desired dose quantity must be converted to the unit of measurement of the dose on hand before the drug dosage is determined. The method chosen to convert a unit of measurement is based on personal preference. Refer to Units 4 and 5 to review methods of conversion before completing this section.

The following steps are required to determine drug dosage when the units of measurement are different:
Step 1: Convert the dose quantities to the same unit of measurement. For consistency, it is best to convert to the unit of measurement of the drug on hand.
Step 2: Determine the amount of medication to administer to the patient, using the drug dosage formula.

EXAMPLES

PROBLEM   *Oral solid medication:*
           The provider orders 0.5 gram of medication po.
           The medication label reads 250 mg/tablet.
           How much medication should be administered to the patient?

Step 1: The dosage ordered must be converted to the unit of measurement of the medication on hand. In this problem, 0.5 gram must be converted to milligrams. The ratio and proportion method of conversion is used to make the conversion.

1 gram = _____ mg
1 gram : 1000 mg = 0.5 gram : x mg
$500 = 1x$
$x = 500$ mg

Answer	0.5 gram = 500 mg

The medication ordered is in the same unit of measurement as the medication on hand.
Step 2: Determine the amount of medication to administer to the patient using the drug dosage formula.

$$\frac{D}{H} \times V = x$$

$$\frac{500 \text{ mg}}{250 \text{ mg}} \times 1 \text{ tablet}$$

$(500 \div 250 = 2) \times 1 \text{ tablet} = x$

$2 \times 1 \text{ tablet} = x$

$x = 2$ tablets

Answer	A dose of 2 tablets is administered to the patient.

PROBLEM   *Oral liquid medication:*
           The provider orders 0.5 gram of a medication po.
           The medication label reads 125 mg/5 mL.
           How much medication should be administered to the patient?

Step 1: Convert 0.5 gram to milligrams using ratio and proportion:

0.5 gram = _____ mg

1 gram : 1000 mg = 0.5 gram : x mg

$1x$ = 500 mg

x = 500 mg

Answer	0.5 gram = 500 mg

Step 2: Determine the amount of medication to administer to the patient using the drug dosage formula.

$$\frac{D}{H} \times V = x$$

$$\frac{500 \text{ mg}}{125 \text{ mg}} \times 5 \text{ mL} = x$$

$(500 \div 125 = 4) \times 5 \text{ mL} = x$

$4 \times 5 \text{ mL} = x$

x = 20 mL

Answer	A dose of 20 mL of medication is administered to the patient.

Oral Administration: Practice Problems

Directions: Determine the drug dosage to be administered for each of the following oral medication orders, and document your answer below. In the space provided, indicate the drug category based on action for each medication using a drug reference.

Oral Solid Medications

1. The provider orders Inderal 160 mg po.
   Medication label:

Inderal
propranolol
80 mg/capsule

   How much medication should be administered? _____

   Drug category: _____

2. The provider orders Tagamet 600 mg po.
   Medication label:

Tagamet
cimetidine
300 mg/tablet

   How much medication should be administered? _____

   Drug category: _____

3. The provider orders Amoxil 0.5 g po.
   Medication label:

Amoxil
amoxicillin
250 mg/capsule

   How much medication should be administered? _____

   Drug category: _____

4. The provider orders Lasix 80 mg po.
   Medication label:

Lasix furosemide 40 mg/tablet

   How much medication should be administered? _____

   Drug category: _____

5. The provider orders Lomotil 5 mg po.
   Medication label:

Lomotil diphenoxylate/atropine 2.5 mg/tablet

   How much medication should be administered? _____

   Drug category: _____

6. The provider orders Zithromax 0.5 g po.
   Medication label:

Zithromax azithromycin 250 mg/tablet

   How much medication should be administered? _____

   Drug category: _____

7. The provider orders Calan 120 mg po.
   Medication label:

Calan verapamil 40 mg/tablet

   How much medication should be administered? _____

   Drug category: _____

8. The provider orders Xanax 0.5 mg po.
   Medication label:

Xanax alprazolam 0.25 mg/tablet

   How much medication should be administered? _____

   Drug category: _____

9. The provider orders Phenergan 25 mg po.
   Medication label:

Phenergan
promethazine
12.5 mg/tablet

   How much medication should be administered? _____

   Drug category: _____

10. The provider orders Procardia XL 30 mg po.
    Medication label:

Procardia
nifedipine
10 mg/tablet

    How much medication should be administered? _____

    Drug category: _____

Oral Liquid Medications

1. The provider orders Sumycin Suspension 250 mg po.
   Medication label:

Sumycin Suspension
tetracycline
125 mg/5 mL

   How much medication should be administered? _____

   Drug category: _____

2. The provider orders Tagamet liquid 300 mg po.
   Medication label:

Tagamet
cimetidine liquid
300 mg/5 mL

   How much medication should be administered? _____

   Drug category: _____

3. The provider orders Tylenol Elixir 60 mg po.
   Medication label:

Tylenol Elixir
acetaminophen
120 mg/5 mL

   How much medication should be administered? _____

   Drug category: _____

4. The provider orders Amoxil Suspension 0.5 g po.
   Medication label:

Amoxil Suspension
amoxicillin
125 mg/5 mL

   How much medication should be administered? _____

   Drug category: _____

5. The provider orders Gantanol Suspension 1 g po.
   Medication label:

Gantanol Suspension
sulfamethoxazole
500 mg/5 mL

   How much medication should be administered? _____

   Drug category: _____

B. Parenteral Administration

Medications for parenteral administration must be suspended in solution. The medication label indicates the amount of the drug contained in each milliliter of solution. For example, if a medication label reads 10 mg/mL, there are 10 mg of medication for each 1 mL of liquid volume. Some medications, such as penicillin, insulin, and heparin, are ordered and measured in units (e.g., 300,000 units/mL). This refers to their biologic activity in animal tests or the amount of the drug that is required to produce a particular response.

Parenteral medication is available in several dispensing forms, including ampules, single-dose vials, and multiple-dose vials. After the proper drug dosage has been determined, the medication is drawn into a syringe from the dispensing unit. Most syringes are calibrated in milliliters (mL).

Determining drug dosage for parenteral administration is calculated in a similar manner as that for oral liquid medication. The first problem illustrates the determination of drug dosage when the medication is ordered in a different unit of measurement from the dose on hand, requiring two calculation steps.

EXAMPLES

PROBLEM   The provider orders 0.5 g of a medication IM.
The medication label reads 250 mg/2 mL.
How much medication should be administered?

Step 1: Convert 0.5 gram to milligrams.
0.5 gram = _____ mg
1000 mg : 1 g = x mg : 0.5 g
$1x = 500$
$x = 500$ mg

Answer	0.5 mg = 500 mg

Step 2: Determine the amount of medication to administer to the patient:

$$\frac{D}{H} \times V = x$$

$$\frac{500 \text{ mg}}{250 \text{ mg}} \times 2 \text{ mL} = x$$

$(500 \div 250 = 2) \times 2 \text{ mL} = x$
$2 \times 2 \text{ mL} = x$
$x = 4 \text{ mL}$

Answer	A dose of 4 mL of medication is administered to the patient.

553

The next problem illustrates the determination of drug dosage with a medication ordered in units. Notice that the dose ordered and the dose on hand are in the same unit of measurement; therefore, conversion of units of measurement is not necessary.

PROBLEM   The provider orders 600,000 units of a medication IM.
The medication label reads 300,000 units/mL.
How much medication should be administered?

$$\frac{D}{H} \times V = x$$

$$\frac{600,000 \text{ units}}{300,000 \text{ units}} \times 1 \text{ mL} = x$$

$$(600,000 \div 300,000 = 2) \times 1 \text{ mL} = x$$

$$x = 2 \text{ mL}$$

Answer	A dose of 2 mL of medication is administered to the patient.

Parenteral Administration: Practice Problems

Determine the drug dosage to be administered for each of the following parenteral medication orders, and document your answer. In the space provided, indicate the drug category based on action using a drug reference.

1. The provider orders Vistaril 75 mg IM.
   Medication label:

   > Vistaril
   > hydroxyzine injection
   > 50 mg/mL

   How much medication should be administered? _____

   Drug category: _____

2. The provider orders Cobex (vitamin B_{12}) 200 mcg IM.
   Medication label:

   > Cobex
   > cyanocobalamin injection
   > 100 mcg/mL

   How much medication should be administered? _____

   Drug category: _____

3. The provider orders Depo-Medrol 40 mg IM.
   Medication label:

   > Depo-Medrol
   > methylprednisolone injection
   > 80 mg/mL

   How much medication should be administered? _____

   Drug category: _____

4. The provider orders Wycillin 600,000 units IM.
   Medication label:

   > Wycillin
   > porcine penicillin G injection
   > 300,000 units/mL

   How much medication should be administered? _____

   Drug category: _____

5. The provider orders Rocephin 1000 mg IM.
   Medication label:

Rocephin
ceftriaxone injection
1 g/mL

   How much medication should be administered? _____

   Drug category: _____

6. The provider orders INFeD 100 mg IM.
   Medication label:

INFeD
iron dextran injection
50 mg/mL

   How much medication should be administered? _____

   Drug category: _____

7. The provider orders Bicillin 1.2 million units IM.
   Medication label:

Bicillin
benzathine penicillin G injection
600,000 units/mL

   How much medication should be administered? _____

   Drug category: _____

8. The provider orders Depo-Provera 150 mg IM.
   Medication label:

Depo-Provera
medroxyprogesterone
150 mg/mL

   How much medication should be administered? _____

   Drug category: _____

9. The provider orders Pronestyl 0.25 g IM.
   Medication label:

Pronestyl
procainamide injection
500 mg/mL

   How much medication should be administered? _____

   Drug category: _____

10. The provider orders Compazine 7 mg IM.
    Medication label:

Compazine
prochlorperazine injection
5 mg/mL

    How much medication should be administered? _____

    Drug category: _____

Table 11-1 Metric System Conversion of Equivalent Values

WEIGHT
1000 micrograms = 1 milligram
1000 milligrams = 1 gram
1000 grams = 1 kilogram

VOLUME
1000 milliliters = 1 liter
1000 liters = 1 kiloliter
1 milliliter = 1 cubic centimeter

Table 11-2 Household System: Conversion of Equivalent Values

ABBREVIATIONS
drop: gtt
teaspoon: tsp
tablespoon: T
ounce: oz
cup: c

VOLUME
60 drops = 1 teaspoon
3 teaspoons = 1 tablespoon
6 teaspoons = 1 ounce
2 tablespoons = 1 ounce
6 ounces = 1 teacup
8 ounces = 1 glass
8 ounces = 1 cup

Table 11-3 Conversion Chart for Household and Metric Equivalents (Volume)

Household		Metric
1 drop	=	0.06 mL
15 drops	=	1 mL (cc)
1 teaspoon	=	5 (4) mL
1 tablespoon	=	15 mL
2 tablespoons	=	30 mL
1 ounce	=	30 mL
1 teacup	=	180 mL
1 glass	=	240 mL

12 Cardiopulmonary Procedures

CHAPTER ASSIGNMENTS

√ After Completing	Date Due	Study Guide Pages	STUDY GUIDE ASSIGNMENTS (CTA = Critical Thinking Activity)	Possible Points	Points You Earned
		561	?≡ Pretest	10	
		562-563	✎Term Key Term Assessment A. Definitions B. Word Parts (Add 1 point for each key term)	21 15	
		563-571	✐ Evaluation of Learning questions	64	
		571	CTA A. Chest Leads	5	
			e Evolve Activity: Find That Lead (Record points earned)		
		571	CTA B: ECG Cycle	10	
			e Evolve Site: It's a Cycle (Record points earned)		
			e Evolve Site: It's an Artifact (Record points earned)		
		572	CTA C: Myocardial Infarction	20	
		575	CTA D: Crossword Puzzle	29	
			e Evolve Site: Apply Your Knowledge questions	10	
			e Evolve Site: Video Evaluation	33	
		561	?≡ Posttest	10	
			ADDITIONAL ASSIGNMENTS		
			Total points		

√ When Assigned by Your Instructor	Study Guide Pages	Practices Required	LABORATORY ASSIGNMENTS (Procedure Number and Name)	Score*
	576	3	**e** **Practice for Competency** 12-1: Running a 12-Lead, Three-Channel Electrocardiogram Textbook reference: pp. 470-473	
	579-581		**Evaluation of Competency** 12-1: Running a 12-Lead, Three-Channel Electrocardiogram	*
	576	3	**Practice for Competency** 12-2: Applying a Holter Monitor Textbook reference: pp. 476-479	
	583-585		**Evaluation of Competency** 12-2: Applying a Holter Monitor	*
	577	3	**e** **Practice for Competency** 12-3: Spirometry Testing Textbook reference: p. 487-489	
	587-589		**Evaluation of Competency** 12-3: Spirometry Testing	*
	577-578	3	**e** **Practice for Competency** 12-4: Measuring Peak Flow Rate Textbook reference: pp. 494-495	
	591-593		**Evaluation of Competency** 12-4: Measuring Peak Flow Rate	*
			ADDITIONAL ASSIGNMENTS	

Notes

Name: _____   Date: _____

True or False

_____ 1. The cardiac cycle represents one complete heartbeat.

_____ 2. The portion of the ECG between two waves is known as a segment.

_____ 3. A standard electrocardiogram consists of 10 leads.

_____ 4. An electrolyte facilitates the transmission of electrical impulses.

_____ 5. Leads V_1 through V_6 are known as the augmented leads.

_____ 6. Electrodes that are too loose can cause a 60-cycle interference artifact.

_____ 7. When running an ECG, the medical assistant should work on the left side of the patient.

_____ 8. An electrocardiographic (ECG) result that is within normal limits is said to indicate a normal sinus rhythm.

_____ 9. The purpose of a pulmonary function test is to assess cardiac functioning.

_____ 10. During an asthma attack, the bronchial tubes constrict, swell, and become clogged with mucus.

📄 **POSTTEST**

True or False

_____ 1. An electrocardiogram is a recording of the electrical activity of the heart.

_____ 2. The amplifier is a device placed on the skin that picks up electrical impulses released by the heart.

_____ 3. The P wave represents the contraction of the ventricles.

_____ 4. If the electrocardiograph is standardized, the standardization mark will be 20 mm high.

_____ 5. A muscle artifact can be identified by its fuzzy, irregular baseline.

_____ 6. A spirometer measures how much air is exhaled from the lungs and how fast it is exhaled.

_____ 7. Spirometry can be used to assess a patient with emphysema.

_____ 8. Quick-relief asthma medication is used to prevent asthma symptoms.

_____ 9. The amount of supplemental oxygen prescribed for a patient is known as the flow rate.

_____ 10. A nasal cannula interferes with a patient's ability to talk, eat, and drink.

A. Definitions

Directions: Match each key term with its definition.

_____ D _____ 1. Artifact

_____ N _____ 2. Atherosclerosis

_____ B _____ 3. Baseline

_____ F _____ 4. Cardiac cycle

_____ O _____ 5. Dysrhythmia

_____ I _____ 6. ECG cycle

_____ G _____ 7. Electrocardiogram

_____ C _____ 8. Electrocardiograph

_____ P _____ 9. Flow rate

_____ J _____ 10. Electrode

_____ A _____ 11. Electrolyte

_____ Q _____ 12. Hypoxemia

_____ R _____ 13. Hypoxia

_____ H _____ 14. Interval

_____ L _____ 15. Ischemia

_____ E _____ 16. Normal sinus rhythm

_____ S _____ 17. Oxygen therapy

_____ T _____ 18. Peak flow rate

_____ K _____ 19. Segment

_____ M _____ 20. Spirometer

_____ U _____ 21. Wheezing

A. A chemical substance that promotes conduction of an electrical current

B. The flat, horizontal line that separates the various waves of the ECG cycle

C. The instrument used to record the electrical activity of the heart

D. Additional electrical activity picked up by the electrocardiograph that interferes with the normal appearance of the ECG cycles

E. Refers to an electrocardiogram that is within normal limits

F. One complete heartbeat

G. The graphic representation of the electrical activity of the heart

H. The length of one or more waves and a segment

I. The graphic representation of a heartbeat

J. A conductor of electricity, which is used to promote contact between the body and the electrocardiograph

K. The portion of the ECG between two waves

L. Deficiency of blood in a body part

M. An instrument for measuring air taken into and expelled from the lungs

N. Buildup of fibrous plaques of fatty deposits and cholesterol on the inner walls of an artery that causes narrowing, obstruction, and hardening of the artery

O. An irregular heart rate or rhythm

P. The number of liters of oxygen per minute that come out of an oxygen delivery system

Q. A decrease in the oxygen saturation of the blood

R. A reduction in the oxygen supply to the tissues of the body

S. The administration of supplemental oxygen at concentrations greater than room air to treat or prevent hypoxemia

T. The maximum volume of air that can be exhaled when a patient blows into a peak flow meter as forcefully and as rapidly as possible

U. A continuous, high-pitched whistling musical sound heard particularly during exhalation and sometimes during inhalation

B. Word Parts

Directions: Indicate the meaning of each word part in the space provided. List as many medical terms as possible that incorporate the word part in the space provided.

Word Part	Meaning of Word Part	Medical Terms That Incorporate Word Part
1. ather/o		
2. -sclerosis		
3. cardi/o		
4. electr/o		
5. dys-		
6. -gram		
7. -graph		
8. hypo-		
9. ox/i		
10. -emia		
11. -ia		
12. isch/o		
13. spir/o		
14. -meter		
15. -metry		

EVALUATION OF LEARNING

Directions: Fill in each blank with the correct answer.

1. What is the purpose of electrocardiography?

   _____

   _____

   _____

2. Trace the path blood takes through the heart, starting with the right atrium.

   _____

   _____

   _____

3. What is the function of the coronary arteries?

   _____

   _____

4. What is the function of the SA node?

_____

_____

5. Why is the impulse initiated by the SA node delayed momentarily by the AV node?

_____

6. What is the cardiac cycle?

_____

7. Label the following on the ECG cycle:

P wave	P–R segment
QRS complex	S–T segment
T wave	P–R interval
Q–T interval	

8. Explain what each component of the ECG cycle represents.

P wave _____

QRS complex _____

T wave _____

P–R segment _____

S–T segment _____

P–R interval _____

Q–T interval _____

9. Why is the R wave taller than the P wave on the ECG graph cycle?

_____

_____

10. Why does atrial repolarization not appear as a separate wave on the ECG cycle?

_____

_____

11. Why is the baseline flat following the U wave?

_____

_____

12. What changes can occur on an ECG due to the following?

    a. Coronary artery disease: _____

    b. Myocardial infarction: _____

13. What is the purpose of standardizing the electrocardiograph?

_____

_____

_____

14. How high should the standardization mark be when the electrocardiograph is standardized?

_____

15. What is a lead, and what information does it provide?

_____

_____

16. What is the function of an electrode?

_____

_____

17. What is the function of each of the following?

    a. Amplifier: _____

    b. Galvanometer: _____

    c. Thermal print head: _____

18. Which electrode is used as a ground reference? _____

19. Why must an electrolyte be used when recording an electrocardiogram?

_____

_____

_____

20. Why should the expiration date on an electrode pouch be checked?

_____

_____

21. How should electrodes be stored?

_____

_____

565

22. Diagram the bipolar leads on the following illustration:

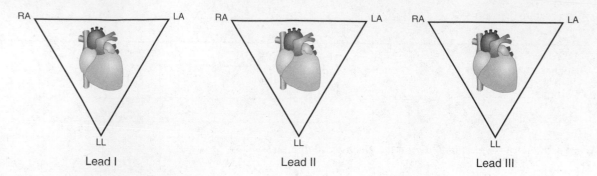

Lead I   Lead II   Lead III

23. Locate and label the locations of the chest electrodes on the following illustration:

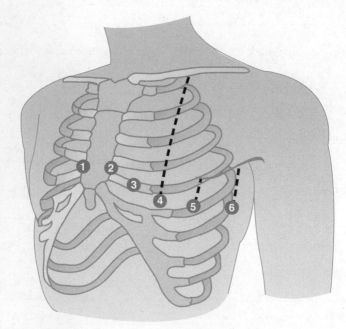

24. What patient preparation is required for an ECG?

_____

_____

25. What maintenance should be performed on an ECG machine?

_____

_____

26. At what speed does the paper move while recording a normal electrocardiogram?

_____

27. What is the difference between a three-channel and a single-channel electrocardiograph?

_____

_____

_____

28. What is the purpose of each of the following electrocardiograph capabilities?

    a. Interpretive capability

    _____

    _____

    b. EMR connectivity

    _____

    _____

    c. Teletransmission

    _____

    _____

29. Why should artifacts be eliminated if they occur in an ECG recording?

    _____

    _____

    _____

30. What is the function of an artifact filter?

    _____

31. List three possible causes of muscle artifacts.

    _____

    _____

    _____

32. List three possible causes of wandering baseline.

    _____

    _____

33. List three possible causes of 60-cycle interference artifacts.

    _____

    _____

    _____

34. List four uses of Holter monitor electrocardiography.

    _____

    _____

    _____

    _____

35. Explain the use of the patient diary in Holter monitor electrocardiography.

_____

_____

_____

36. List five guidelines that should be relayed to the patient undergoing Holter monitor electrocardiography.

_____

_____

_____

_____

_____

37. List the distinguishing characteristics of each of the following cardiac arrhythmias.

    a. Paroxysmal supraventricular tachycardia

    _____

    _____

    b. Atrial fibrillation

    _____

    _____

    c. Premature ventricular contraction

    _____

    _____

    d. Ventricular fibrillation

    _____

    _____

38. What is the purpose of a pulmonary function test?

_____

39. What are the indications for performing spirometry?

_____

_____

_____

40. What patient preparation is required for spirometry?

_____

_____

_____

41. What is the purpose of postbronchodilator spirometry?

_____

_____

42. What are the characteristics of asthma?

_____

_____

43. What are five examples of allergens that may trigger an asthma attack?

_____

_____

44. What are five examples of environmental irritants, activities, or events that may trigger an asthma attack?

_____

_____

45. What happens to the bronchial tubes during an asthma attack?

_____

_____

46. What is the purpose of long-term-control asthma medication?

_____

_____

47. What is the purpose of quick-relief asthma medication?

_____

_____

48. What is the purpose of a peak flow meter?

_____

_____

49. What is the difference between a low-range and full-range peak flow meter?

_____

_____

50. What is the purpose of peak flow measurements?

_____

_____

_____

569

51. Why is oxygen needed by the body?

_____

_____

52. What occurs when the body cannot maintain an adequate oxygen level?

_____

_____

53. What conditions may require home oxygen therapy?

_____

_____

54. What information is included on a prescription for home oxygen therapy?

_____

_____

55. What are the advantages and disadvantages of compressed oxygen gas?

a. Advantages:

_____

_____

b. Disadvantages:

_____

_____

56. What is liquid oxygen?

_____

_____

57. What are the advantages and disadvantages of liquid oxygen?

a. Advantages:

_____

_____

b. Disadvantages:

_____

_____

58. What is an oxygen concentrator?

_____

_____

59. What is the primary advantage of using a nasal cannula to administer oxygen?

_____

_____

60. List two reasons for using a face mask to administer oxygen therapy.

_____

_____

61. What are the symptoms of a low oxygen level in the body?

_____

_____

62. How much tubing should be used with an oxygen delivery system and why?

_____

_____

63. What occurs if oxygen comes in contact with a fire?

_____

_____

64. How should oxygen be stored?

_____

_____

CRITICAL THINKING ACTIVITIES

A. Chest Leads

Practice locating the six chest leads on five individuals. Select individuals of both genders and of varying ages and body contours. Document each person's name here after you have successfully located the chest leads. Document any problems you encountered locating the leads.

1. _____

2. _____

3. _____

4. _____

5. _____

B. ECG Cycle

Attach part of an ECG from a recording. Identify and label the various waves, intervals, and segments making up an ECG cycle on two of the leads.

C. Myocardial Infarction

You are working for a cardiologist. Your provider is concerned about the increase in the numbers of patients having heart attacks. He asks you to design a colorful, creative, and informative brochure on heart attacks using the brochure provided on the following page. This brochure will be published and placed in the waiting room to provide patients with education about heart attacks. Heart disease Internet sites can be used to complete this activity.

FAQ
ON:

Q: A:

Q: A:

Q: A:

Q: A:

Q: A:

Q: A:

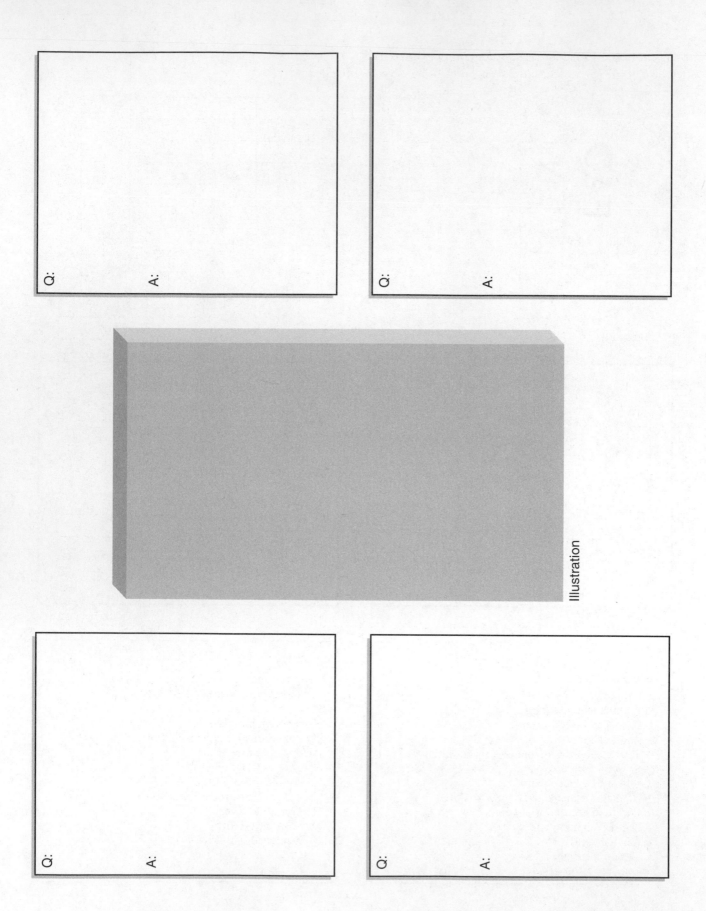

Illustration

Q: A:

Q: A:

D. Crossword Puzzle: Cardiopulmonary Procedures

Directions: Complete the crossword puzzle using the clues provided.

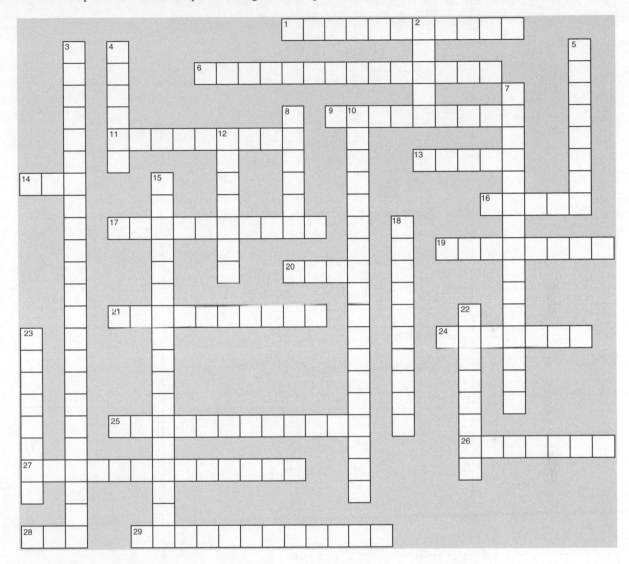

Across
1. Rhythm not normal
6. Drug that opens air passages
9. Asthma allergen trigger
11. Damaged alveoli disease
13. Atria contract
14. Take a deep breath and blow it all out!
16. Mighty big artery
17. Lower heart chambers
19. Keep this blanket away from a Holter
20. Fourth intercostal to the left
21. "How well can you breathe?" test
24. Leads I, II, III
25. O_2 administration device
26. Delivers asthma med
27. Drug for angina
28. ECG std mark in mm
29. Inflammation of heart's lining

Down
2. The ventricles are recovering
3. Serious rhythm disturbance
4. Not with a Holter on
5. Not enough blood
7. Coronary artery plaque condition
8. Pacemaker of the heart
10. Separates O_2 out of air
12. Primary cause of COPD
15. "Too loose" electrodes cause this
18. Heart muscle layer
22. Left-side heart valve
23. High-pitched whistling sound

Procedure 12-1: 12-Lead Electrocardiogram

Practice the procedure for running a 12-lead electrocardiogram, and document the procedure in the chart provided.

Procedure 12-2: Holter Monitor

1. Activity diary. Complete the patient information section on the Holter Activity Diary below.
2. Holter monitor. Practice the procedure for applying the Holter monitor, and document the procedure in the chart provided.

HOLTER MONITOR

PATIENT ACTIVITY DIARY

☐ 10 Hr.   ☐ 12 Hr.   ☐ 24 Hr.   ☐ 26 Hr.

Patient's Name: _____

Patient's Address: _____

_____

Age: _____ Sex: _____ Phone: _____

Date of Birth: _____ Soc. Sec. #: _____

Medication: _____

Doctor: _____ Phone: _____

Hospital: _____ Room: _____

Date of Recording: _____ Started: _____ AM PM

Serial Numbers

Recorder: _____

Battery: _____

Connected by: _____

_____

Procedure 12-3: Spirometry

Practice the procedure for performing a spirometry test, and document the procedure in the chart provided.

Procedure 12-4: Peak Flow Rate Measurement

Practice the procedure for measuring peak flow rate, and document the procedure in the chart provided.

CHART	
Date	

PEAK FLOW CHART

Name _____

DATE															
TIME															
800															
750															
700															
650															
600															
550															
500															
450															
400															
350															
300															
250															
200															
150															
100															
50															
Peak Flow Number															

Procedure 12-1: Running a 12-Lead, Three-Channel Electrocardiogram

Name: _____   Date: _____

Evaluated by: _____   Score: _____

Performance Objective

Outcome:	Record a 12-lead electrocardiogram.
Conditions:	Using a three-channel electrocardiograph.
Standards:	Given ECG paper and disposable electrodes.
	Time: 15 minutes. Student completed procedure in _____ minutes.
	Accuracy: Satisfactory score on the Performance Evaluation Checklist.

Performance Evaluation Checklist

Trial 1	Trial 2	Point Value	Performance Standards
		•	Worked in a quiet atmosphere away from sources of electrical interference.
		•	Sanitized hands.
		•	Checked the expiration date of the electrodes.
		▷	Explained what may occur if the electrodes are outdated.
		•	Greeted the patient and introduced yourself.
		•	Identified the patient and explained the procedure.
		•	Instructed the patient that he or she will need to lie still, breathe normally, and not talk during the procedure.
		▷	Explained why the patient should lie still and not talk.
		•	Asked the patient to remove appropriate clothing.
		•	Assisted the patient into a supine position on the table.
		•	Made sure that the patient's arms and legs were adequately supported on the table.
		•	Draped the patient properly.
		•	Positioned the electrocardiograph with the power cord pointing away from the patient and not passing under the table.
		•	Worked on the left side of the patient.
		•	Prepared the patient's skin for application of the disposable electrodes.
		▷	Explained why the patient's skin must be prepared properly.
		•	Applied the limb electrodes.
		•	Properly located each chest position and applied the chest electrodes.
		▷	Explained why the tabs of the electrodes should be positioned correctly.
		•	Connected the lead wires to the electrodes.

Trial 1	Trial 2	Point Value	Performance Standards
		•	Arranged the lead wires to follow body contour.
		▷	Explained why the lead wires should follow body contour.
		•	Plugged the patient's cable into the machine and properly supported the cable.
		•	Turned on the electrocardiograph.
		•	Entered the patient's data using the soft-touch keypad.
		▷	Stated the purpose of entering the patient's data.
		•	Reminded the patient to lie still, and pressed the AUTO button to run the recording.
		•	Checked to make sure the standardization mark is 10 mm high.
		•	Checked to make sure the R wave has a positive deflection.
		▷	Stated what would cause the R wave to have a negative deflection.
		•	Checked the recording for artifacts and corrected them if they occurred.
		•	Informed the patient that he or she can move and talk.
		•	Turned off the electrocardiograph.
		•	Disconnected the lead wires.
		•	Removed and discarded the disposable electrodes.
		•	Assisted the patient from the table.
		•	Sanitized hands.
		•	Documented the procedure correctly.
		•	Placed the recording in the appropriate place to be reviewed by the provider.
		•	Returned equipment to proper place.
			Demonstrated the following affective behavior(s) during this procedure:
		Ⓐ	Incorporated critical thinking skills when performing patient assessment.
		Ⓐ	Showed awareness of a patient's concerns related to the procedure being performed.
		Ⓐ	Explained to a patient the rationale for performance of a procedure.
		★	Completed the procedure within 15 minutes.
			Totals

CHART	
Date	

Evaluation of Student Performance

EVALUATION CRITERIA			COMMENTS
Symbol	**Category**	**Point Value**	
★	Critical Step	16 points	
•	Essential Step	6 points	
Ⓐ	Affective Competency	6 points	
▷	Theory Question	2 points	

Score calculation: 100 points

− _____ points missed

_____ Score

Satisfactory score: 85 or above

CAAHEP Competencies Achieved

Psychomotor (Skills)
☑ I. 2. a. Perform electrocardiography.
☑ I. 8. Instruct and prepare a patient for a procedure or a treatment.
☑ V. 3. Use medical terminology correctly and pronounced accurately to communicate information to providers and patients.
☑ VI. 8. Perform routine maintenance of administrative or clinical equipment.

Affective (Behavior)
☑ I. 1. Incorporate critical thinking skills when performing patient assessment.
☑ I. 3. Show awareness of a patient's concerns related to the procedure being performed.
☑ V. 4. Explain to a patient the rationale for performance of a procedure.

ABHES Competencies Achieved

☑ 2. c. Identify diagnostic and treatment modalities as they relate to each body system.
☑ 7. g. Display professionalism through written and verbal communications.
☑ 8. e. Perform specialty procedures including but not limited to minor surgery, cardiac, respiratory, OB-GYN, neurological, and gastroenterology.

Notes

Procedure 12-2: Applying a Holter Monitor

Name: _____   Date: _____

Evaluated by: _____   Score: _____

Performance Objective

Outcome:	Apply a Holter monitor.
Conditions:	Using a Holter monitor with an internal memory card.
Standards:	Given the following: battery, disposable pouch and lanyard or a belt clip, disposable electrodes, razor, antiseptic wipes, gauze pads, abrasive pad, nonallergenic tape, and a patient diary.
	Time: 20 minutes. Student completed procedure in _____ minutes.
	Accuracy: Satisfactory score on the Performance Evaluation Checklist.

Performance Evaluation Checklist

Trial 1	Trial 2	Point Value	Performance Standards
		•	Assembled equipment.
		•	Installed a new battery.
		•	Checked the expiration date of the electrodes.
		•	Connected the Holter monitor to the computer.
		•	Entered the patient's demographic data into the computer and downloaded this information to the monitor.
		•	Sanitized hands.
		•	Greeted the patient and introduced yourself.
		•	Identified the patient and explained the procedure.
		•	Instructed the patient in the guidelines for wearing a Holter monitor.
		•	Asked the patient to remove clothing from the waist up.
		•	Positioned the patient in a sitting position.
		•	Located the chest electrode placement sites.
		•	Shaved the patient's chest at each electrode site, if needed.
		•	Rubbed the patient's skin with an alcohol wipe and allowed it to dry.
		•	Slightly abraded the skin.
		▷	Explained why the skin should be abraded.
		•	Attached a lead wire to the snap of each electrode.
		•	Properly applied the electrodes with an attached lead wire.
		▷	Explained why the electrodes should be firmly attached.
		•	Plugged the patient cable into the monitor and turned on the monitor.

583

Trial 1	Trial 2	Point Value	Performance Standards
		•	Checked the ECG signal quality.
		▷	Stated why the signal quality should be clear and strong.
		•	Placed tape over each electrode.
		•	Checked to make sure the date and time displayed on the monitor are accurate.
		•	Started the monitor.
		•	Placed the pouch around the patient's neck and inserted the monitor in the pouch.
		•	Instructed the patient to get dressed.
		•	Completed the patient information section of the diary.
		•	Documented the starting time in the patient diary.
		•	Provided the patient with instructions on completing the diary.
		•	Instructed the patient when to return for removal of the monitor.
		•	Sanitized hands.
		•	Documented the procedure correctly.
			Demonstrated the following affective behavior(s) during this procedure:
		Ⓐ	Incorporated critical thinking skills when performing patient assessment.
		Ⓐ	Showed awareness of a patient's concerns related to the procedure being performed.
		Ⓐ	Explained to a patient the rationale for performance of a procedure.
		★	Completed the procedure within 20 minutes.
			Totals

CHART	
Date	

Evaluation of Student Performance

EVALUATION CRITERIA			COMMENTS
Symbol	**Category**	**Point Value**	
★	Critical Step	16 points	
•	Essential Step	6 points	
Ⓐ	Affective Competency	6 points	
▷	Theory Question	2 points	

Score calculation: 100 points

− _____ points missed

_____ Score

Satisfactory score: 85 or above

CAAHEP Competencies Achieved

Psychomotor (Skills)
☑ I. 2. a. Perform electrocardiography.
☑ I. 8. Instruct and prepare a patient for a procedure or a treatment.
☑ V. 3. Use medical terminology correctly and pronounced accurately to communicate information to providers and patients.
☑ VI. 8. Perform routine maintenance of administrative or clinical equipment.

Affective (Behavior)
☑ I. 1. Incorporate critical thinking skills when performing patient assessment.
☑ I. 3. Show awareness of a patient's concerns related to the procedure being performed.
☑ V. 4. Explain to a patient the rationale for performance of a procedure.

ABHES Competencies Achieved

☑ 2. c. Identify diagnostic and treatment modalities as they relate to each body system.
☑ 7. g. Display professionalism through written and verbal communications.
☑ 8. e. Perform specialty procedures including but not limited to minor surgery, cardiac, respiratory, OB-GYN, neurological, and gastroenterology.

Notes

Procedure 12-3: Spirometry Testing

Name: _____   Date: _____

Evaluated by: _____   Score: _____

Performance Objective

Outcome:	Perform a spirometry test.
Conditions:	Using a spirometer.
Standards:	Given the following: disposable tubing, disposable mouthpiece, disposable nose clips, waste container.
	Time: 20 minutes. Student completed procedure in _____ minutes.
	Accuracy: Satisfactory score on the Performance Evaluation Checklist.

Performance Evaluation Checklist

Trial 1	Trial 2	Point Value	Performance Standards
		•	Sanitized hands.
		•	Assembled and prepared equipment.
		•	Calibrated the spirometer.
		▷	Stated the reason for calibrating the spirometer.
		•	Applied a disposable mouthpiece to the mouthpiece holder.
		•	Greeted the patient and introduced yourself.
		•	Identified the patient and explained the procedure.
		•	Asked the patient if he or she had prepared properly.
		•	Asked the patient to remove heavy or restrictive clothing, to loosen tight clothing, and to discard gum.
		▷	Explained why tight clothing should be loosened.
		•	Measured the patient's weight and height.
		▷	Explained the reason for measuring weight and height.
		•	Asked the patient to sit near the machine.
		•	Entered the patient's data into the computer database of the spirometer.
			Described and demonstrated the breathing maneuver:
		•	Relax and take the deepest breath possible.
		•	Place the mouthpiece in your mouth and seal your lips tightly around it.
		•	Blow out as hard as you can for as long as possible.
		•	Do not block the opening of the mouthpiece with your tongue.
		•	Remove the mouthpiece from your mouth.

Trial 1	Trial 2	Point Value	Performance Standards
		▷	Explained why the lips should be tightly sealed around the mouthpiece.
		•	Told the patient the instructions would be repeated during the test.
		•	Encouraged the patient to remain calm.
		•	Gently applied the nose clips.
		▷	Stated the purpose of the nose clips.
		•	Handed the mouthpiece to the patient.
		•	Began the test and actively coached the patient.
		•	Informed the patient of modifications needed if the breathing maneuver was not performed correctly.
		•	Continued the test until three acceptable efforts were obtained.
		•	Gently removed the nose clips from the patient's nose.
		•	Removed the mouthpiece from its holder.
		•	Disposed of the nose clips and mouthpiece in a waste container.
		•	Allowed the patient to remain seated for a few minutes.
		•	Sanitized your hands.
		•	Printed the report and labeled it.
		•	Documented the procedure correctly.
		•	Placed the spirometry report in an appropriate location for review by the provider.
		•	Cleaned the spirometer according to the manufacturer's instructions.
			Demonstrated the following affective behavior(s) during this procedure:
		Ⓐ	Incorporated critical thinking skills when performing patient assessment.
		Ⓐ	Showed awareness of a patient's concerns related to the procedure being performed.
		Ⓐ	Explained to a patient the rationale for performance of a procedure.
		★	Completed the procedure within 20 minutes.
			Totals

CHART	
Date	

Evaluation of Student Performance

EVALUATION CRITERIA			COMMENTS
Symbol	**Category**	**Point Value**	
★	Critical Step	16 points	
•	Essential Step	6 points	
Ⓐ	Affective Competency	6 points	
▷	Theory Question	2 points	

Score calculation: 100 points

− _____ points missed

_____ Score

Satisfactory score: 85 or above

CAAHEP Competencies Achieved

Psychomotor (Skills)
☑ I. 2. d. Perform pulmonary function testing.
☑ I. 8. Instruct and prepare a patient for a procedure or a treatment.
☑ I. 10. Perform a quality control measure.
☑ V. 3. Use medical terminology correctly and pronounced accurately to communicate information to providers and patients.
☑ VI. 8. Perform routine maintenance of administrative or clinical equipment.

Affective (Behavior)
☑ I. 1. Incorporate critical thinking skills when performing patient assessment.
☑ I. 3. Show awareness of a patient's concerns related to the procedure being performed.
☑ V. 4. Explain to a patient the rationale for performance of a procedure.

ABHES Competencies Achieved

☑ 2. c. Identify diagnostic and treatment modalities as they relate to each body system.
☑ 7. g. Display professionalism through written and verbal communications.
☑ 8. e. Perform specialty procedures including but not limited to minor surgery, cardiac, respiratory, OB-GYN, neurological, and gastroenterology.
☑ 9. a. Practice quality control

Notes

Procedure 12-4: Measuring Peak Flow Rate

Name: _____   Date: _____

Evaluated by: _____   Score: _____

Performance Objective

Outcome:	Measure a patient's peak flow rate.
Conditions:	Using a spirometer.
Standards:	Given the following: disposable mouthpiece, waste container.
	Time: 15 minutes. Student completed procedure in _____ minutes.
	Accuracy: Satisfactory score on the Performance Evaluation Checklist.

Performance Evaluation Checklist

Trial 1	Trial 2	Point Value	Performance Standards
		•	Sanitized hands.
		•	Assembled and prepared equipment.
		•	Moved the sliding indicator to the bottom of the scale.
		▷	Stated why the indicator must be moved to the bottom of the scale.
		•	Applied a disposable mouthpiece to the mouthpiece holder.
		▷	Stated the purpose of the disposable mouthpiece.
		•	Greeted the patient and introduced yourself.
		•	Identified the patient and explained the procedure.
		•	Asked the patient to remove heavy or restrictive clothing, to loosen tight clothing, and to discard any gum.
			Described and demonstrated the breathing maneuver:
		•	Relax and take the deepest breath possible.
		•	Place the mouthpiece in your mouth and seal your lips tightly around it.
		•	Blow out as hard and fast as you can.
		•	Try to move the marker as high as you can on the scale.
		•	Do not block the opening of the mouthpiece with your tongue.
		•	Remove the mouthpiece from your mouth.
		•	Told the patient the instructions would be repeated during the test.
		•	Encouraged the patient to remain calm during the procedure.
		▷	Explained why the patient should remain calm.
		•	Placed a new disposable mouthpiece on the peak flow meter.

591

Trial 1	Trial 2	Point Value	Performance Standards
		•	Slid the marker to the bottom of the numbered scale.
		•	Handed the peak flow meter to the patient.
		•	Instructed the patient to stand up straight and look straight ahead.
		•	Began the test and actively coached the patient.
		•	Noted the number where the indicator stopped on the scale and jotted it down on a piece of paper.
		•	Informed the patient of modifications needed if the breathing maneuver was not performed correctly.
		•	Continued the test until three acceptable efforts were obtained.
		▷	Explained why three acceptable efforts must be obtained.
		•	The numbers from the three tests were about the same.
		▷	Stated the significance of the three numbers being about the same.
		•	Took the peak flow meter from the patient.
		•	Removed the mouthpiece from its holder and discarded it in a waste container.
		•	Sanitized your hands.
		•	Noted the highest of the three peak flow measurements.
		•	Documented the procedure correctly.
		•	Cleaned the peak flow meter.
		▷	Explained how to clean the peak flow meter.
			Demonstrated the following affective behavior(s) during this procedure:
		Ⓐ	Incorporated critical thinking skills when performing patient assessment.
		Ⓐ	Showed awareness of a patient's concerns related to the procedure being performed.
		Ⓐ	Explained to a patient the rationale for performance of a procedure.
		★	Completed the procedure within 15 minutes.
			Totals

CHART	
Date	

Evaluation of Student Performance

EVALUATION CRITERIA			COMMENTS
Symbol	**Category**	**Point Value**	
★	Critical Step	16 points	
•	Essential Step	6 points	
Ⓐ	Affective Competency	6 points	
▷	Theory Question	2 points	

Score calculation: 100 points

     − _____ points missed

       _____ Score

Satisfactory score: 85 or above

CAAHEP Competencies Achieved

Psychomotor (Skills)

☑ I. 2. d. Perform pulmonary function testing.
☑ I. 8. Instruct and prepare a patient for a procedure or a treatment.
☑ V. 3. Use medical terminology correctly and pronounced accurately to communicate information to providers and patients.
☑ VI. 8. Perform routine maintenance of administrative or clinical equipment.

Affective (Behavior)

☑ I. 1. Incorporate critical thinking skills when performing patient assessment.
☑ I. 3. Show awareness of a patient's concerns related to the procedure being performed.
☑ V. 4. Explain to a patient the rationale for performance of a procedure.

ABHES Competencies Achieved

☑ 2. c. Identify diagnostic and treatment modalities as they relate to each body system.
☑ 7. g. Display professionalism through written and verbal communications.
☑ 8. e. Perform specialty procedures including but not limited to minor surgery, cardiac, respiratory, OB-GYN, neurological, and gastroenterology.

13 Colon Procedures and Male Reproductive Health

√ After Completing	Date Due	Study Guide Pages	STUDY GUIDE ASSIGNMENTS (CTA = Critical Thinking Activity)	Possible Points	Points You Earned
		599	Pretest	10	
		600	Key Term Assessment A. Definitions B. Word Parts (Add 1 point for each key term)	10 10	
		601-605	Evaluation of Learning questions	40	
		605	CTA A: FOBT Patient Preparation	10	
		606	CTA B: Capsule Endoscopy	25	
		607	CTA C: Dear Gabby	10	
		608	CTA D: Crossword Puzzle	24	
			Evolve Site: Apply Your Knowledge questions	12	
			Evolve Site: Video Evaluation	18	
		599	Posttest	10	
			ADDITIONAL ASSIGNMENTS		
			Total points		

Chapter **13** **Colon Procedures and Male Reproductive Health**

√ When Assigned by Your Instructor	Study Guide Pages	Practices Required	LABORATORY ASSIGNMENTS (Procedure Number and Name)	Score*
	609-610	5	**Practice for Competency** 13-1 and 13-2: Fecal Occult Blood Testing: Guaiac Slide Test Method and Developing the Hemoccult Slide Test Textbook reference: pp. 509-513	
	611-614		**Evaluation of Competency** 13-1 and 13-2: Fecal Occult Blood Testing: Guaiac Slide Test Method and Developing the Hemoccult Slide Test	*
	609-610	5	**Practice for Competency** 13-A: Testicular Self-Examination Instructions Textbook reference: p. 519-520	
	615-616		**Evaluation of Competency** 13-A: Testicular Self-Examination Instructions	*
			ADDITIONAL ASSIGNMENTS	

Chapter **13** Colon Procedures and Male Reproductive Health

Notes

Name: _____   Date: _____

True or False

_____ 1. Hemorrhoids can cause visible red blood to appear on the outside of the stool.

_____ 2. Nonvisible blood in the stool is called occult blood.

_____ 3. Colorectal cancer is a common form of cancer in individuals older than 50 years.

_____ 4. A blue color appearing on a Hemoccult test result is interpreted as a negative result.

_____ 5. If a Hemoccult test result is positive, the provider may order a colonoscopy.

_____ 6. The patient is placed in the prone position for a colonoscopy.

_____ 7. The function of the prostate gland is to produce sperm.

_____ 8. Most prostate cancers are slow growing.

_____ 9. A normal prostate gland feels firm and hard.

_____ 10. The most common sign of testicular cancer is a small, hard, painless lump on the testicle.

? POSTTEST

True or False

_____ 1. Melena means that the stool appears hard and dry.

_____ 2. Consuming red meat may cause a false-positive result on a fecal occult guaiac slide test.

_____ 3. Ibuprofen should be avoided for 7 days before beginning a fecal occult guaiac slide test.

_____ 4. The Hemoccult test should be stored at room temperature after applying a stool specimen to it.

_____ 5. Patient preparation for a sigmoidoscopy includes partial bowel preparation.

_____ 6. After use, a sigmoidoscope must be autoclaved for 20 minutes.

_____ 7. Colonoscopy is performed for the early detection of colorectal cancer.

_____ 8. There are often no symptoms in the early stages of prostate cancer.

_____ 9. A prostate-specific antigen (PSA) level of 20 is within normal range.

_____ 10. Testicular cancer occurs most commonly between the ages of 15 and 34.

Chapter **13** Colon Procedures and Male Reproductive Health

A. Definitions

Directions: Match each key term with its definition.

_____ 1. Biopsy

_____ 2. Colonoscope

_____ 3. Colonoscopy

_____ 4. Endoscope

_____ 5. Insufflate

_____ 6. Melena

_____ 7. Occult blood

_____ 8. Peroxidase

_____ 9. Sigmoidoscope

_____ 10. Sigmoidoscopy

A. The visualization of the rectum and the entire colon using a colonoscope

B. Blood occurring in such a small amount that it is not visually detectable by the unaided eye

C. The surgical removal and examination of tissue from the living body

D. The visual examination of the rectum and sigmoid colon using a sigmoidoscope

E. The darkening of the stool caused by the presence of blood in an amount of 50 mL or more

F. An instrument that consists of a tube and an optical system that is used for direct visual inspection of organs or cavities

G. A substance that is able to transfer oxygen from hydrogen peroxide to oxidize guaiac, causing the guaiac to turn blue

H. An endoscope that is specially designed for passage through the anus to permit visualization of the rectum and sigmoid colon

I. To blow a powder, vapor, or gas (such as air) into a body cavity

J. An endoscope that is specially designed for passage through the anus to permit visualization of the rectum and the entire length of the colon

B. Word Parts

Directions: Indicate the meaning of each word part in the space provided. List as many medical terms as possible that incorporate the word part in the space provided.

Word Part	Meaning of Word Part	Medical Terms That Incorporate Word Part
1. bi/o		
2. -opsy		
3. colon/o		
4. -scopy		
5. -scope		
6. endo-		
7. -oxia		
8. -ase		
9. ox/i		
10. sigmoid/o		

Directions: Fill in each blank with the correct answer.

1. What are the three parts of the large intestine?

   _____

2. What are the functions of the large intestine?

   _____

   _____

3. What is the function of the anal sphincter muscles?

   _____

   _____

4. What is the function of the mucus secreted by the large intestine?

   _____

   _____

5. List five causes of blood in the stool.

   _____

   _____

   _____

   _____

6. Define the term melena, and explain what causes it.

   _____

   _____

   _____

   _____

7. What is the primary reason for screening patients for the presence of fecal occult blood?

   _____

   _____

8. What are the symptoms of colorectal cancer?

   _____

   _____

9. Why must three stool specimens be obtained for the fecal occult guaiac slide test?

_____

_____

_____

10. List two reasons for placing the patient on a high-fiber diet when testing for fecal occult blood.

_____

_____

11. What medications and vitamin supplements must be discontinued before guaiac slide testing?

_____

_____

12. List two factors that could cause false-positive test results on a guaiac slide test.

_____

_____

13. List three examples of diagnostic tests that may be performed if the guaiac slide test result is positive.

_____

_____

_____

14. Why is it important to perform quality-control methods when developing the guaiac slide test?

_____

_____

15. How should the guaiac slide test be stored?

_____

_____

16. What factors can cause a failure of the expected control results to occur on a guaiac slide test?

_____

_____

17. List the advantages of the fecal immunochemical test (FIT) compared with the guaiac slide test.

_____

_____

_____

18. How does a fecal DNA test function to detect colorectal cancer?

_____

_____

19. What is the purpose of performing a sigmoidoscopy?

_____

_____

_____

20. Describe the following patient preparation required for a sigmoidoscopy:

   a. The day before the procedure and continuing until the examination is completed:

   _____

   _____

   b. The evening before the procedure:

   _____

   _____

   c. The day of the procedure:

   _____

   _____

21. What is the purpose of performing a digital rectal examination (DRE) before a sigmoidoscopy?

_____

_____

_____

22. What is the purpose of insufflating air into the colon during a sigmoidoscopy?

_____

_____

23. What is the purpose of suctioning during sigmoidoscopy?

_____

_____

24. What is the recommended position of the patient during flexible fiberoptic sigmoidoscopy?

_____

25. What parts of the colon are viewed during a colonoscopy?

_____

_____

26. What is the purpose of a full bowel preparation before a colonoscopy?

_____

_____

27. How should a patient consume the liquid laxative solution when preparing the bowel for a colonoscopy?

_____

_____

28. Where is the prostate gland located?

_____

_____

29. What are the symptoms of prostate cancer?

_____

_____

_____

30. How is the digital rectal examination used for the early detection of prostate cancer?

_____

_____

31. What conditions can cause an elevated PSA level?

_____

_____

32. What is the PSA level for each of the following?

    a. Normal range _____

    b. Slightly elevated range _____

    c. Moderately elevated range _____

    d. Highly elevated _____

33. What patient preparation is required for a PSA test?

_____

_____

34. What tests may be ordered by the provider if the patient has positive prostate screening results?

_____

_____

35. What is the definition of the term screening?

_____

_____

36. What is the American Cancer Society recommendation for the PSA test and the DRE?

_____

_____

_____

37. When does testicular cancer most commonly occur?

_____

38. When is the best time for a male to perform a testicular self-examination (TSE) and why?

_____

_____

39. What are the risk factors for testicular cancer?

_____

_____

_____

40. What is the most common sign of testicular cancer?

_____

_____

CRITICAL THINKING ACTIVITIES

A. FOBT Patient Preparation

Frank Morrison has been given a Hemoccult slide kit for fecal occult blood testing (FOBT). In the space provided, plan breakfast, lunch, and dinner for him following the FOBT patient preparation guidelines on pages 505-506 of your textbook.

_____

_____

_____

_____

_____

_____

B. Capsule Endoscopy

Perform an Internet search for capsule endoscopy. Search for textual information and videos of this procedure. Based on your research, answer the following questions regarding this procedure.

1. What is capsule endoscopy?

_____

_____

_____

_____

_____

2. What conditions can be diagnosed using capsule endoscopy?

_____

_____

_____

3. What patient preparation is required for this procedure?

_____

_____

_____

4. What are the advantages of capsule endoscopy?

_____

_____

_____

5. What are the disadvantages of capsule endoscopy?

_____

_____

_____

_____

C. Dear Gabby

Gabby broke her wrist while ice skating and wants you to fill in for her. In the space provided, respond to the following letter using the knowledge you have acquired in this chapter.

Dear Gabby:

I am 15 years old, and my mom just took me to a new doctor for a sports physical examination. I am going to play football this fall at my high school. Before this, I had always gone to the doctor I had since I was little, but I had to switch because I am getting older. After the doctor did my physical, he told me that I needed to examine my testicles every month and that the medical assistant would be in to explain how this is done.

Gabby, I was totally shocked, and you can bet I got out of that office before she had a chance to do that. I am too embarrassed to ask my parents about this. Gabby, what is going on? I am only 15 years old. Are my parents taking me to a quack, and should I report this to someone?

Signed,

Don't Know What to Do

_____

_____

_____

_____

_____

_____

_____

_____

_____

D. Crossword Puzzle: Colon Procedures and Male Reproductive Health

Directions: Complete the crossword puzzle using the clues provided.

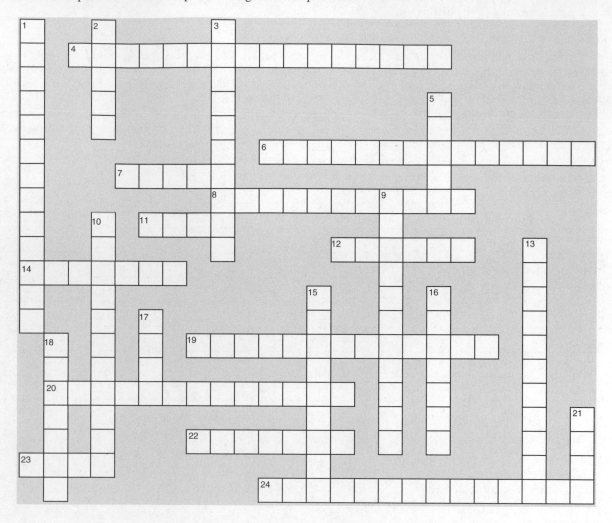

Across
4 Normally increases PSA level
6 Symptom of CRC
7 Majority of large intestine
8 Used to visualize entire colon
11 Color of positive Hemoccult
12 Black and tarlike stool
14 Can cause false-positive on FOBT
19 Increases risk of CRC
20 Secretes fluid that transports sperm
22 Age to start TSE
23 Patient position for sigmoidoscopy
24 Cause of failed FOBT control

Down
1 Results in an empty colon
2 CRC increases after this age
3 Leading cause of cancer deaths
5 CRC often starts from this
9 Colon abnormality detection gold standard
10 Can cause blood in the stool
13 Hidden blood
15 How to clean sigmoidoscope
16 Prostate CA screening test
17 Protect FOBT from this
18 Med to avoid during FOBT
21 May be done after elevated PSA

Procedures 13-1 and 13-2: Fecal Occult Blood Testing: Guaiac Slide Test Method

1. Patient instructions. Instruct the patient in the specimen collection procedure for a fecal occult blood test (e.g., Hemoccult). Document these instructions in the chart provided.
2. Developing the test. Develop a fecal occult blood test, and document the results in the chart provided.

Procedure 13-A: Testicular Self-Examination

Instruct an individual about the procedure for testicular self-examination, and document the procedure in the chart provided.

CHART	
Date	

609

CHART	
Date	

Procedures 13-1 and 13-2: Fecal Occult Blood Testing: Guaiac Slide Test Method and Developing the Fecal Occult Blood Test

Name: _____ Date: _____

Evaluated by: _____ Score: _____

Performance Objective

Outcome:	Instruct an individual in the specimen collection procedure for a Hemoccult slide test and develop the test.
Conditions:	Given the following: Hemoccult slide testing kit, disposable gloves, developing solution, reference card, and a waste container.
Standards:	Time: 15 minutes. Student completed procedures in _____ minutes.
	Accuracy: Satisfactory score on the Performance Evaluation Checklist.

Performance Evaluation Checklist

Trial 1	Trial 2	Point Value	Performance Standards
			Instructions for the Hemoccult slide test
		•	Obtained the Hemoccult slide testing kit.
		•	Checked the expiration date on the slides.
		▷	Described what may occur if the slides are outdated.
		•	Greeted the patient and introduced yourself.
		•	Identified the patient and explained the purpose of the test.
		•	Informed the patient when the test should not be performed.
		•	Instructed the patient in the proper preparation required for the test.
		•	Encouraged the patient to adhere to the diet modifications.
		▷	Explained why the patient should follow the diet modifications.
		•	Provided the patient with the Hemoccult slide test kit.
		•	Instructed the patient in completion of the information on the front flap of each card.
		•	Provided instructions on the proper care and storage of the slides.
		▷	Explained why the slides must be stored properly.
			Instructed the patient in the initiation of the test
		•	Began the diet modifications.
		•	Collected a stool specimen from the first bowel movement after the 3-day preparatory period.

Trial 1	Trial 2	Point Value	Performance Standards
			Instructed the patient in the collection of the stool specimen
		•	Filled in the collection date on the front flap.
		•	Used a clean, dry container to collect the stool specimen.
		•	Collected the stool sample before it came in contact with toilet bowl water.
		•	Used the wooden applicator to obtain a specimen from one part of the stool.
		•	Opened the front flap of the first cardboard slide.
		•	Spread a thin smear of the specimen over the filter paper in the square labeled A.
		•	Obtained another specimen from a different area of the stool by using the other end of the applicator.
		•	Spread a thin smear of the specimen over the filter paper in the square labeled B.
		•	Closed the front flap of the cardboard slide and filled in the date.
		•	Discarded the applicator in a waste container.
		▷	Explained why a sample is collected from two different parts of the stool.
		•	Instructed the patient to place the slides in a regular envelope to air-dry overnight.
		•	Instructed the patient to continue the testing period on 3 different days until all three specimens have been obtained.
		•	Instructed the patient to place the cardboard slides in the foil envelope and return them to the medical office.
		•	Provided the patient with an opportunity to ask questions.
		•	Made sure the patient understood the instructions.
		•	Documented the procedure correctly.
			Developing the Hemoccult slide test
		•	Assembled equipment.
		•	Checked the expiration date on the developing solution bottle.
		▷	Explained how the solution should be stored.
		•	Sanitized hands and applied gloves.
		•	Opened the back flap of the cardboard slides.
		•	Applied 2 drops of the developing solution to the guaiac test paper underlying the back of each smear.
		•	Did not allow the developing solution to come in contact with skin or eyes.
		•	Read results within 60 seconds.
		★	Results were identical to the evaluator's results.
		▷	Explained why the slides should be read within 60 seconds.

Trial 1	Trial 2	Point Value	Performance Standards
		•	Performed the quality control procedure on each slide.
		•	Read the quality control results after 10 seconds.
		▷	Described what is observed during a normal positive and negative control reaction.
		▷	Stated the purpose of the quality control procedure.
		•	Properly disposed of the slides in a regular waste container.
		•	Removed gloves and sanitized hands.
		•	Documented the results correctly.
			Demonstrated the following affective behavior(s) during this procedure:
		Ⓐ	Explained to a patient the rationale for performance of a procedure.
		Ⓐ	Showed awareness of a patient's concerns related to the procedure being performed.
		Ⓐ	Showed awareness of patient's concerns regarding a dietary change.
		★	Completed the procedure within 15 minutes.
			Totals

CHART	
Date	

Evaluation of Student Performance

EVALUATION CRITERIA			COMMENTS
Symbol	**Category**	**Point Value**	
★	Critical Step	16 points	
•	Essential Step	6 points	
Ⓐ	Affective Competency	6 points	
▷	Theory Question	2 points	

Score calculation: 100 points

−_____ points missed

_____ Score

Satisfactory score: 85 or above

CAAHEP Competencies Achieved

Psychomotor (Skills)

☑ i. 10. Perform a quality control measure.

☑ II. 2. Differentiate between normal and abnormal test results.

☑ IV. 1. Instruct a patient according to patient's special dietary needs.

☑ V. 4. Coach patients regarding (a) office policies, (b) health maintenance, (c) disease prevention, (d) treatment plan.

Affective (Behavior)

☑ I. 3. Show awareness of a patient's concerns related to the procedure being performed.

☑ IV. 1. Show awareness of patient's concerns regarding a dietary change.

☑ V. 4. Explain to a patient the rationale for performance of a procedure.

ABHES Competencies Achieved

☑ 7. g. Display professionalism through written and verbal communication.

☑ 8. e. Perform specialty procedures including but not limited to minor surgery, cardiac, respiratory, OB-GYN, neurological, gastroenterology.

☑ 9. a. Practice quality control.

☑ 9. e. (2). Instruct patients in the collection of fecal specimens.

Procedure 13-A: Testicular Self-Examination Instructions

Name: _____ Date: _____

Evaluated by: _____ Score: _____

Performance Objective

Outcome:	Instruct an individual in the procedure for performing a testicular self-examination (TSE).
Conditions:	None.
Standards:	Time: 10 minutes. Student completed procedure in _____ minutes.
	Accuracy: Satisfactory score on the Performance Evaluation Checklist.

Performance Evaluation Checklist

Trial 1	Trial 2	Point Value	Performance Standards
		•	Greeted the patient and introduced yourself.
		•	Identified the patient and explained that you will be instructing the patient in a TSE.
		•	Explained the purpose of the examination and when to perform it.
			Instructed the patient as follows:
		•	Take a warm bath or shower.
		•	Stand in front of a mirror.
		•	Inspect for any swelling of the skin of the scrotum.
		•	Place the index and middle fingers of both hands on the underside of one testicle and the thumbs on top of the testicle.
		•	Apply a small amount of pressure, and gently roll the testicle between the thumbs and fingers of both hands.
		•	Palpate for lumps, swelling, or any change in the size, shape, or consistency of the testicle.
		▷	Stated the normal characteristics of a testicle.
		•	Locate the epididymis so that you do not confuse it with a lump.
		▷	Stated the characteristics and function of the epididymis.
		•	Repeat the examination on the other testicle.
		•	Report any abnormalities to the provider.
		▷	Stated examples of abnormalities that should be reported.
		•	Documented the procedure correctly.

Trial 1	Trial 2	Point Value	Performance Standards
			Demonstrated the following affective behavior(s) during this procedure:
		Ⓐ	Explained to a patient the rationale for performance of a procedure.
		Ⓐ	Demonstrated (a) empathy, (b) active listening, (c) nonverbal communication.
		Ⓐ	Demonstrated respect for individual diversity, including (a) gender, (b) race, (c) religion, (d) age, (e) economic status, (f) appearance.
		★	Completed the procedure within 10 minutes.
			Totals

CHART	
Date	

Evaluation of Student Performance

EVALUATION CRITERIA			COMMENTS
Symbol	**Category**	**Point Value**	
★	Critical Step	16 points	
•	Essential Step	6 points	
Ⓐ	Affective Competency	6 points	
▷	Theory Question	2 points	

Score calculation: 100 points

− _____ points missed

____ Score

Satisfactory score: 85 or above

CAAHEP Competencies Achieved

Psychomotor (Skills)
☑ V. 4. Coach patients regarding (a) office policies, (b) health maintenance, (c) disease prevention, (d) treatment plan.

Affective (Behavior)
☑ V. 1. Demonstrate (a) empathy, (b) active listening, (c) nonverbal communication.
☑ V. 3. Demonstrate respect for individual diversity, including (a) gender, (b) race, (c) religion, (d) age, (e) economic status, (f) appearance.
☑ V. 4. Explain to a patient the rationale for performance of a procedure.

ABHES Competencies Achieved

☑ 7. g. Display professionalism through written and verbal communication.
☑ 8. h. Teach self-examination, disease management and health promotion.

Radiology and Diagnostic Imaging

√ After Completing	Date Due	Study Guide Pages	STUDY GUIDE ASSIGNMENTS (CTA = Critical Thinking Activity)	Possible Points	Points You Earned
		621	Pretest	10	
		622	Key Term Assessment A. Definitions B. Word Parts	13 15	
		623-627	Evaluation of Learning questions	42	
		627	CTA A: Lower Gastrointestinal Tract	5	
		628	CTA B: Intravenous Pyelogram	5	
		628-629	CTA C: Magnetic Resonance Imaging	7	
		630	CTA D: Crossword Puzzle	22	
			Evolve Site: Apply Your Knowledge questions	10	
		621	Posttest	10	
			ADDITIONAL ASSIGNMENTS		
			Total points		

√ When Assigned by Your Instructor	Study Guide Pages	Practices Required	LABORATORY ASSIGNMENTS (Procedure Number and Name)	Score*
	631-632	3	**Practice for Competency** 14-A: Preparation for Radiology Examinations Textbook reference: pp. 525-530	
	633-634		**Evaluation of Competency** 14-A: Preparation for Radiology Examinations	*
	631-632	3	**Practice for Competency** 14-B: Preparation for Diagnostic Imaging Procedures Textbook reference: pp. 530-536	
	635-636		**Evaluation of Competency** 14-B: Preparation for Diagnostic Imaging Procedures	*
			ADDITIONAL ASSIGNMENTS	

Notes

Name: _____   Date: _____

True or False

_____ 1. A radiologist is a medical doctor specializing in the diagnosis and treatment of disease using radiation and other imaging techniques.

_____ 2. The permanent record of the picture produced on x-ray film is a sonogram.

_____ 3. The purpose of a contrast medium is to make a structure visible on a radiograph.

_____ 4. With an anteroposterior view, x-rays are directed from the back toward the front of the body.

_____ 5. Mammography can be used to detect breast calcifications.

_____ 6. An upper gastrointestinal (GI) examination assists in diagnosing kidney stones.

_____ 7. An IVP is a radiograph of the kidneys, ureters, and bladder.

_____ 8. Ultrasonography allows for continuous viewing of a structure.

_____ 9. Obstetric ultrasound can be used to determine gestational age.

_____10. A patient must remove all metal before undergoing MRI.

📋 POSTTEST

True or False

_____ 1. Wilhelm Roentgen discovered x-rays in 1895.

_____ 2. Bone is an example of a radiolucent structure.

_____ 3. An instrument used to view internal organs directly is a fluoroscope.

_____ 4. The patient should be instructed not to move during a radiographic examination to prevent confusing shadows on the film.

_____ 5. The breasts are compressed during mammography to prevent radiation burns.

_____ 6. After an upper GI study is performed, the barium causes the stool to be loose and watery.

_____ 7. Gas must be removed from the colon before a lower GI study to prevent blurring of the radiograph.

_____ 8. Before performing an IVP, the patient must be asked whether he or she is allergic to penicillin.

_____ 9. Computed tomography produces a series of cross-sectional images.

_____10. A radioactive material is introduced into the body before a nuclear medicine imaging procedure is performed.

A. Definitions

Directions: Match each key term with its definition.

_____ 1. Contrast medium

_____ 2. Echocardiogram

_____ 3. Enema

_____ 4. Fluoroscope

_____ 5. Fluoroscopy

_____ 6. Radiograph

_____ 7. Radiography

_____ 8. Radiologist

_____ 9. Radiology

_____10. Radiolucent

_____11. Radiopaque

_____12. Sonogram

_____13. Ultrasonography

A. A permanent record of a picture of an internal body organ or structure produced on radiographic film

B. A physician who specializes in the diagnosis and treatment of disease using radiation and other imaging techniques

C. A substance used to make a particular structure visible on a radiograph

D. The record obtained with ultrasonography

E. An injection of fluid into the rectum to aid in the elimination of feces from the colon

F. The branch of medicine that deals with the use of radiation and other imaging techniques in the diagnosis and treatment of disease

G. An instrument used to view internal organs and structures directly

H. Describing a structure that obstructs the passage of x-rays

I. The taking of permanent records of internal body organs and structures by passing x-rays through the body to act on a specially sensitized film

J. Describing a structure that permits the passage of x-rays

K. Examination of a patient with a fluoroscope

L. An ultrasound examination of the heart

M. The use of high-frequency sound waves to produce an image of an organ or tissue

B. Word Parts

Directions: Indicate the meaning of each word part in the space provided. List as many medical terms as possible that incorporate the word part in the space provided.

Word Part	Meaning of Word Part	Medical Terms That Incorporate Word Part
1. ech/o		
2. cardi/o		
3. -gram		
4. fluor/o		
5. -scope		
6. -scopy		
7. radi/o		
8. -graph		
9. -graphy		
10. -ologist		
11. -ology		
12. -lucent		
13. -opaque		
14. son/o		
15. ultra-		

Directions: Fill in each blank with the correct answer.

1. Who discovered x-rays?

   _____

2. What is the function of x-rays?

   _____

   _____

3. What are the two ways in which radiographs can be taken?

   _____

4. What are the advantages of digital radiology?

   _____

   _____

5. Why is it important for a patient to prepare properly for a radiographic examination?

   _____

   _____

6. What is the function of a radiopaque contrast medium?

   _____

   _____

7. What are the various ways in which contrast medium can be administered to a patient?

   _____

   _____

8. How is a patient positioned to obtain an anteroposterior view?

   _____

   _____

9. What is the purpose of mammography?

   _____

   _____

10. Why should the patient be instructed not to wear lotions, powders, or deodorants when having a mammogram?

   _____

   _____

11. Why must the breasts be compressed during mammography?

_____

_____

12. What is the purpose of a bone density scan?

_____

_____

13. What is osteoporosis?

_____

_____

14. Who is at particular risk for osteoporosis?

_____

15. What patient preparation is required for a bone density scan?

_____

_____

16. What information is provided by DXA bone density measurements?

_____

_____

_____

_____

17. What is the purpose of the upper GI radiographic examination?

_____

_____

_____

18. Why must the GI tract be free of food and fluid before an upper GI radiographic examination is performed?

_____

_____

19. How can the patient prevent constipation after an upper GI examination?

_____

_____

20. A lower GI radiographic examination assists in the diagnosis of what conditions?

_____

_____

21. Why is it important to remove gas and fecal material from the colon before a lower GI radiographic examination is performed?

_____

_____

22. What is the advantage of the air used with a double-contrast barium enema?

_____

_____

23. What is an intravenous pyelogram (IVP)?

_____

_____

24. An IVP assists in the diagnosis of what conditions?

_____

_____

25. What may the patient experience during an IVP when the iodine enters the bloodstream?

_____

_____

26. Define the following:

a. Angiocardiogram

_____

_____

b. Bronchogram

_____

_____

c. Cerebral angiogram

_____

_____

d. Coronary angiogram

_____

_____

e. Cystogram

_____

_____

27. What are the primary uses of ultrasonography?

_____

_____

28. What are the advantages of ultrasonography?

_____

_____

_____

29. What can be determined during an echocardiogram?

_____

_____

30. What is the purpose of the gel used with ultrasonography?

_____

_____

31. What is the purpose of performing obstetric ultrasound?

_____

_____

_____

32. Doppler ultrasound assists in the diagnosis of what conditions?

_____

_____

33. What type of image is produced by computed tomography?

_____

_____

34. What are the primary uses of computed tomography?

_____

_____

_____

35. What type of patient preparation is required for computed tomography?

_____

_____

_____

_____

36. What are the primary uses of magnetic resonance imaging (MRI)?

_____

_____

_____

37. What items must the patient remove before having an MRI scan?

_____

_____

38. What material is used with a nuclear medicine diagnostic imaging procedure?

_____

39. What is the function of a gamma camera used in nuclear medicine?

_____

_____

40. What is the purpose of a bone scan?

_____

_____

41. A nuclear cardiac stress test assists in the evaluation of what heart condition?

_____

_____

42. A PET scan is used to assist in the diagnosis of what conditions?

_____

_____

CRITICAL THINKING ACTIVITIES

A. Lower Gastrointestinal Tract

Trent Douglas has been having pain in his lower abdomen and occult blood in his stool. Dr. Hartman tells you to schedule him for a lower GI radiographic examination at Grant Hospital. In the space provided, explain how you would instruct Mr. Douglas to prepare for this examination. Include the patient preparation and the reason for each of the measures.

_____

_____

_____

_____

_____

_____

_____

B. Intravenous Pyelogram

Dr. Tristen instructs you to schedule Ellie Ray for an intravenous pyelogram (IVP) at Grant Hospital. After you have explained to Ms. Ray the instructions for preparing for the examination, she asks you the following questions. Respond to them in the space provided.

1. What body structures will be "x-rayed" during the examination?

    _____

    _____

    _____

2. Why must gas and fecal material be removed from the intestines?

    _____

    _____

    _____

3. Why will iodine be injected into my veins?

    _____

    _____

    _____

4. Will I feel anything when the iodine is injected?

    _____

    _____

    _____

5. What is done if an individual is allergic to iodine?

    _____

    _____

C. Magnetic Resonance Imaging

Jason Zindra, a college baseball player, has been experiencing pain in his left shoulder joint. Dr. Baker schedules him for magnetic resonance imaging (MRI) of the left shoulder. Jason asks you the following questions regarding this procedure. Respond to them in the space provided.

1. Is this a safe procedure?

    _____

    _____

2. Will there be any pain involved with this procedure?

    _____

    _____

3. Will I be exposed to x-rays?

_____

_____

4. What should I wear to the test?

_____

_____

5. May I wear my watch during the procedure to keep track of the time?

_____

_____

6. Does the MRI machine make any noise?

_____

_____

7. Will the technician be in the room with me?

_____

_____

D. Crossword Puzzle: Radiology and Diagnostic Imaging

Directions: Complete the crossword puzzle using the clues provided.

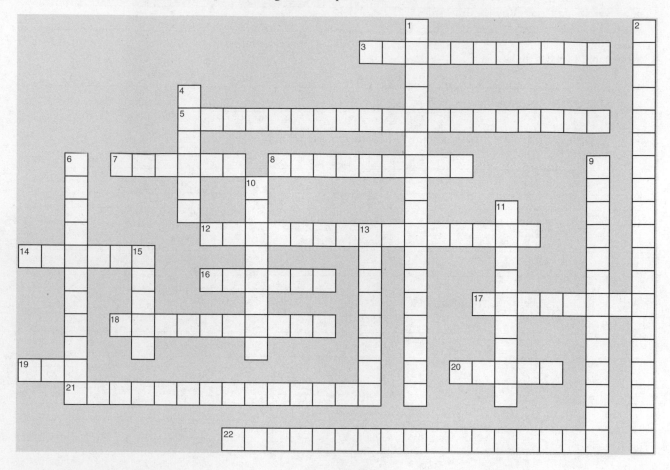

Across
- **3** Radiograph of the lungs
- **5** Can tell if it's twins
- **7** X-rays directed from back to front
- **8** Radiograph of urinary bladder
- **12** Detects "presence" of osteoporosis
- **14** Lower GI contrast medium
- **16** Produces cross-sectional images
- **17** Discovered x-rays
- **18** Obstructs x-rays
- **19** Used to diagnose kidney stones
- **20** Color of radiolucent structure
- **21** US of heart
- **22** Radiograph of coronary arteries

Down
- **1** Helps diagnose blood flow blockages
- **2** Radiograph of uterus and fallopian tubes
- **4** IVP contrast medium
- **6** Used to directly view internal organs
- **9** Radiograph of bile ducts
- **10** Detects stress fractures
- **11** Breast radiograph
- **13** US recording
- **15** Remove during an MRI

Procedure 14-A: Radiology Examinations

Instruct a patient in the proper preparation required for each of the following types of radiographic examinations: mammogram, bone density scan, upper GI, lower GI, and intravenous pyelogram. Document the procedure in the chart provided.

Procedure 14-B: Diagnostic Imaging Procedures

Instruct a patient in the proper preparation required for each of the following types of diagnostic imaging procedures: ultrasonography, computed tomography, magnetic resonance imaging, and nuclear medicine. Document the procedure in the chart provided.

CHART	
Date	

631

CHART	
Date	

Chapter **14** **Radiology and Diagnostic Imaging**

Procedure 14-A: Preparation for Radiology Examinations

Name: _____ Date: _____

Evaluated by: _____ Score: _____

Performance Objective

Outcome:	Instruct a patient in the proper preparation required for each of the following radiographic examinations: mammogram, upper GI, lower GI, and intravenous pyelogram.
Conditions:	Given the following: a patient instruction sheet for each radiographic examination.
Standards:	Time: 15 minutes. Student completed procedures in _____ minutes.
	Accuracy: Satisfactory score in the Performance Evaluation Checklist.

Performance Evaluation Checklist

Trial 1	Trial 2	Point Value	Performance Standards
		•	Greeted and identified the patient.
		•	Introduced yourself.
			Instructed the patient in the proper preparation for each of the following radiographic examinations:
		•	Mammogram
		•	Bone density scan
		•	Upper GI
		•	Lower GI
		•	Intravenous pyelogram
		•	Documented the procedure correctly.
			Demonstrated the following affective behavior(s) during this procedure:
		Ⓐ	Explained to a patient the rationale for performance of a procedure.
		Ⓐ	Showed awareness of a patient's concerns related to the procedure being performed.
		★	Completed the procedure within 15 minutes.
			Totals

CHART	
Date	

Evaluation of Student Performance

EVALUATION CRITERIA			COMMENTS
Symbol	Category	Point Value	
★	Critical Step	16 points	
•	Essential Step	6 points	
Ⓐ	Affective Competency	6 points	
▷	Theory Question	2 points	

Score calculation: 100 points

− _____ points missed

_____ Score

Satisfactory score: 85 or above

CAAHEP Competencies Achieved

Psychomotor (Skills)

☑ I. 8. Instruct and prepare a patient for a procedure or a treatment.
☑ IV. 1. Instruct a patient according to patient's special dietary needs.
☑ V. 11. Report relevant information concisely and accurately.

Affective (Behavior)

☑ I. 3. Show awareness of a patient's concerns related to the procedure being performed.
☑ V. 4. Explain to a patient the rationale for performance of a procedure.

ABHES Competencies Achieved

☑ 2. c. Identify diagnostic and treatment modalities as they relate to each body system.
☑ 7. g. Display professionalism through written and verbal communication.

Procedure 14-B: Preparation for Diagnostic Imaging Procedures

Name: _____ Date: _____

Evaluated by: _____ Score: _____

Performance Objective

Outcome:	Instruct a patient in the proper preparation required for each of the following diagnostic imaging procedures: ultrasonography, computed tomography, magnetic resonance imaging, and nuclear medicine.
Conditions:	Given the following: a patient instruction sheet for each diagnostic imaging procedure.
Standards:	Time: 15 minutes. Student completed procedure in _____ minutes.
	Accuracy: Satisfactory score in the Performance Evaluation Checklist.

Performance Evaluation Checklist

Trial 1	Trial 2	Point Value	Performance Standards
		•	Greeted and identified the patient.
		•	Introduced yourself.
			Instructed patient in the proper preparation for each of the following diagnostic imaging procedures:
		•	Ultrasonography
		•	Computed tomography
		•	Magnetic resonance imaging
		•	Nuclear medicine
		•	Documented the procedure correctly.
			Demonstrated the following affective behavior(s) during this procedure:
		Ⓐ	Explained to a patient the rationale for performance of a procedure.
		Ⓐ	Showed awareness of a patient's concerns related to the procedure being performed.
		★	Completed the procedure within 15 minutes.
			Totals

CHART	
Date	

Evaluation of Student Performance

EVALUATION CRITERIA			COMMENTS
Symbol	**Category**	**Point Value**	
★	Critical Step	16 points	
•	Essential Step	6 points	
Ⓐ	Affective Competency	6 points	
▷	Theory Question	2 points	

Score calculation: 100 points

− _____ points missed

_____ Score

Satisfactory score: 85 or above

CAAHEP Competencies Achieved

Psychomotor (Skills)
☑ I. 8. Instruct and prepare a patient for a procedure or a treatment.
☑ V. 11. Report relevant information concisely and accurately.

Affective (Behavior)
☑ I. 3. Show awareness of a patient's concerns related to the procedure being performed.
☑ V. 4. Explain to a patient the rationale for performance of a procedure.

ABHES Competencies Achieved

☑ 2. c. Identify diagnostic and treatment modalities as they relate to each body system.
☑ 7. g. Display professionalism through written and verbal communication.

15 Introduction to the Clinical Laboratory

CHAPTER ASSIGNMENTS

√ After Completing	Date Due	Study Guide Pages	STUDY GUIDE ASSIGNMENTS (CTA = Critical Thinking Activity)	Possible Points	Points You Earned
		641	📄 Pretest	10	
		642	🔑 Term Key Term Assessment	22	
		643-648	📋 Evaluation of Learning questions	45	
		648	CTA A: Laboratory Directory Information	10	
		648-649	CTA B: Specimen Requirements	15	
		649	CTA C: Identifying Abnormal Values	10	
		649-650	CTA D: Laboratory Report	25	
		651-651	CTA E: Laboratory Directory	9	
		651	CTA F: Testing Kit Product Insert (3 points for each section)	42	
		652	CTA G: Crossword Puzzle	29	
			🅔 Evolve Site: Road to Recovery: Laboratory Test Categories (Record points earned)		
			🅔 Evolve Site: Apply Your Knowledge questions	10	
		641	📄 Posttest	10	
			ADDITIONAL ASSIGNMENTS		
			Total points		

√ When Assigned by Your Instructor	Study Guide Pages	Practices Required	LABORATORY ASSIGNMENTS (Procedure Number and Name)	Score*
	653	2	**Practice for Competency** 15-A: Operate an Emergency Eyewash Station Textbook reference: pp. 544-545	
	657-659		**Evaluation of Competency** 15-A: Operate an Emergency Eyewash Station	*
	654-656	3	**Practice for Competency** 15-1: Collecting a Specimen for Transport to an Outside Laboratory Textbook reference: pp. 562-564	
	661-662		**Evaluation of Competency** 15-1: Collecting a Specimen for Transport to an Outside Laboratory	*

Notes

Name: _____ Date: _____

True or False

_____ 1. When the body is in homeostasis, an imbalance exists in the body.

_____ 2. A routine test is performed to assist in the early detection of disease.

_____ 3. The laboratory request form provides the outside laboratory with information needed to test the specimen.

_____ 4. The clinical diagnosis is indicated on a laboratory request to correlate laboratory data with the needs of the provider.

_____ 5. The purpose of a laboratory report is to indicate the patient's diagnosis.

_____ 6. A patient who is fasting in preparation for a laboratory test is permitted to drink diet soda.

_____ 7. A small sample taken from the body to represent the nature of the whole is known as a specimen.

_____ 8. A laboratory report marked QNS means that the patient did not prepare properly.

_____ 9. Fecal occult blood testing is an example of a CLIA-waived test.

_____ 10. The purpose of quality control is to prevent accidents in the laboratory.

? POSTTEST

True or False

_____ 1. Laboratory tests are most frequently ordered by the provider to assist in the diagnosis of pathologic conditions.

_____ 2. A laboratory directory indicates the patient preparation required for laboratory tests.

_____ 3. Laboratory tests called profiles contain a number of different tests.

_____ 4. A lipid profile includes a test for glucose.

_____ 5. The purpose of patient preparation for a laboratory test is to ensure that the test results fall within the reference range.

_____ 6. A comprehensive metabolic profile requires that the patient fast.

_____ 7. Antibiotics taken by the patient before the collection of a throat specimen for culture may produce a false-positive result.

_____ 8. The purpose of CLIA is to prevent exposure of employees to bloodborne pathogens.

_____ 9. If a POL is performing moderate-complexity tests, CLIA requires that two levels of controls be run daily.

_____ 10. The study of blood and blood-forming tissues is known as serology.

Directions: Match each key term with its definition.

_____ 1. Analyte

_____ 2. Calibration

_____ 3. Clinical diagnosis

_____ 4. Control

_____ 5. Fasting

_____ 6. Homeostasis

_____ 7. In vivo

_____ 8. Laboratory test

_____ 9. Nonwaived test

_____ 10. Plasma

_____ 11. Product insert

_____ 12. Profile

_____ 13. Qualitative test

_____ 14. Quality control

_____ 15. Quantitative test

_____ 16. Reagent

_____ 17. Reference range

_____ 18 Routine test

_____ 19. Serum

_____ 20. Specimen

_____ 21. Test system

_____ 22. Waived test

A. Liquid part of the blood, consisting of a clear, yellowish fluid that comprises approximately 55% of the total blood volume

B. State in which body systems are functioning normally and the internal environment of the body is in equilibrium; the body is in a healthy state

C. Array of laboratory tests for identifying a disease state or evaluating a particular organ or organ system

D. Printed document supplied by the manufacturer with a laboratory test product that contains information on the proper storage and use of the product

E. Solution that is used to monitor a test system to ensure the reliability and accuracy of the test results

F. Test that indicates whether a substance is present in the specimen being tested and provides an approximate indication of the amount of the substance present

G. Application of methods to ensure that test results are reliable and valid and that errors are detected and eliminated

H. Occurring in the living body or organism

I. Test that indicates the exact amount of a chemical substance that is present in the body, with the results being reported in measurable units

J. Substance that is being identified or measured in a laboratory test

K. Substance that produces a reaction with a patient specimen that allows detection or measurement of the substance by the test system

L. A certain established and acceptable parameter of reference range within which the laboratory test results of a healthy individual are expected to fall

M. Tentative diagnosis of a patient's condition obtained through the evaluation of the health history and the physical examination, without the benefit of laboratory or diagnostic tests

N. Abstaining from food or fluids (except water) for a specified amount of time before the collection of a specimen

O. Laboratory test that meets the CLIA criteria for being a simple procedure that is easy to perform and has a low risk of erroneous test results

P. Laboratory test performed routinely on apparently healthy patients to assist in the early detection of disease

Q. Clear, straw-colored part of the blood (plasma) that remains after the solid elements and the clotting factor fibrinogen have been separated from it

R. Mechanism to check the precision and accuracy of a test system, such as an automated analyzer

S. Small sample of something taken to show the nature of the whole

T. Clinical analysis and study of materials, fluids, or tissues obtained from patients to assist in the diagnosis and treatment of disease

U. Setup that includes all of the test components required to perform a laboratory test, such as testing devices, controls, and testing reagents

V. Complex laboratory test that does not meet the CLIA criteria for waiver and is subject to the CLIA regulations

Directions: Fill in each blank with the correct answer.

1. What is the general purpose of a laboratory test?

_____

_____

_____

2. Define each of the following categories of laboratory tests.

   a. Hematology:

   _____

   _____

   b. Clinical chemistry:

   _____

   _____

   c. Immunology and blood banking:

   _____

   _____

   d. Urinalysis:

   _____

   _____

   e. Microbiology:

   _____

   _____

3. List five specific uses of laboratory test results.

   _____

   _____

   _____

   _____

   _____

4. What is the purpose of performing a routine test?

   _____

   _____

5. What is the purpose of CLIA?

   _____

   _____

643

6. What requirements must be followed regarding a refrigerator used to store specimens and testing components?

_____

_____

7. What is the purpose of an emergency eyewash station?

_____

_____

8. Why is it important to flush the eyes immediately after they have been exposed to a hazardous substance?

_____

_____

9. What temperature range is usually required for storing testing materials and performing laboratory tests?

_____

10. What information is included in a laboratory directory?

_____

_____

_____

11. What is the purpose of a laboratory request?

_____

_____

12. What is the reason for indicating the following information on the laboratory request form?

a. Patient's age and gender:

_____

_____

b. Date and time of collection of the specimen:

_____

_____

c. Source of the specimen:

_____

_____

d. Provider's clinical diagnosis:

_____

_____

e. Medications the patient is taking:

_____

_____

13. How does a laboratory report the results when a laboratory request is marked STAT?

_____

_____

_____

14. What tests are included in the following profiles?

    a. Comprehensive metabolic profile:

_____

_____

    b. Hepatic function profile:

_____

_____

    c. Prenatal profile:

_____

_____

15. What information is included on laboratory reports?

_____

_____

_____

_____

16. Why must the test results of specimens tested by an outside laboratory be compared with the reference ranges supplied by the laboratory?

_____

_____

17. How are laboratory reports delivered to the medical office?

_____

_____

18. If a laboratory request form is completed on a computer, how is it transmitted to the laboratory?

_____

_____

19. Why do some laboratory tests require advance patient preparation?

_____

_____

20. Why is it important to explain the reason for the advance preparation to the patient?

_____

645

21. Why are fasting specimens usually collected in the morning?

_____

_____

22. What is a specimen?

_____

_____

23. List 10 examples of specimens.

_____

_____

_____

_____

_____

24. What reference source should be used to locate the specimen collection and handling requirements for the following?

a. Specimen transported to an outside laboratory:

_____

b. Specimen tested in the medical office:

_____

25. Why must the appropriate container be used to collect a specimen?

_____

_____

26. What is a unique identifier?

_____

_____

27. What two methods can be used to label a specimen?

_____

_____

28. Why is it important to properly identify a patient?

_____

29. Why must a specimen be properly handled and stored?

_____

_____

30. List the CLIA-waived tests that are most frequently performed in the medical office.

_____

646

31. What is included in a laboratory testing kit?

_____

_____

32. What may occur if a testing kit is outdated?

_____

_____

33. What is a unitized testing device?

_____

_____

34. Describe a CLIA-waived automated analyzer.

_____

_____

35. What is the purpose of quality control?

_____

_____

36. What are the storage requirements for most testing systems?

_____

_____

37. What should be written on the label of a control that is stable only for a certain period of time after opening it?

_____

_____

38. What is an internal control?

_____

39. An internal control checks for what conditions?

_____

40. What is the purpose of an external control?

_____

_____

41. What types of results are produced by the following controls?

a. Low-level control:

_____

b. High-level control:

_____

42. What may cause a control to fail to produce expected results?

_____

_____

43. What may cause invalid test results to occur when testing a specimen with a testing kit?

_____

_____

44. What is the difference between qualitative test results and quantitative test results?

_____

_____

45. List 10 laboratory safety guidelines that should be followed in the medical office to prevent accidents.

_____

_____

_____

_____

_____

CRITICAL THINKING ACTIVITIES

A. Laboratory Directory Information

Look at a laboratory directory (from an outside medical laboratory), and list the categories of information included in it (e.g., normal range of laboratory tests).

_____

_____

_____

_____

_____

_____

B. Specimen Requirements

Refer to Table 15-2 in your textbook, and list the specimen requirements for each of the following tests:

1. ALT _____

2. Bilirubin, total _____

3. Blood group (ABO) and Rh Type _____

648

4. BUN, serum _____

5. Calcium _____

6. CBC (with differential) _____

7. CRP _____

8. Glucose, plasma _____

9. LD _____

10. PT/INR _____

11. RPR _____

12. Sedimentation rate (ESR) _____

13. Thyroxine (T$_4$) _____

14. Triglycerides _____

15. Urinalysis _____

C. Identifying Abnormal Values

Refer to the laboratory report in your textbook (see Figure 15-7), and circle any abnormal values using a red pen.

D. Laboratory Report

Refer to the laboratory report in your textbook (see Figure 15-7). Using the normal values listed on this report, determine whether the following tests fall within normal ranges or whether they are high or low. Mark each test according to the following: **N** = normal, **H** = high, **L** = low. Your patient is an adult female.

1. Glucose: 140 mg/dL _____

2. BUN: 15 mg/dL _____

3. Creatinine: 1.7 mg/dL _____

4. Calcium: 10.2 mg/dL _____

5. Magnesium: 0.4 mmol/L _____

6. Sodium: 156 mmol/L _____

7. Potassium: 5.5 mmol/L _____

8. Chloride: 84 mmol/L _____

9. Carbon dioxide: 18 mmol/L _____

10. Uric acid: 5.2 mg/dL _____

11. Total protein: 4.0 g/dL _____

12. Albumin: 3.5 g/dL _____

13. Total bilirubin: 0.8 mg/dL _____

14. Alkaline phosphatase: 80 U/L _____

15. LD: 132 U/L _____

16. AST: 24 U/L _____

17. ALT: 44 U/L _____

18. Total cholesterol: 260 mg/dL _____

19. HDL cholesterol: 57 mg/dL _____

20. LDL cholesterol: 165 mg/dL _____

21. WBC: 15.5 ($\times$ 10³/mm³) _____

22. Hemoglobin: 10.4 g/dL _____

23. Hematocrit: 34% _____

24. Prothrombin time: 10 seconds _____

25. Neutrophils: 84% _____

E. Laboratory Directory

Your provider has ordered a triglyceride test on a patient that will be analyzed at an outside laboratory. You are required to collect the specimen and prepare it for transport to the outside laboratory. Using Figure 15-11 in your textbook as a reference, respond to the following questions in the space provided.

1. What is the amount and type of specimen required for this test?

_____

2. What patient preparation is required for this test?

_____

_____

3. What collection supplies are required for this test?

_____

4. What collection techniques must be performed after collecting the specimen?

_____

_____

5. How should you store the specimen while awaiting pickup by the laboratory?

_____

_____

6. What would cause the laboratory to reject the specimen?

_____

_____

7. What are the limitations of this test?

_____

_____

_____

8. When would be the best time to collect this specimen (AM or PM)? Explain the reason for your answer.

_____

_____

_____

9. When the laboratory report is returned, the triglyceride test results are 250 mg/dL. How is this interpreted: desirable, borderline high, high, or very high?

_____

F. Testing Kit Product Insert

Obtain a product insert from a CLIA-waived testing kit. The product insert can be obtained from an actual testing kit or from a Google search on the Internet. Provide a brief description of the information included in each section of the product insert in the space provided. Examples of brand names of CLIA-waived testing kits include the following:

Hemoccult fecal occult blood test	QuickVue hCG pregnancy test
ColoScreen fecal occult blood test	OSOM hCG urine pregnancy test
Seracult fecal occult blood test	ICON hCG urine pregnancy test
Hemoccult ICT test	QuickVue In-Line Strep A test
QuickVue iFOB test	OSOM Ultra Strep A test
OSOM mono test	ICON DS Strep A test
Clearview mono test	Acceava Strep A test

Name of Testing Kit: _____

Section	Brief description of information included in this section of the product insert
Intended use	
Summary and explanation	
Principles of the procedure	
Precautions and warnings	
Reagents and materials provided	
Materials not provided	
Storage and stability	
Specimen collection and handling	
Test procedure	
Interpretation and reading results	
Quality control	
Limitations of the procedure	
Expected values	
Performance characteristics	

G. Crossword Puzzle: Introduction to the Clinical Laboratory

Directions: Complete the crossword puzzle using the clues provided.

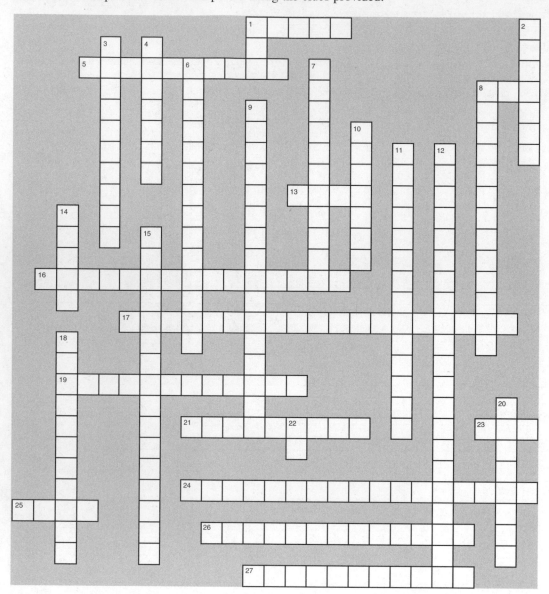

Across

1 For documenting control results
5 Order a laboratory test
8 In-house laboratory
13 As soon as possible
16 Approximate amount of substance present
17 Outside lab reference source
19 Determines CAD risk
21 What are the results?
23 Microscopic analysis of urine (example)
24 Tentative diagnosis
25 To improve quality of lab testing
26 Complex lab test
27 Detects disease early

Down

1 Not enough specimen?
2 A substance being identified
3 Has a low risk of erroneous test results
4 More than one lab test
6 Accurate and reliable test results
7 Healthy body
8 Provides info on performing lab test
9 Is that you?
10 No food or fluid
11 Where healthy test results should fall
12 Which disease is it?
14 Plasma minus fibrinogen
15 A cause of abnormal control results
18 Test system working OK?
20 Sample of the body
22 CLIA requires 3 times per year

Procedure 15-A: Operate and Inspect an Emergency Eyewash Station

Operate and inspect an emergency eyewash station. Document the inspection on the eyewash inspection tag presented below.

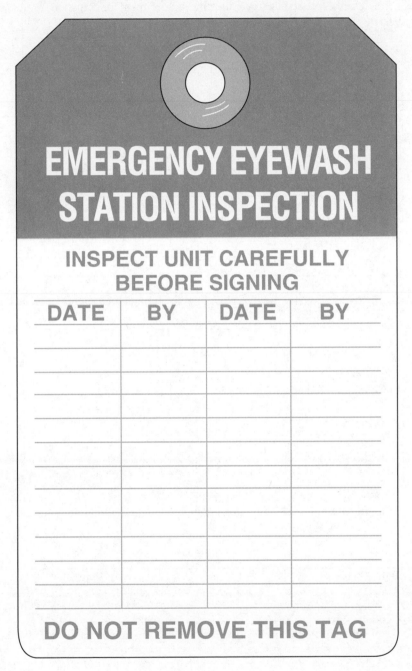

EMERGENCY EYEWASH STATION INSPECTION

INSPECT UNIT CAREFULLY BEFORE SIGNING

DATE	BY	DATE	BY

DO NOT REMOVE THIS TAG

Procedure 15-1: Collecting Specimen for Transport to an Outside Laboratory

1. Laboratory requisition. Complete the Laboratory Request form on page 656 using a classmate as a patient. The tests that have been ordered by the provider include the following: basic metabolic profile, lipid profile, CBC (with differential), and Rheumatoid Arthritis Factor.
2. Specimen collection. Practice the procedure for collecting a specimen for transport to an outside laboratory, and document the procedure in the chart provided.

CHART	
Date	

654

CHART	
Date	

LABORATORY REQUISITION
Biomedical Laboratories, Inc.
100 Main Street
Athens, Georgia 45760

☐ Fax   Send additional copy of report to:
☐ Call   Client Number/Physician's Name   ( ) Phone/Fax number
☐ Mail   Physician's Address   City, State, Zip

Patient's Name (Last)	(First)	(MI)	Sex	Date of Birth MO | DAY | YEAR	Collection Time : AM PM	Fasting YES NO	Collection Date MO | DAY | YEAR

NPI/UPIN	Physician's ID #	Patient's SS #	Patient's ID #	Urine hrs/vol hrs____ vol ____

PATIENT / RESP. PARTY

Physician's Name (Last, First)	Physician's Signature	Patient's Address Phone

Medicare # (Include prefix/suffix)	☐ Primary ☐ Secondary	City State ZIP

Medicaid # State	Physician's Provider #	Name of Responsible Party (if different from patient)

Diagnosis/Signs/Symptoms in ICD-9 Format (Highest Specificity)
REQUIRED

Address of Responsible Party (if different from patient)   APT #

City   State   ZIP

INSURANCE

Patient's Relationship to Responsible Party ☐ 1–Self ☐ 2–Spouse ☐ 3–Child ☐ 4–Other

Performance Lab ☐   Carrier   Group #   Employee #   Mem

Insurance Company Name	Plan	Carrier Code
Subscriber/Member #	Location	Group #
Insurance Address	Physician's Provider #	
City	State ZIP	
Employer's Name or Number	Insured SS # (If not patient)	Worker's Comp ☐ Yes ☐ No

I hereby authorize the release of medical information related to the service subscribed herein and authorize payment directed to LabCorp.
X _____ Patient's Signature   Date

MEDICARE ADVANCE BENEFICIARY NOTICE
I have read the ABN on the reverse. If Medicare denies payment, I agree to pay for the identified test(s).
X _____ Patient's Signature   Date

NOTE: WHEN ORDERING TESTS FOR WHICH MEDICARE OR MEDICAID REIMBURSEMENT WILL BE SOUGHT, PHYSICIANS SHOULD ONLY ORDER TESTS THAT ARE MEDICALLY NECESSARY FOR THE DIAGNOSIS OR TREATMENT OF THE PATIENT. COMPONENTS OF THE ORGAN OR DISEASE PANELS/COMBINATIONS PRINTED BELOW ARE SHOWN ON THE REVERSE SIDE AND MAY ALSO BE ORDERED INDIVIDUALLY BELOW. COMPONENTS MAY BE BILLED SEPARATELY PER CARRIER POLICY.

PROFILES (See reverse for components)

Code	Test	Tube
80049	Basic Metabolic Profile	SST
80054	Comp Metabolic Profile	SST
80051	Electrolyte Profile	SST
80058	Hepatic Profile	SST
80059	Hepatitis Profile	SST
80061	Lipid Profile	SST
80091	Thyroid Profile	SST
80055	Prenatal Profile	RED LAV
80072	Rheumatoid Profile	SST

HEMATOLOGY

Code	Test	Tube
85025	CBC w Diff	LAV
85027	CBC w/o Diff	LAV
85014	Hematocrit	LAV
85018	Hemoglobin	LAV
85595	Platelet Count	LAV
85041	RBC Count	LAV
85048	WBC Count	LAV
85007	WBC Differential	LAV
89190	Nasal Smear, Eosin	Nasal Smear
85060	Pathologist Consult-Peripheral Smear	LAV

ALPHABETICAL/COMBINATION TESTS

Code	Test	Tube
86900 86901	ABO and Rh	LAV
82040	Albumin	SST
84075	Alkaline Phosphatase	SST
84460	ALT (SGPT)	SST
82150	Amylase, Serum	SST
86038	Antinuclear Antibodies	SST
84450	AST (SGOT)	SST
82607 82746	B₁₂ and Folate	SST
82250	Bilirubin, Total	SST

ALPHABETICAL TESTS CON'T

Code	Test	Tube
84520	BUN	SST
82310	Calcium	SST
80156	Carbamazepine (Tegretol®)	SER
82378	CEA	SST
82465	Cholesterol, Total	SST
82565	Creatinine	SST
80162	Digoxin	SER
82670	Estradiol	SST
82728	Ferritin, Serum	SST
82985	Fructosamine	SST
83001	FSH	SST
83001 83002	FSH and LH	SST
82977	GGT	SST
82947	Glucose, Plasma	GRY
82947	Glucose, Serum	SST
82950	Glucose, 2-hr. PP	SST
83036	Glycohemoglobin, Total	LAV
84703	hCG, Beta Subunit, Qual	SST
84702	hCG, Beta Subunit, Quant	SST
83718	HDL Cholesterol	SST
86677	Helicobacter pylori, IgG	SST
86706	Hep B Surface Antibody	SST
87340	Hep B Surface Antigen	SST
86803	Hep C Antibody	SST
83036	Hemoglobin A₁C	LAV
86701	HIV Antibodies	SST
83540	Iron, Total	SST
83540 83550	Iron and IBC	SST
83615	LDH	SST

ALPHABETICAL TESTS CON'T

Code	Test	Tube
83002	LH	SST
83690	Lipase	SER
80178	Lithium (Eskalith®)	SER
83735	Magnesium, Serum	SST
80184	Phenobarbital (Luminal®)	SER
80185	Phenytoin (Dilantin®)	SER
84132	Potassium	SST
84146	Prolactin, Serum	SST
84153	Prostate-Specific Antigen	SST
84066	Prostatic Acid Phos	SST
84155	Protein, Total	SST
85610	Prothrombin Time (PT)	BLU
85610 85730	PT and PTT Activated	BLU
85730	PTT Activated	BLU
86431	Rheumatoid Arthritis Factor	SST
86592	RPR	SST
86762	Rubella Antibodies, IgG	SST
85651	Sed Rate	LAV
84295	Sodium	SST
84403	Testosterone	SST
80198	Theophylline	SER
84436	Thyroxine (T₄)	SST
84478	Triglycerides	SST
84480	Triiodothyronine (T₃)	SST
84443	TSH, High Sensitivity	SST
84550	Uric Acid	SST
81003	Urinalysis Microscopic on Positives	URN
81001	Urinalysis with Microscopic	URN
80164	Valproic Acid (Depakene®)	SER

MICROBIOLOGY (See Reverse Side)

☐ ENDOCERVICAL ☐ THROAT ☐ URINE
☐ STOOL ☐ URETHRAL   INDICATE SOURCE

Code	Test	Transport
87070	Aerobic Bacterial Culture	Bact Trnspt
87490 87590	Chlamydia/GC DNA Probe w/ Confirmation on Positives	Probe Trnspt
87490 87590	Chlamydia/GC DNA Probe Without Confirmation	Probe Trnspt
87490	Chlamydia DNA Probe	Probe Trnspt
87081	Genital, Beta-Hemolytic Strep Cult, Group B	Bact Trnspt
87070	Genital Culture, Routine	Bact Trnspt
87070	Lower Respiratory Culture	Steril Trnspt
87590	N. gonorrhoeae DNA Probe	Probe Trnspt
87015 87211	Ova and Parasites	O & P Kit
87081 X2 87045	Stool Culture	Fecal Trnspt
87081	Throat, Beta-Hemolytic Strep Cult, Group A	Bact Trnspt
87060	Upper Respiratory Culture, Routine	Bact Trnspt
87086	Urine Culture, Routine	Urn Cul Trnspt

Clinical Information/Comments

OTHER TESTS/INDIVIDUAL COMPONENTS
TEST #   TEST NAMES

LAB USE ONLY	STAT ☐ 998074	VENIPUNCTURE ☐ 998085	TRAVEL ☐ 998096	NON LABCORP ☐ 998239	VERBAL ORDER ☐ 998250	CHART ORDER ☐ 998261	HANDWRITTEN ☐ 998272	24 HR TUV ☐ 998283	PST/PSC #

CONTAINERS RECEIVED: SST SPUN | USST UNSPUN | SER SERUM | FRZ TRNSPT | RED RED | LAV LAVENDER | SLD SLIDE | BLU LT. BLUE | GRY GREY | GRN GREEN | RYB RYL BLU | YEL ACD | PLS PLASMA | URN URINE | 24U 24 HR URINE | TA-U TART. ACID | FL FLUID | OT OTHER | BACT TRNSP | O & P KIT | PROBE TRNSP | URN CULT TRNSP | STERIL TRNSP | FECAL TRNSP | VIRAL TRNSP

300-0384

Procedure 15-A: Operating an Emergency Eyewash Station

Name: _____   Date: _____

Evaluated by: _____   Score: _____

Performance Objective

Outcome:	Operate and inspect an emergency eyewash station.
Conditions:	Using an emergency eyewash station.
	Given a disinfectant.
Standards:	Time: 5 minutes. Student completed procedure in _____ minutes.
	Accuracy: Satisfactory score on the Performance Evaluation Checklist.

Performance Evaluation Checklist

Trial 1	Trial 2	Point Value	Performance Standards
			Operate the Emergency Eyewash Station
		•	Immediately proceeded to the emergency eyewash station after the eye(s) came in contact with a hazardous substance.
		•	Asked for assistance, if needed.
		•	Activated the eyewash station using the activation lever or paddle.
		•	Held both eyelids apart with your thumbs and forefingers.
		▷	Stated why the eyelids must be held apart.
		•	Directed the flow of water at an angle to the eyes from the outside edge of the lower eyes toward the inside of the eyes.
		▷	Stated why the water should not be aimed directly onto the eyes.
		•	If necessary, removed contact lenses.
		▷	Stated why contact lenses should be removed.
		•	Continued to hold the eyelids apart and gently rolled your eyeballs from left to right and up and down.
		▷	Stated why the eyeballs should be gently rolled.
		•	Continued to flush the eyes for a full 15 minutes.
		•	Returned the activation lever or paddle to its resting position.
		•	Sought medical attention to determine whether further treatment was required.
		•	Cleaned, disinfected, rinsed, and completely dried the eyewash device.
			Inspect the Emergency Eyewash Station
		•	Made sure the access route to the eyewash station is well lit and free of obstructions.

Trial 1	Trial 2	Point Value	Performance Standards
		▷	Stated what may occur if there is a delay in reaching the eyewash station.
		•	Made sure the eyewash station is well-lit and the area around the eyewash station is free of clutter.
		▷	Stated why the area around the station should be free of clutter.
		•	Made sure the nozzle covers are in place and in good condition.
		▷	Stated the purpose of the nozzle covers.
		•	Made sure the eyewash bowl is clean and free of debris.
		•	Activated the eyewash device using the activation lever or paddle.
		•	Made sure the water flow from the nozzles occurred in one second or less following activation of the eyewash.
		•	Made sure the nozzle covers come off automatically when the eyewash device is activated.
		•	Activated the eyewash station for approximately three minutes to flush out the water supply lines.
		▷	Stated the purpose of flushing the water lines.
		•	Made sure that water flows continuously without the use of the hands.
		•	Made sure the nozzle heads are not clogged and that water flows equally from both nozzle heads.
		•	Cleaned, disinfected, rinsed, and completely dried the eyewash device.
		•	Replaced the nozzle covers on the nozzle heads.
		•	Reported any problems to the appropriate personnel.
		•	Documented the inspection date and signed your initials on the eyewash inspection tag.
		▷	Stated how often the eyewash station should be inspected.
			Demonstrated the following affective behavior(s) during this procedure:
		Ⓐ	Recognized the physical and emotional effects of persons involved in an emergency situation.
		Ⓐ	Demonstrated self-awareness in responding to emergency situations.
		★	Completed the procedure within 20 minutes.
			Totals

Evaluation of Student Performance

EVALUATION CRITERIA			COMMENTS
Symbol	**Category**	**Point Value**	
★	Critical Step	16 points	
•	Essential Step	6 points	
Ⓐ	Affective Competency	6 points	
▷	Theory Question	2 points	

Score calculation: 100 points

−_____ points missed

_____ Score

Satisfactory score: 85 or above

CAAHEP Competencies Achieved

Psychomotor (Skills)

☑ III. 1. Participate in bloodborne pathogen training.
☑ VI. 8. Perform routine maintenance of administrative or clinical equipment.
☑ XII. 2. a. Demonstrate proper use of eyewash equipment.

Affective (Behavior)

☑ XII. 1. Recognize the physical and emotional effects of persons involved in an emergency situation.
☑ XII. 2. Demonstrate self-awareness in responding to emergency situations.

ABHES Competencies Achieved

☑ 8. a. Practice standard precautions and perform disinfection/sterilization techniques.
☑ 8. g. Recognize and respond to medical office emergencies.

Notes

Procedure 15-1: Collecting a Specimen for Transport to an Outside Laboratory

Name: _____   Date: _____

Evaluated by: _____   Score: _____

Performance Objective

Outcome:	Collect a specimen for transport to an outside laboratory.
Conditions:	Given the appropriate supplies for the specimen collection and transport (will be based upon the type of specimen collected).
Standards:	Time: 10 minutes. Student completed procedure in _____ minutes.
	Accuracy: Satisfactory score on the Performance Evaluation Checklist.

Performance Evaluation Checklist

Trial 1	Trial 2	Point Value	Performance Standards
		•	Informed the patient of any advance preparation or special instructions.
		▷	Explained why the patient should prepare properly.
		•	Reviewed the requirements in the laboratory directory for the collection and handling of the specimen.
		•	Completed the laboratory request form.
		•	Sanitized hands.
		•	Assembled equipment and supplies.
		•	Labeled the tubes and containers with the patient's name, date, and initials.
		•	Greeted the patient and introduced yourself. Identified the patient and explained the procedure.
		▷	Stated why it is important to correctly identify the patient.
		•	Determined whether the patient prepared properly for the test.
			Collected the specimen incorporating the following guidelines:
		•	Followed the OSHA Standard.
		•	Collected the specimen using proper technique.
		•	Collected the proper type and amount of specimen required for the test.
		•	Processed the specimen further if required by the outside laboratory.
		•	Placed the lid tightly on the specimen container.
			Prepared the specimen for transport:
		•	Placed the specimen in a biohazard specimen bag.
		•	Placed the lab request in the outside pocket of the bag.
		•	Properly handled and stored the specimen.
		•	Documented the procedure correctly.
			Processed the laboratory report:
		•	Reviewed the laboratory report when it was returned.
		•	Notified the provider of any abnormal results.

Trial 1	Trial 2	Point Value	Performance Standards
		•	Filed the laboratory report in the patient's medical record after review by the provider.
			Demonstrated the following affective behavior(s) during this procedure:
		Ⓐ	Explained to a patient the rationale for performance of a procedure.
		★	Completed the procedure within 10 minutes.
			Totals

CHART

Date	

Evaluation of Student Performance

EVALUATION CRITERIA			COMMENTS
Symbol	**Category**	**Point Value**	
★	Critical Step	16 points	
•	Essential Step	6 points	
Ⓐ	Affective Competency	6 points	
▷	Theory Question	2 points	

Score calculation: 100 points

− _____ points missed

_____ Score

Satisfactory score: 85 or above

CAAHEP Competencies Achieved

Psychomotor (Skills)
☑ I. 10. Perform a quality control measure.
☑ II. 2. Differentiate between normal and abnormal test results.
☑ II. 3. Maintain laboratory test results using flow sheets.

Affective (Behavior)
☑ V. 4. Explain to a patient the rationale for performance of a procedure.

ABHES Competencies Achieved

☑ 9. a. Practice quality control.
☑ 9. d. Collect, label, and process specimens.

16 Urinalysis

CHAPTER ASSIGNMENTS

√ After Completing	Date Due	Study Guide Pages	STUDY GUIDE ASSIGNMENTS (CTA = Critical Thinking Activity)	Possible Points	Points You Earned
		667	?≡ Pretest	10	
		668-669	Term Key Term Assessment A. Definitions B. Word Parts (Add 1 point for each key term)	23 16	
		669-672	Evaluation of Learning questions	36	
		673	CTA A: First-Voided Specimen	2	
		673	CTA B: Clean-Catch Specimen	4	
		673-674	CTA C: Urine Testing Kit Instructions	6	
			e Evolve Site: Chemical Testing of Urine (Record points earned)		
		675	CTA D: Crossword Puzzle	20	
			e Evolve Site: Road to Recovery: Urinalysis Terminology (Record points earned)		
			e Evolve Site: Apply Your Knowledge questions	10	
			e Evolve Site: Video Evaluation	25	
		667	?≡ Posttest	10	
			ADDITIONAL ASSIGNMENTS		
			Total points		

√ When Assigned by Your Instructor	Study Guide Pages	Practices Required	LABORATORY ASSIGNMENTS (Procedure Number and Name)	Score*
	677	3	**Practice for Competency** 16-1: Clean-Catch Midstream Specimen Collection Instructions Textbook reference: pp. 581-582	
	683-685		**Evaluation of Competency** 16-1: Clean-Catch Midstream Specimen Collection Instructions	*
	677	3	**Practice for Competency** 16-2: Collection of a 24-Hour Urine Specimen Textbook reference: pp. 582-584	
	687-689		**Evaluation of Competency** 16-2: Collection of a 24-Hour Urine Specimen	*
	677	5	**Practice for Competency** 16-A: Assessing Color and Appearance of a Urine Specimen Textbook reference: pp. 584-585	
	691-692		**Evaluation of Competency** 16-A: Assessing Color and Appearance of a Urine Specimen	*
	677	5	**Practice for Competency** 16-3: Chemical Testing of Urine with the Multistix 10 SG Reagent Strip Textbook reference: pp. 593-595	
	693-695		**Evaluation of Competency** 16-3: Chemical Testing of Urine with the Multistix 10 SG Reagent Strip	*
	677	2	**Practice for Competency** 16-4: Prepare a Urine Specimen for Microscopic Examination: Kova Method Textbook reference: pp. 605-608	
	697-699		**Evaluation of Competency** 16-4: Prepare a Urine Specimen for Microscopic Examination: Kova Method	*
	677	2	**Practice for Competency** 16-5: Performing a Rapid Urine Culture Test Textbook reference: pp. 611-612	
	701-702		**Evaluation of Competency** 16-5: Performing a Rapid Urine Culture Test	*

√ When Assigned by Your Instructor	Study Guide Pages	Practices Required	LABORATORY ASSIGNMENTS (Procedure Number and Name)	Score*
	677	2	**e** **Practice for Competency** 16-6: Performing a Urine Pregnancy Test Textbook reference: pp. 612-614	
	703-705		**Evaluation of Competency** 16-6: Performing a Urine Pregnancy Test	*
			ADDITIONAL ASSIGNMENTS	

Name: _____ Date: _____

True or False

_____ 1. Approximately 95% of urine consists of water.

_____ 2. Frequency is the condition of having to urinate often.

_____ 3. An excessive increase in urine output is called polyuria.

_____ 4. A clean-catch midstream urine specimen is required for a urine culture.

_____ 5. Urinalysis consists of a physical, chemical, and microscopic examination of urine.

_____ 6. A urine specimen that is light yellow indicates that bacteria are present in the specimen.

_____ 7. The pH of most urine specimens is neutral.

_____ 8. Blood may normally be present in the urine due to menstruation.

_____ 9. Hematuria refers to the presence of blood in the urine.

_____ 10. HCG is a hormone that is present in the urine and blood of a pregnant woman.

? POSTTEST

True or False

_____ 1. Urea is a waste product derived from the breakdown of water.

_____ 2. A normal adult excretes approximately 250 mL of urine each day.

_____ 3. Vomiting can result in oliguria.

_____ 4. The distal urethra normally contains microorganisms.

_____ 5. A 24-hour urine specimen may be collected to assist in the diagnosis of a UTI.

_____ 6. If a urine specimen is allowed to stand for more than 1 hour at room temperature, the pH becomes more acidic.

_____ 7. If a freshly voided specimen is cloudy, the patient may have a urinary tract infection.

_____ 8. The normal specific gravity of urine ranges from 1.003 to 1.030.

_____ 9. Dysuria is the inability to control urination at night.

_____ 10. Casts are formed in the urinary bladder.

A. Definitions

Directions: Match each key term with its definition.

_____ 1. Anuria

_____ 2. Bilirubinuria

_____ 3. Dysuria

_____ 4. Frequency

_____ 5. Glycosuria

_____ 6. Hematuria

_____ 7. Ketonuria

_____ 8. Ketosis

_____ 9. Micturition

_____ 10. Nephron

_____ 11. Nocturia

_____ 12. Nocturnal enuresis

_____ 13. Oliguria

_____ 14. pH

_____ 15. Polyuria

_____ 16. Proteinuria

_____ 17. Pyuria

_____ 18. Retention

_____ 19. Specific gravity

_____ 20. Urgency

_____ 21. Urinalysis

_____ 22. Urinary incontinence

_____ 23. Void

A. Decreased or scanty output of urine
B. The presence of protein in the urine
C. Inability of an individual to control urination at night during sleep (bedwetting)
D. The presence of bilirubin in the urine
E. Increased output of urine
F. The presence of pus in the urine
G. The presence of glucose in the urine
H. The physical, chemical, and microscopic analysis of urine
I. The presence of ketone bodies in the urine
J. Act of voiding urine
K. An accumulation of large amounts of ketone bodies in the tissues and body fluids
L. The weight of a substance compared with the weight of an equal volume of a substance known as the standard
M. The unit that describes the acidity or alkalinity of a solution
N. The functional unit of the kidney
O. The inability to empty the bladder; urine is being produced normally but is not being voided
P. The immediate need to urinate
Q. To empty the bladder
R. Failure of the kidneys to produce urine
S. Difficult or painful urination
T. The condition of having to urinate often
U. Blood present in the urine
V. Excessive (voluntary) urination during the night
W. The inability to retain urine

B. Word Parts

Directions: Indicate the meaning of each word part in the space provided. List as many medical terms as possible that incorporate the word part in the space provided.

Word Part	Meaning of Word Part	Medical Terms That Incorporate Word Part
1. an-		
2. ur/o		
3. -ia		
4. bilirubin/o		
5. dys-		
6. glyc/o		
7. hemat/o		
8. keton/o		
9. -osis		
10. noct/i		
11. olig/o		
12. poly-		
13. py/o		
14. supra-		
15. pub/o		
16. -ic		

EVALUATION OF LEARNING

Directions: Fill in each blank with the correct answer.

1. List two functions of the urinary system.

_____

_____

2. What is the function of the urinary bladder?

_____

_____

3. How does the function of the urethra differ in the male and female?

_____

_____

669

4. What is the urinary meatus?

_____

5. Most of the urine (95%) is composed of what substance?

_____

_____

6. List two conditions that may cause polyuria.

_____

_____

7. List two conditions that may cause oliguria.

_____

_____

8. What type of urine specimen is required for the detection of a urinary tract infection (UTI)?

_____

9. Why is a first-voided morning specimen often preferred for urine testing?

_____

_____

10. A 24-hour urine specimen is often used to diagnose what condition?

_____

11. Why should a patient not void directly into a 24-hour urine specimen container that contains a preservative?

_____

12. List three changes that may take place in a urine specimen if it is allowed to stand at room temperature for more than 1 hour.

_____

_____

13. Why does concentrated urine tend to be dark yellow?

_____

_____

14. List two factors that may cause a urine specimen to become cloudy.

_____

_____

15. A urine specimen that has been allowed to stand at room temperature for a long period of time will have what type of odor?

_____

16. What is the purpose of testing the specific gravity of urine?

_____

17. What is the normal range for the specific gravity of urine?

_____

18. What is the difference between qualitative and quantitative test results?

_____

_____

_____

19. What may cause an increase in the pH of urine?

_____

_____

20. Why does urine become more alkaline if it is not preserved?

_____

_____

21. What may cause glycosuria?

_____

_____

22. What conditions may cause proteinuria?

_____

_____

23. What may cause ketosis?

_____

_____

24. What conditions may cause bilirubin to appear in the urine?

_____

_____

25. What may cause blood to appear in the urine?

_____

_____

26. Why should a nitrite test not be performed on a urine specimen that has been left standing at room temperature?

_____

_____

671

27. How should urine reagent strips be stored?

_____

_____

28. What is the purpose of performing a microscopic examination of the urine?

_____

_____

_____

29. Why is a first-voided urine specimen recommended for a microscopic examination of the urine?

_____

_____

30. What effect does concentrated urine have on red blood cells in it?

_____

_____

31. What is a urinary cast?

_____

_____

32. What is the name of the vaginal infection caused by yeast?

_____

_____

33. List two reasons for performing a urine culture test.

_____

_____

34. List three reasons for performing a pregnancy test.

_____

_____

35. What is the name of the hormone that is present in the urine and blood only of a pregnant woman?

_____

36. List five guidelines that should be followed when performing a pregnancy test.

_____

_____

_____

_____

CRITICAL THINKING ACTIVITIES

A. First-Voided Specimen

You have instructed Jim Pratt to collect a first-voided morning urine specimen, which is to be brought to the medical office for testing. Mr. Pratt asks the following questions. Respond to them in the spaces provided.

1. Why is a first-voided specimen desired?

_____

_____

2. Why must the specimen be preserved until it is brought to the medical office?

_____

_____

B. Clean-Catch Specimen

You have just instructed Ann Berger to obtain a clean-catch midstream specimen at the medical office. Mrs. Berger asks the following questions. Respond to them in the spaces provided.

1. What is the purpose of cleansing the urinary meatus?

_____

_____

2. Why must a front-to-back motion be used to clean the urinary meatus?

_____

_____

3. Why must a small amount of urine first be voided into the toilet?

_____

_____

4. Why should the inside of the specimen cup not be touched?

_____

_____

C. Urine Testing Kit Instructions

Obtain the package insert instructions that come with any type of commercially prepared diagnostic kit for the chemical testing of urine (e.g., Multistix 10 SG). Using the instructions, answer the following questions in the spaces provided. (*Note:* A package insert for Multistix 10 SG can be obtained on the Internet by performing a search for *Multistix 10 SG product insert.*)

1. What is the brand name of the test?

_____

2. This test assists in the diagnosis of what conditions?

_____

_____

_____

673

3. What type of urine specimen is recommended for this test?

_____

_____

_____

4. This test is used to detect the presence of what substances?

_____

_____

_____

5. Explain the proper storage and handling of this test.

_____

_____

_____

6. List any substances or techniques that may interfere with obtaining an accurate reading (e.g., not reading the test at the prescribed time).

_____

_____

_____

D. Crossword Puzzle: Urinalysis

Directions: Complete the crossword puzzle using the clues provided.

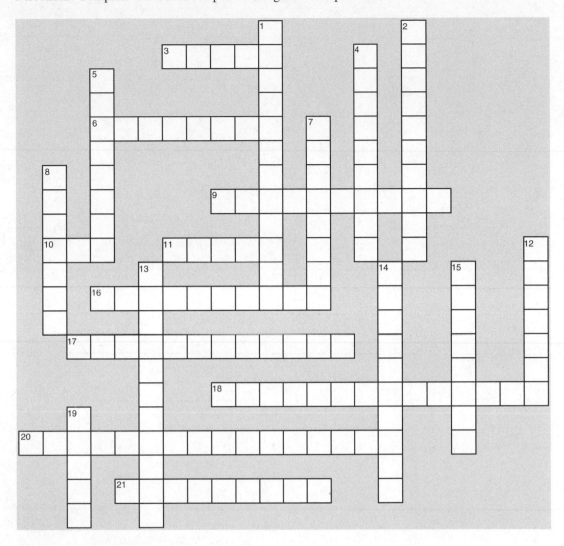

Across

3 UTI bacteria
6 Deteriorates urine strips
9 Tx for UTI
10 Makes preg test +
11 Neutral pH **seven**
16 Physical, chemical, and microscopic
17 Normal cause of hematuria
18 Security for urine drug testing
20 Measures exact amount
21 Cause of bilirubinuria

Down

1 24-hour spec dx can cause this
2 Cause of ketonuria
4 Yellow urine pigment
5 Cause of oliguria
7 Cause of glycosuria
8 Kidney unit
12 Sym of UTI
13 Spec for preg test
14 Spec for C & S
15 This drug causes polyuria
19 Most of urine

Notes

PRACTICE FOR COMPETENCY

Procedure 16-1: Clean-Catch Midstream Specimen Collection Instructions

Instruct an individual in the procedure for collecting a clean-catch midstream specimen, and document the procedure in the chart provided.

Procedure 16-2: 24-Hour Urine Specimen

Instruct an individual in the procedure for collecting a 24-hour urine specimen, and document the procedure in the chart provided.

Procedure 16-A: Color and Appearance of a Urine Specimen

Assess the color and appearance of a urine specimen, and document the results in the chart provided.

Procedure 16-3: Chemical Testing of Urine Using the Multistix 10 SG Reagent Strip

a. Perform a Multistix 10 SG quality control testing procedure, and document the results on the quality control log on page 679.
b. Perform a chemical assessment of a urine specimen using a Multistix 10 SG reagent strip. Document the results on the laboratory report form provided. Circle any abnormal results.

Procedure 16-4: Prepare a Urine Specimen for Microscopic Examination of Urine

Practice the procedure for preparing a urine specimen for a microscopic analysis of the urine sediment. Examine the specimen, and document the results in the chart provided.

Procedure 16-5: Rapid Urine Culture Test

Perform a rapid urine culture test, and document the results in the chart provided.

Procedure 16-6: Urine Pregnancy Test

Perform a urine pregnancy test, and document the results in the chart provided.

CHART	
Date	

CHART	
Date	

URINALYSIS QUALITY CONTROL LOG

Name of Test: _____ Date: _____	Name of Control: _____ Lot #: _____ Exp. Date: _____	Technician: _____
TEST	**EXPECTED RESULT** (specified in product insert accompanying the control)	**CONTROL RESULT**
Glucose		
Bilirubin		
Ketone		
Specific gravity		
Blood		
pH		
Protein		
Urobilinogen		
Nitrite		
Leukocytes		

Multistix® 10 SG Reagent Strips for Urinalysis

PATIENT

DATE   TIME

Test							
LEUKOCYTES	NEGATIVE ☐		TRACE ☐	SMALL + ☐	MODERATE ++ ☐	LARGE +++ ☐	
NITRITE	NEGATIVE ☐		POSITIVE ☐	POSITIVE ☐	(Any degree of uniform pink color is found)		
UROBILINOGEN	NORMAL 0.2 ☐	NORMAL 1 ☐	mg/dL 2 ☐	4 ☐	8 ☐	(1mg = approx. 1 BU)	
PROTEIN	NEGATIVE ☐	TRACE ☐	mg/dL 30 * ☐	100 ++ ☐	300 +++ ☐	2000 OR MORE ☐	
pH	5.0 ☐	6.0 ☐	6.5 ☐	7.0 ☐	7.5 ☐	8.0 ☐	8.5 ☐
BLOOD	NEGATIVE ☐	NON-HEMOLYZED TRACE ☐	NON-HEMOLYZED MODERATE ☐	HEMOLYZED TRACE ☐	SMALL + ☐	MODERATE ++ ☐	LARGE +++ ☐
SPECIFIC GRAVITY	1.000 ☐	1.006 ☐	1.010 ☐	1.015 ☐	1.020 ☐	1.025 ☐	1.030 ☐
KETONE	NEGATIVE ☐	mg/dL	TRACE 5 ☐	SMALL 15 ☐	MODERATE 40 ☐	LARGE 80 ☐	LARGE 160 ☐
BILIRUBIN	NEGATIVE ☐		SMALL + ☐	MODERATE ++ ☐	LARGE +++ ☐		
GLUCOSE	NEGATIVE ☐	g/L (%) mg/dL	1/10 (tr.) 100 ☐	1/6 250 ☐	1/2 500 ☐	1 1000 ☐	2 or more 2000 or more ☐

(Modified and printed with permission of Siemens Medical Solutions Diagnostic, Tarrytown, NY 10591.)

Multistix® 10 SG Reagent Strips for Urinalysis

PATIENT

DATE   TIME

Test							
LEUKOCYTES	NEGATIVE ☐		TRACE ☐	SMALL + ☐	MODERATE ++ ☐	LARGE +++ ☐	
NITRITE	NEGATIVE ☐		POSITIVE ☐	POSITIVE ☐	(Any degree of uniform pink color is found)		
UROBILINOGEN	NORMAL 0.2 ☐	NORMAL 1 ☐	mg/dL 2 ☐	4 ☐	8 ☐	(1mg = approx. 1 BU)	
PROTEIN	NEGATIVE ☐	TRACE ☐	mg/dL 30 * ☐	100 ++ ☐	300 +++ ☐	2000 OR MORE ☐	
pH	5.0 ☐	6.0 ☐	6.5 ☐	7.0 ☐	7.5 ☐	8.0 ☐	8.5 ☐
BLOOD	NEGATIVE ☐	NON-HEMOLYZED TRACE ☐	NON-HEMOLYZED MODERATE ☐	HEMOLYZED TRACE ☐	SMALL + ☐	MODERATE ++ ☐	LARGE +++ ☐
SPECIFIC GRAVITY	1.000 ☐	1.006 ☐	1.010 ☐	1.015 ☐	1.020 ☐	1.025 ☐	1.030 ☐
KETONE	NEGATIVE ☐	mg/dL	TRACE 5 ☐	SMALL 15 ☐	MODERATE 40 ☐	LARGE 80 ☐	LARGE 160 ☐
BILIRUBIN	NEGATIVE ☐		SMALL + ☐	MODERATE ++ ☐	LARGE +++ ☐		
GLUCOSE	NEGATIVE ☐	g/L (%) mg/dL	1/10 (tr.) 100 ☐	1/6 250 ☐	1/2 500 ☐	1 1000 ☐	2 or more 2000 or more ☐

(Modified and printed with permission of Siemens Medical Solutions Diagnostic, Tarrytown, NY 10591.)

Multistix® 10 SG Reagent Strips for Urinalysis

PATIENT

DATE   TIME

Analyte							
LEUKOCYTES	NEGATIVE ☐		TRACE ☐	SMALL + ☐	MODERATE ++ ☐	LARGE +++ ☐	
NITRITE	NEGATIVE ☐		POSITIVE ☐	POSITIVE ☐	(Any degree of uniform pink color is found)		
UROBILINOGEN	NORMAL 0.2 ☐	NORMAL 1 ☐	mg/dL 2 ☐	4 ☐	8 ☐	(1mg = approx. 1 BU)	
PROTEIN	NEGATIVE ☐	TRACE ☐	mg/dL 30 * ☐	100 ++ ☐	300 +++ ☐	2000 OR MORE ☐	
pH	5.0 ☐	6.0 ☐	6.5 ☐	7.0 ☐	7.5 ☐	8.0 ☐	8.5 ☐
BLOOD	NEGATIVE ☐	NON-HEMOLYZED TRACE ☐	NON-HEMOLYZED MODERATE ☐	HEMOLYZED TRACE ☐	SMALL + ☐	MODERATE ++ ☐	LARGE +++ ☐
SPECIFIC GRAVITY	1.000 ☐	1.006 ☐	1.010 ☐	1.015 ☐	1.020 ☐	1.025 ☐	1.030 ☐
KETONE	NEGATIVE ☐	mg/dL	TRACE 5 ☐	SMALL 15 ☐	MODERATE 40 ☐	LARGE 80 ☐	LARGE 160 ☐
BILIRUBIN	NEGATIVE ☐		SMALL + ☐	MODERATE ++ ☐	LARGE +++ ☐		
GLUCOSE	NEGATIVE ☐	g/L (%) mg/dL	1/10 (tr.) 100 ☐	1/6 250 ☐	1/2 500 ☐	1 1000 ☐	2 or more 2000 or more ☐

(Modified and printed with permission of Siemens Medical Solutions Diagnostic, Tarrytown, NY 10591.)

Multistix® 10 SG Reagent Strips for Urinalysis

PATIENT

DATE   TIME

Analyte							
LEUKOCYTES	NEGATIVE ☐		TRACE ☐	SMALL + ☐	MODERATE ++ ☐	LARGE +++ ☐	
NITRITE	NEGATIVE ☐		POSITIVE ☐	POSITIVE ☐	(Any degree of uniform pink color is found)		
UROBILINOGEN	NORMAL 0.2 ☐	NORMAL 1 ☐	mg/dL 2 ☐	4 ☐	8 ☐	(1mg = approx. 1 BU)	
PROTEIN	NEGATIVE ☐	TRACE ☐	mg/dL 30 * ☐	100 ++ ☐	300 +++ ☐	2000 OR MORE ☐	
pH	5.0 ☐	6.0 ☐	6.5 ☐	7.0 ☐	7.5 ☐	8.0 ☐	8.5 ☐
BLOOD	NEGATIVE ☐	NON-HEMOLYZED TRACE ☐	NON-HEMOLYZED MODERATE ☐	HEMOLYZED TRACE ☐	SMALL + ☐	MODERATE ++ ☐	LARGE +++ ☐
SPECIFIC GRAVITY	1.000 ☐	1.006 ☐	1.010 ☐	1.015 ☐	1.020 ☐	1.025 ☐	1.030 ☐
KETONE	NEGATIVE ☐	mg/dL	TRACE 5 ☐	SMALL 15 ☐	MODERATE 40 ☐	LARGE 80 ☐	LARGE 160 ☐
BILIRUBIN	NEGATIVE ☐		SMALL + ☐	MODERATE ++ ☐	LARGE +++ ☐		
GLUCOSE	NEGATIVE ☐	g/L (%) mg/dL	1/10 (tr.) 100 ☐	1/6 250 ☐	1/2 500 ☐	1 1000 ☐	2 or more 2000 or more ☐

(Modified and printed with permission of Siemens Medical Solutions Diagnostic, Tarrytown, NY 10591.)

Notes

Procedure 16-1: Clean-Catch Midstream Specimen Collection Instructions

Name: _____   Date: _____

Evaluated by: _____   Score: _____

Performance Objective

Outcome:	Instruct a patient in the procedure for collecting a clean-catch midstream urine specimen.
Conditions:	Given the following: sterile specimen container, personal antiseptic towelettes, and tissues.
Standards:	Time: 10 minutes. Student completed procedure in _____ minutes.
	Accuracy: Satisfactory score on the Performance Evaluation Checklist.

Performance Evaluation Checklist

Trial 1	Trial 2	Point Value	Performance Standards
		•	Sanitized hands.
		•	Greeted the patient and introduced yourself.
		•	Identified the patient and explained the procedure.
		•	Assembled equipment.
		•	Labeled specimen container.
			Instructed the female patient by telling her to:
		•	Wash hands and open antiseptic towelettes.
		•	Remove the lid from the specimen container without touching the inside of the container or lid.
		•	Pull down undergarments and sit on the toilet.
		•	Expose the urinary meatus by spreading the labia apart with one hand.
		•	Cleanse each side of the urinary meatus with a front-to-back motion using a separate towelette on each side of the meatus.
		▷	Explained why a front-to-back motion should be used.
		•	After use, discard each towelette into the toilet.
		•	Cleanse directly across the meatus using a third towelette and discard it.
		•	Void a small amount of urine into the toilet, while continuing to hold the labia apart.
		▷	Explained the purpose of voiding into the toilet.
		•	Without stopping the urine flow, collect the next amount of urine by voiding into the sterile container.
		•	Fill the container approximately half full with urine without touching the inside of the container.

Trial 1	Trial 2	Point Value	Performance Standards
		▷	Stated why the inside of the container should not be touched.
		•	Void the last amount of urine into the toilet.
		•	Replace the specimen container lid.
		•	Wipe the area dry with a tissue, flush the toilet, and wash hands.
			Instructed the male patient by telling him to:
		•	Wash hands, open antiseptic towelettes, and remove the lid from the specimen container.
		•	Pull down undergarments and stand in front of toilet.
		•	Retract the foreskin of the penis if uncircumcised.
		•	Cleanse the area around the meatus and the urethral opening by wiping each side of the meatus with a separate antiseptic towelette.
		•	Cleanse directly across the meatus using a third antiseptic towelette.
		•	Discard each towelette into the toilet after use.
		•	Void a small amount of urine into the toilet.
		•	Collect the next amount of urine by voiding into the sterile container without touching the inside of the container.
		•	Fill the container approximately half full with urine.
		•	Void the last amount of urine into the toilet.
		•	Replace the lid on the specimen container.
		•	Wipe the area dry with a tissue, flush the toilet, and wash hands.
			Performed the following:
		•	Provided the patient with instructions on what to do with the specimen.
		•	Documented the procedure correctly.
		•	Tested the specimen or prepared it for transport to an outside laboratory.
			Demonstrated the following affective behavior(s) during this procedure:
		Ⓐ	Explained to a patient the rationale for performance of a procedure.
		★	Completed the procedure within 10 minutes.
			Totals

CHART	
Date	

Evaluation of Student Performance

EVALUATION CRITERIA			COMMENTS
Symbol	**Category**	**Point Value**	
★	Critical Step	16 points	
•	Essential Step	6 points	
Ⓐ	Affective Competency	6 points	
▷	Theory Question	2 points	

Score calculation: 100 points

− _____ points missed

_____ Score

Satisfactory score: 85 or above

CAAHEP Competencies Achieved

Psychomotor (Skills)
☑ V. 11. Report relevant information concisely and accurately.

Affective (Behavior)
☑ V. 4. Explain to a patient the rationale for performance of a procedure.

ABHES Competencies Achieved

☑ 7. g. Display professionalism through written and verbal communications.
☑ 9. e. (1). Instruct patient in the collection of clean-catch midstream urine specimen.

Notes

Procedure 16-2: Collection of a 24-Hour Urine Specimen

Name: _____   Date: _____

Evaluated by: _____   Score: _____

Performance Objective

Outcome:	Instruct a patient in the procedure for collecting a 24-hour urine specimen.
Conditions:	Given a large urine specimen container, written instructions, and a laboratory requisition.
Standards:	Time: 10 minutes. Student completed procedure in _____ minutes.
	Accuracy: Satisfactory score on the Performance Evaluation Checklist.

Performance Evaluation Checklist

Trial 1	Trial 2	Point Value	Performance Standards
		•	Sanitized hands.
		•	Greeted and introduced yourself.
		•	Identified the patient and explained the procedure.
		•	Assembled equipment.
		•	Labeled the specimen container.
			Instructed the patient in the collection of the specimen:
		•	Empty your bladder when you get up in the morning.
		•	Write the date and start time on the container label.
		•	The next time you need to urinate, void into the collecting container.
		•	Pour the urine into the large specimen container.
		•	Tightly screw the lid onto the container.
		•	Store the container in the refrigerator or in an ice chest.
		•	Repeat these steps each time you urinate.
		•	Collect all of your urine in a 24-hour period, and store it in the designated container.
		•	Urinate in the collection container before having a bowel movement.
		▷	Stated when the patient must start the collection process again from the beginning.
		•	On the following morning, get up at the same time.
		•	Void into the collection container for the last time, and pour the urine into the large specimen container.
		•	Put the lid on the container tightly.
		•	Write the date and time the test ended on the container label.

Trial 1	Trial 2	Point Value	Performance Standards
		•	Return the urine specimen container to the office the same morning as completing the test.
		•	Provided the patient with the 24-hour specimen container, a collecting container, and written instructions.
		•	Provided the patient with a Material Safety Data Sheet (MSDS) if the specimen container contains a preservative.
		▷	Stated the purpose of the MSDS.
		•	Documented instructions given to the patient in his or her medical record.
			Processing the specimen:
		•	Asked the patient whether there were any problems when he or she returned the specimen container.
		▷	Explained what should be done if the specimen was undercollected or overcollected.
		•	Prepared the specimen for transport to the laboratory.
		•	Completed a laboratory request form.
		•	Documented the results correctly.
			Demonstrated the following affective behavior(s) during this procedure:
		Ⓐ	Explain to a patient the rationale for performance of a procedure.
		★	Completed the procedure within 5 minutes.
			Totals

CHART	
Date	

Evaluation of Student Performance

EVALUATION CRITERIA			COMMENTS
Symbol	**Category**	**Point Value**	
★	Critical Step	16 points	
•	Essential Step	6 points	
Ⓐ	Affective Competency	6 points	
▷	Theory Question	2 points	

Score calculation: 100 points
− _____ points missed
_____ Score

Satisfactory score: 85 or above

CAAHEP Competencies Achieved

Psychomotor (Skills)
☑ V. 11. Report relevant information concisely and accurately.

Affective (Behavior)
☑ V. 4. Explain to a patient the rationale for performance of a procedure.

ABHES Competencies Achieved

☑ 7. g. Display professionalism through written and verbal communications.
☑ 9. d. Collect, label, and process specimens.

Notes

Procedure 16-A: Assessing Color and Appearance of a Urine Specimen

Name: _____   Date: _____

Evaluated by: _____   Score: _____

Performance Objective

Outcome:	Assess the color and appearance of a urine specimen.
Conditions:	Given a transparent container and a urine specimen.
Standards:	Time: 5 minutes. Student completed procedure in _____ minutes.
	Accuracy: Satisfactory score on the Performance Evaluation Checklist.

Performance Evaluation Checklist

Trial 1	Trial 2	Point Value	Performance Standards
			Color
		•	Sanitized hands and applied gloves.
		•	Transferred the urine specimen to a transparent container.
		•	Assessed the color of the urine specimen.
		★	The assessment was identical to the evaluator's assessment.
		•	Documented the results correctly.
			Appearance
		•	Assessed the appearance of the urine specimen in the transparent container.
		★	The assessment was identical to the evaluator's assessment.
		•	Documented the results correctly.
		•	Properly disposed of the urine specimen.
		•	Sanitized hands and removed gloves.
			Demonstrated the following affective behavior(s) during this procedure:
		Ⓐ	Incorporated critical thinking skills when performing patient assessment.
		Ⓐ	Reassured a patient of the accuracy of the test results.
		★	Completed the procedure within 5 minutes.
			Totals

CHART	
Date	

Evaluation of Student Performance

EVALUATION CRITERIA			COMMENTS
Symbol	**Category**	**Point Value**	
★	Critical Step	16 points	
•	Essential Step	6 points	
Ⓐ	Affective Competency	6 points	
▷	Theory Question	2 points	

Score calculation: 100 points

− _____ points missed

_____ Score

Satisfactory score: 85 or above

CAAHEP Competencies Achieved

Psychomotor (Skills)
☑ I. 11. c. Obtain specimen and perform CLIA-waived urinalysis.
☑ II. 2. Differentiate between normal and abnormal test results.

Affective (Behavior)
☑ I. 1. Incorporate critical thinking skills when performing patient assessment.
☑ II. 1. Reassure a patient of the accuracy of the test results.

ABHES Competencies Achieved

☑ 9. b. (1). Perform selected CLIA-waived tests that assist with diagnosis and treatment; urinalysis.

Procedure 16-3: Chemical Testing of Urine with the Multistix 10 SG Reagent Strip

Name: _____   Date: _____

Evaluated by: _____   Score: _____

Performance Objective

Outcome:	Perform a chemical assessment of a urine specimen.
Conditions:	Given the following: disposable gloves, Multistix 10 SG reagent strips, urine container, laboratory report form, and a waste container.
Standards:	Time: 5 minutes. Student completed procedure in _____ minutes.
	Accuracy: Satisfactory score on the Performance Evaluation Checklist.

Performance Evaluation Checklist

Trial 1	Trial 2	Point Value	Performance Standards
		•	If necessary, performed a quality control testing procedure.
		▷	Stated when a quality control procedure should be performed.
		•	Obtained a freshly voided urine specimen from the patient.
		▷	Explained why the container used to collect the specimen should be clean.
		•	Sanitized hands.
		•	Assembled equipment.
		•	Checked the expiration date of the reagent strips.
		▷	Stated why the expiration date should be checked.
		•	Applied gloves.
		•	Removed a reagent strip from the container and recapped it immediately.
		▷	Explained why the container should be recapped immediately.
		•	Did not touch the test areas with fingers.
		▷	Explained why the test areas should not be touched with fingers.
		•	Mixed the urine specimen thoroughly.
		•	Removed the lid and completely immersed the reagent strip in the urine specimen.
		•	Removed the strip immediately and ran the edge against the rim of the urine container. Started the timer.
		▷	Explained why excess urine should be removed from the strip.
		•	Held the reagent strip in a horizontal position and placed it as close as possible to the corresponding color blocks on the color chart.
		▷	Explained why the strip should be held in a horizontal position.

Trial 1	Trial 2	Point Value	Performance Standards
		•	Read the results at the exact reading times specified on the color chart.
		▷	Explained why the results must be read at specified times.
		★	The results were identical to the evaluator's results.
		•	Disposed of the strip in a regular waste container.
		•	Removed gloves and sanitized hands.
		•	Documented the results correctly.
			Demonstrated the following affective behavior(s) during this procedure:
		Ⓐ	Incorporated critical thinking skills when performing patient assessment.
		Ⓐ	Reassured a patient of the accuracy of the test results.
		★	Completed the procedure within 5 minutes.
			Totals

CHART	
Date	

Evaluation of Student Performance

EVALUATION CRITERIA			COMMENTS
Symbol	**Category**	**Point Value**	
★	Critical Step	16 points	
•	Essential Step	6 points	
Ⓐ	Affective Competency	6 points	
▷	Theory Question	2 points	

Score calculation: 100 points
− _____ points missed
_____ Score

Satisfactory score: 85 or above

CAAHEP Competencies Achieved

Psychomotor (Skills)
☑ I. 10. Perform a quality control measure.
☑ I. 11. c. Obtain specimen and perform CLIA-waived urinalysis.
☑ II. 2. Differentiate between normal and abnormal test results.

Affective (Behavior)
☑ I. 1. Incorporate critical thinking skills when performing patient assessment.
☑ II. 1. Reassure a patient of the accuracy of the test results.

ABHES Competencies Achieved

☑ 9. a. Practice quality control.
☑ 9. b. Perform selected CLIA-waived tests that assist with diagnosis and treatment: (1) urinalysis, (6) kit testing.

Multistix® 10 SG Reagent Strips for Urinalysis

PATIENT

DATE   TIME

LEUKOCYTES	NEGATIVE ☐		TRACE ☐	SMALL ☐ +	MODERATE ☐ ++	LARGE ☐ +++
NITRITE	NEGATIVE ☐		POSITIVE ☐	POSITIVE ☐	(Any degree of uniform pink color is found)	
UROBILINOGEN	NORMAL ☐ 0.2	NORMAL ☐ 1	mg/dL ☐ 2	4 ☐	8 ☐ (1mg = approx. 1 BU)	
PROTEIN	NEGATIVE ☐	TRACE ☐	mg/dL ☐ 30 ^	100 ☐ ++	300 ☐ +++	2000 OR MORE ☐
pH	5.0 ☐	6.0 ☐	6.5 ☐	7.0 ☐	7.5 ☐	8.0 ☐	8.5 ☐
BLOOD	NEGATIVE ☐	NON-HEMOLYZED TRACE ☐	NON-HEMOLYZED MODERATE ☐	HEMOLYZED TRACE ☐	SMALL ☐ +	MODERATE ☐ ++	LARGE ☐ +++
SPECIFIC GRAVITY	1.000 ☐	1.006 ☐	1.010 ☐	1.015 ☐	1.020 ☐	1.025 ☐	1.030 ☐
KETONE	NEGATIVE ☐	mg/dL	TRACE ☐ 5	SMALL ☐ 15	MODERATE ☐ 40	LARGE ☐ 80	LARGE ☐ 160
BILIRUBIN	NEGATIVE ☐		SMALL ☐ +	MODERATE ☐ ++	LARGE ☐ +++	
GLUCOSE	NEGATIVE ☐	g/L (%) mg/dL	1/10 (tr.) ☐ 100	1/6 ☐ 250	1/2 ☐ 500	1 ☐ 1000	2 or more ☐ 2000 or more

(Modified and printed with permission of Siemens Medical Solutions Diagnostic, Tarrytown, NY 10591.)

Multistix® 10 SG Reagent Strips for Urinalysis

PATIENT

DATE   TIME

LEUKOCYTES	NEGATIVE ☐		TRACE ☐	SMALL ☐ +	MODERATE ☐ ++	LARGE ☐ +++
NITRITE	NEGATIVE ☐		POSITIVE ☐	POSITIVE ☐	(Any degree of uniform pink color is found)	
UROBILINOGEN	NORMAL ☐ 0.2	NORMAL ☐ 1	mg/dL ☐ 2	4 ☐	8 ☐ (1mg = approx. 1 BU)	
PROTEIN	NEGATIVE ☐	TRACE ☐	mg/dL ☐ 30 *	100 ☐ ++	300 ☐ +++	2000 OR MORE ☐
pH	5.0 ☐	6.0 ☐	6.5 ☐	7.0 ☐	7.5 ☐	8.0 ☐	8.5 ☐
BLOOD	NEGATIVE ☐	NON-HEMOLYZED TRACE ☐	NON-HEMOLYZED MODERATE ☐	HEMOLYZED TRACE ☐	SMALL ☐ +	MODERATE ☐ ++	LARGE ☐ +++
SPECIFIC GRAVITY	1.000 ☐	1.006 ☐	1.010 ☐	1.015 ☐	1.020 ☐	1.025 ☐	1.030 ☐
KETONE	NEGATIVE ☐	mg/dL	TRACE ☐ 5	SMALL ☐ 15	MODERATE ☐ 40	LARGE ☐ 80	LARGE ☐ 160
BILIRUBIN	NEGATIVE ☐		SMALL ☐ +	MODERATE ☐ ++	LARGE ☐ +++	
GLUCOSE	NEGATIVE ☐	g/L (%) mg/dL	1/10 (tr.) ☐ 100	1/6 ☐ 250	1/2 ☐ 500	1 ☐ 1000	2 or more ☐ 2000 or more

(Modified and printed with permission of Siemens Medical Solutions Diagnostic, Tarrytown, NY 10591.)

Procedure 16-4: Prepare a Urine Specimen for Microscopic Examination of Urine: Kova Method

Name: _____   Date: _____

Evaluated by: _____   Score: _____

Performance Objective

Outcome:	Prepare a urine specimen for microscopic analysis by the provider.
Conditions:	Given the following: disposable gloves; first-voided morning urine specimen; Kova urine centrifuge tube, cap, pipet, slide, and stain; test tube rack; urine centrifuge; mechanical stage microscope; and waste container.
Standards:	Time: 15 minutes. Student completed procedure in _____ minutes.
	Accuracy: Satisfactory score on the Performance Evaluation Checklist.

Performance Evaluation Checklist

Trial 1	Trial 2	Point Value	Performance Standards
		•	Sanitized hands.
		•	Assembled equipment.
		•	Applied gloves.
		•	Mixed the urine specimen with a pipet.
		▷	Stated the purpose of mixing the specimen.
		•	Poured the urine specimen into a urine centrifuge tube to the 12-mL mark.
		•	Capped the tube.
		•	Centrifuged the specimen for 5 minutes.
		▷	Stated the purpose of centrifuging the specimen.
		•	Removed the tube from the centrifuge without disturbing the sediment.
		•	Removed the cap.
		•	Inserted a Kova pipet into the urine tube and seated it firmly.
		•	Poured off the supernatant fluid.
		•	Removed the pipet from the tube.
		•	Added one drop of Kova stain to the tube.
		▷	Stated the purpose of the stain.
		•	Placed the pipet back in the tube and mixed the specimen thoroughly.
		•	Placed the urine tube in the test tube rack.
		•	Transferred a sample of the specimen to the Kova slide.
		•	Did not overfill or underfill the well of the Kova slide.

Trial 1	Trial 2	Point Value	Performance Standards
		•	Placed the pipet in the urine tube.
		•	Allowed the specimen to sit for 1 minute.
		▷	Explained the purpose of allowing the specimen to sit 1 minute.
		•	Placed the slide on the stage of the microscope.
		•	Properly focused the specimen for the provider.
		•	Removed the slide from the stage when the provider was finished examining the specimen.
		•	Disposed of the slide and pipet in a regular waste container.
		•	Rinsed the remaining urine down the sink.
		•	Capped the empty urine tube and disposed of it in a regular waste container.
		•	Removed gloves and sanitized hands.
			Demonstrated the following affective behavior(s) during this procedure:
		Ⓐ	Explained to a patient the rationale for performance of a procedure.
		★	Completed the procedure within 15 minutes.
			Totals

CHART

Date	

Evaluation of Student Performance

EVALUATION CRITERIA			COMMENTS
Symbol	**Category**	**Point Value**	
★	Critical Step	16 points	
•	Essential Step	6 points	
Ⓐ	Affective Competency	6 points	
▷	Theory Question	2 points	

Score calculation: 100 points

− _____ points missed

_____ Score

Satisfactory score: 85 or above

CAAHEP Competencies Achieved

Psychomotor (Skills)
☑ I. 9. Assist provider with patient exam.

Affective (Behavior)
☑ V. 4. Explain to a patient the rationale for performance of a procedure.

ABHES Competencies Achieved

☑ 8. c. Assist provider with general/physical examination.

Notes

Procedure 16-5: Performing a Rapid Urine Culture Test

Name: _____   Date: _____

Evaluated by: _____   Score: _____

Performance Objective

Outcome:	Perform a rapid urine culture test.
Conditions:	Given the following: disposable gloves, rapid urine culture kit, clean-catch midstream urine specimen, incubator, and biohazard waste container.
Standards:	Time: 5 minutes. Student completed procedure in _____ minutes.
	Accuracy: Satisfactory score on the Performance Evaluation Checklist.

Performance Evaluation Checklist

Trial 1	Trial 2	Point Value	Performance Standards
			Preparing the specimen
		•	Sanitized hands.
		•	Assembled equipment.
		•	Checked the expiration date on the rapid culture test.
		•	Labeled the vial with the patient's name, date of birth, and date and time of inoculation.
		•	Applied gloves.
		•	Removed the slide from the vial.
		•	Did not touch the culture media.
		•	Completely immersed the slide in the urine specimen.
		•	Allowed the excess urine to drain from the slide.
		•	Immediately replaced the slide in the vial.
		•	Screwed the cap on loosely.
		•	Placed the vial upright in an incubator.
		▷	Explained why the slide should not remain in the incubator for more than 24 hours.
			Reading test results
		•	Applied gloves.
		•	Removed the vial from the incubator.
		•	Removed the slide from the vial.
		•	Compared the slide with the reference chart.
		•	Read and interpreted the results.

Trial 1	Trial 2	Point Value	Performance Standards
		★	The results were identical to the evaluator's results.
		•	Returned the slide to the vial and screwed on the cap.
		•	Disposed of the test in a biohazard waste container.
		•	Removed gloves and sanitized hands.
		•	Documented the results correctly.
			Demonstrated the following affective behavior(s) during this procedure:
		Ⓐ	Explain to a patient the rationale for performance of a procedure.
		★	Completed the procedure within 5 minutes.
			Totals

CHART

Date	

Evaluation of Student Performance

EVALUATION CRITERIA			COMMENTS
Symbol	**Category**	**Point Value**	
★	Critical Step	16 points	
•	Essential Step	6 points	
Ⓐ	Affective Competency	6 points	
▷	Theory Question	2 points	

Score calculation: 100 points

− _____ points missed

_____ Score

Satisfactory score: 85 or above

CAAHEP Competencies Achieved

Psychomotor (Skills)
☑ II. 2. Differentiate between normal and abnormal test results.

Affective (Behavior)
☑ V. 4. Explain to a patient the rationale for performance of a procedure.

ABHES Competencies Achieved

☑ 9. d. Collect, label, and process specimens.

702

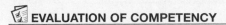 **Procedure 16-6: Performing a Urine Pregnancy Test**

Name: _____ Date: _____

Evaluated by: _____ Score: _____

Performance Objective

Outcome:	Perform a urine pregnancy test.
Conditions:	Given the following: disposable gloves, urine pregnancy testing kit, first-voided morning urine specimen, waste container.
Standards:	Time: 5 minutes. Student completed procedure in _____ minutes.
	Accuracy: Satisfactory score on the Performance Evaluation Checklist.

Performance Evaluation Checklist

Trial 1	Trial 2	Point Value	Performance Standards
		•	Sanitized hands.
		•	Assembled equipment.
		•	Checked the expiration date on the pregnancy test.
		▷	Explained why the expiration date should be checked.
		•	If necessary, ran controls on the pregnancy test.
		▷	Stated when controls should be run.
		•	Applied gloves.
		•	Mixed the urine specimen.
		•	Removed the test cassette from its pouch.
		•	Placed the test cassette on a clean, dry, level surface.
		•	Added 3 drops of urine to the well on the test cassette.
		•	Disposed of the pipet in a regular waste container.
		•	Waited 3 minutes and read the results.
		•	Interpreted the test results.
		★	The results were identical to the evaluator's results.
		▷	Described the appearance of a positive and a negative test result.
		▷	Explained what should be done if a blue control line does not appear.
		•	Disposed of the test cassette in a regular waste container.
		•	Removed gloves and sanitized hands.
		•	Documented the results correctly.

Trial 1	Trial 2	Point Value	Performance Standards
			Demonstrated the following affective behavior(s) during this procedure:
		Ⓐ	Incorporated critical thinking skills when performing patient assessment.
		Ⓐ	Reassured a patient of the accuracy of the test results.
		★	Completed the procedure within 5 minutes.
			Totals

CHART

Date	

Evaluation of Student Performance

EVALUATION CRITERIA			COMMENTS
Symbol	**Category**	**Point Value**	
★	Critical Step	16 points	
•	Essential Step	6 points	
Ⓐ	Affective Competency	6 points	
▷	Theory Question	2 points	

Score calculation: 100 points

− _____ points missed

_____ Score

Satisfactory score: 85 or above

CAAHEP Competencies Achieved

Psychomotor (Skills)

☑ I. 10. Perform a quality control measure.
☑ I. 11. c. Obtain specimen and perform CLIA-waived urinalysis.
☑ II. 2. Differentiate between normal and abnormal test results.

Affective (Behavior)

☑ I. 1. Incorporate critical thinking skills when performing patient assessment.
☑ II. 1. Reassure a patient of the accuracy of the test results.
☑ V. 4. Explain to a patient the rationale for performance of a procedure.

ABHES Competencies Achieved

☑ 9. a. Practice quality control.
☑ 9. b. Perform selected CLIA-waived tests that assist with diagnosis and treatment: (6) kit testing.

17 Phlebotomy

CHAPTER ASSIGNMENTS

√ After Completing	Date Due	Study Guide Pages	STUDY GUIDE ASSIGNMENTS (CTA = Critical Thinking Activity)	Possible Points	Points You Earned
		711	? Pretest	10	
		712	Term Key Term Assessment A. Definitions B. Word Parts (Add 1 point for each key term)	16 13	
		713-717	Evaluation of Learning questions	41	
		717	CTA A: Antecubital Veins	5	
			e Evolve Site: Got Blood? (Record points earned)		
		718-719	CTA B: Venipuncture-Vacuum Tube Method	15	
		719-720	CTA C: Venipuncture Situations	7	
		720	CTA D: Skin Puncture	8	
		721	CTA E: Crossword Puzzle	29	
			e Evolve Site: Apply Your Knowledge questions	10	
			e Evolve Site: Video Evaluation	42	
		711	? Posttest	10	
			ADDITIONAL ASSIGNMENTS		
			Total points		

Notes

√ When Assigned By Your Instructor	Study Guide Pages	Practices Required	LABORATORY ASSIGNMENTS (Procedure Number and Name)	Score*
	723	5	**e** **Practice for Competency** 17-1: Venipuncture—Vacuum Tube Method Textbook reference: pp. 633-639	
	725-728		**e** **Evaluation of Competency** 17-1: Venipuncture—Vacuum Tube Method	*
	723	5	**e** **Practice for Competency** 17-2: Venipuncture—Butterfly Method Textbook reference: pp. 641-646	
	729-732		**e** **Evaluation of Competency** 17-2: Venipuncture—Butterfly Method	*
	723	3	**e** **Practice for Competency** 17-3: Separating Serum from a Blood Specimen Textbook reference: pp. 650-652	
	733-735		**e** **Evaluation of Competency** 17-3: Separating Serum from a Blood Specimen	*
	723	3	**e** **Practice for Competency** 17-4: Skin Puncture—Disposable Semiautomatic Lancet Device Textbook reference: pp. 656-658	
	737-739		**e** **Evaluation of Competency** 17-4: Skin Puncture—Disposable Semiautomatic Lancet Device	*
	723	3	**e** **Practice for Competency** 17-A: Skin Puncture—Reusable Semiautomatic Lancet Device Textbook reference: p. 655	
	741-743		**e** **Evaluation of Competency** 17-A: Skin Puncture—Reusable Semiautomatic Lancet Device	*
			ADDITIONAL ASSIGNMENTS	

Notes

Name: _Leanna Bartlett_   Date: _2/11/2020_

True or False

___F___ 1. An individual who collects blood specimens is known as a vampire.

___T___ 2. The purpose of applying a tourniquet when performing venipuncture is to make the patient's veins stand out.

___F___ 3. The tourniquet should be left on the patient's arm for at least 2 minutes before performing a venipuncture.

___F___ 4. Serum is obtained from whole blood that has been centrifuged.

___F___ 5. A 25-gauge needle is recommended for performing venipuncture.

___F___ 6. The size of the evacuated tube used to obtain a venous blood specimen depends on the size of the patient's veins.

___F___ 7. A correct order of draw for the vacuum tube method of venipuncture is red, lavender, gray, and green.

___F___ 8. Veins are most likely to collapse in patients with large veins and thick walls.

___T___ 9. Hemolysis of a blood specimen results in inaccurate test results.

___F___ 10. When obtaining a capillary specimen, the first drop of blood should be used for the test.

?≡ **POSTTEST**

True or False

___F___ 1. Venous reflux can be prevented by filling the evacuated tube to the exhaustion of the vacuum.

___T___ 2. If the tourniquet is applied too tightly, inaccurate test results may occur.

___T___ 3. The median cubital vein is the best vein to use for venipuncture.

___T___ 4. On standing, a blood specimen to which an anticoagulant has been added separates into plasma, buffy coat, and blood cells.

___T___ 5. Whole blood is obtained by using a tube containing an anticoagulant.

___T___ 6. An evacuated glass tube with a lavender stopper contains EDTA.

___T___ 7. A red-stoppered tube is used to collect a blood specimen for most blood chemistries.

___T___ 8. Not filling a tube to the exhaustion of the vacuum can result in hemolysis of the blood specimen.

___F___ 9. If the needle is removed from the arm before removing the tourniquet, the evacuated tube will not fill completely.

___F___ 10. If a fibrin clot forms in the serum layer of a blood specimen, it will lead to inaccurate test results.

KEY TERM ASSESSMENT

A. Definitions

Directions: Match each key term with its definition.

H	1. Antecubital space	A. The liquid part of blood, consisting of a clear, straw-colored fluid that makes up approximately 55% of the blood volume
B	2. Anticoagulant	B. A substance that inhibits blood clotting
G	3. Buffy coat	C. Health professional trained in the collection of blood specimens
E	4. Evacuated tube	D. The breakdown of blood cells
N	5. Hematoma	E. A closed glass or plastic tube that contains a premeasured vacuum
J	6. Hemoconcentration	F. The temporary cessation or slowing of the venous blood flow
D	7. Hemolysis	G. A thin, light-colored layer of white blood cells and platelets that lies between a top layer of plasma and a bottom layer of red blood cells when an anticoagulant has been added to a blood specimen
I	8. Osteochondritis	H. The surface of the arm in front of the elbow
M	9. Osteomyelitis	I. Inflammation of bone and cartilage
C	10. Phlebotomist	J. An increase in the concentration of the nonfilterable blood components
L	11. Phlebotomy	K. Plasma from which the clotting factor fibrinogen has been removed
A	12. Plasma	L. Incision of a vein for the removal of blood
K	13. Serum	M. Inflammation of the bone or bone marrow as a result of bacterial infection
O	14. Venipuncture	N. A swelling or mass of coagulated blood caused by a break in a blood vessel
P	15. Venous reflux	O. Puncturing of a vein
F	16. Venous stasis	P. The backflow of blood (from an evacuated tube) into the patient's vein

B. Word Parts

Directions: Indicate the meaning of each word part in the space provided. List as many medical terms as possible that incorporate the word part in the space provided.

Word Part	Meaning of Word Part	Medical Terms That Incorporate Word Part
1. ante-	before	Antecubital Space
2. anti-	against	Anticoagulation
3. hemat/o	blood	Hematoma
4. -oma	tumor or swelling	Hematoma
5. hem/o	blood	Hemoconcentration
6. -lysis	breakdown	Hemolysis
7. oste/o	bone	Osteochondritis
8. myel/o	bone Marrow	Osteomyelitis
9. -itis	inflammation	
10. phleb/o	vein	Phlebotomist
11. -otomy	incision	Phlebotomy
12. ven/o	vein	Venipuncture
13. -ous	pertaining to	Venous reflux

Directions: Fill in each blank with the correct answer.

1. List the three major areas of blood collection included in phlebotomy.

_____

_____

_____

2. What is the purpose of performing a venipuncture?

_____

_____

3. List methods that can be used to perform a venipuncture.

_____

_____

_____

4. What are the advantages of using the vacuum tube method of venipuncture?

_____

_____

5. When would the butterfly method of venipuncture be preferred over the vacuum tube method?

_____

_____

_____

6. What reference source should be consulted for collection and handling requirements in the following situations?

   a. The specimen is being transported to an outside laboratory for testing:

   _____

   b. The specimen is being tested in the medical office:

   _____

7. Why should a patient be identified using two forms of identification?

_____

_____

8. What is a unique identifier?

_____

9. Explain how to prevent venous reflux.

_____

_____

10. What is the purpose of the tourniquet?

_____

_____

11. Why are the antecubital veins preferred for performing a venipuncture?

_____

_____

_____

12. After locating a suitable vein for venipuncture, what three qualities should be determined with respect to the vein?

_____

_____

_____

13. List four techniques that can be used to make veins more prominent.

_____

_____

_____

_____

14. Why should the veins of the hand be used only as a last resort when performing a venipuncture?

_____

_____

_____

15. How is a serum specimen obtained?

_____

_____

16. How is a whole blood specimen obtained?

_____

_____

17. List the three layers into which blood separates when it is mixed with an anticoagulant.

_____

_____

18. List the layers into which blood separates when an anticoagulant is not added to it.

_____

_____

19. List six OSHA safety precautions that must be followed when performing a venipuncture and separating serum or plasma from whole blood.

_____

_____

_____

_____

_____

20. What are the ranges for the gauge and length of the needle used for the vacuum tube method of venipuncture?

_____

_____

21. What is the purpose of the flange on the plastic holder of the vacuum tube system?

_____

_____

22. What type of additive is present in each of the following evacuated tubes?

Red _____

Red/gray speckled _____

Lavender _____

Light blue _____

Green _____

Gray _____

Royal blue _____

23. What color stopper must be used to collect the blood specimen for each of the tests listed?

Complete blood count _____

Prothrombin time _____

Glucose tolerance test _____

Most blood chemistry tests _____

Blood gas determinations _____

Lead testing _____

24. Why is it important to use the correct order of draw when performing a venipuncture?

_____

_____

25. Why is it important to mix a tube containing an anticoagulant immediately after drawing it?

_____

_____

26. What are the ranges for the gauge and length of needle used for the butterfly method of venipuncture?

_____

_____

27. How can a vein be prevented from rolling when performing a venipuncture on the cephalic or basic veins?

_____

_____

28. What is typically observed when performing a venipuncture on a vein that collapses?

_____

_____

29. What are three ways in which a hematoma may occur?

_____

_____

_____

30. List four ways to prevent a blood specimen from becoming hemolyzed.

_____

_____

_____

_____

31. List examples of substances dissolved in the serum of blood.

_____

_____

_____

32. What is the purpose of performing laboratory tests on serum?

_____

_____

_____

33. List the proper size tube that must be used to obtain the following serum specimens:

2 mL of serum _____

6 mL of serum _____

4 mL of serum _____

34. What is a fibrin clot, and why should it be avoided in a serum specimen?

_____

_____

_____

35. How does a serum separator tube function in the collection of a serum specimen?

_____

_____

_____

36. What is the preferred site for a skin puncture for the following individuals?

a. Adult _____

b. Infant _____

37. Why is it important not to penetrate the skin too deeply when performing a skin puncture?

_____

_____

38. How does the medical assistant determine the blade length to use to perform a skin puncture?

_____

_____

39. What are two examples of microcollection devices?

_____

_____

40. Why should a finger puncture not be performed on the index finger?

_____

_____

41. Why should the first drop of blood be wiped away when performing a finger puncture?

_____

_____

CRITICAL THINKING ACTIVITIES

A. Antecubital Veins

Practice palpating the antecubital veins on at least five classmates. Use a tourniquet applied to each person's arm, and ask the individual to clench his or her fist. Document the individual's name and which vein would be considered the best to use on each person when performing venipuncture.

NAME	SUITABLE VEIN
1.	
2.	
3.	
4.	
5.	

717

Chapter **17** **Phlebotomy**

B. Venipuncture—Vacuum Tube Method

Using the principles outlined in the vacuum tube venipuncture procedure, state what can happen under the following circumstances:

1. An evacuated tube is used that is past its expiration date.

   _____

   _____

2. The vacuum tube is not labeled.

   _____

   _____

3. The tourniquet is not applied tightly enough.

   _____

   _____

4. The tourniquet is left on for more than 1 minute.

   _____

   _____

5. The area that has just been cleansed with an antiseptic is not allowed to dry before the venipuncture is made.

   _____

   _____

6. The evacuated tube is inserted past the indentation in the plastic holder before the vein is entered.

   _____

   _____

7. An angle of less than 15 degrees is used when performing venipuncture.

   _____

   _____

8. An angle of more than 15 degrees is used when performing venipuncture.

   _____

   _____

9. The needle is moved after inserting it.

   _____

   _____

10. Venous reflux occurs when using an EDTA evacuated tube.

   _____

   _____

11. The vacuum tube is removed before it has filled to the exhaustion of the vacuum.

_____

_____

12. The needle is removed from the arm before the tourniquet has been removed.

_____

_____

13. A gauze pad is not placed slightly above the puncture site before removing the needle.

_____

_____

14. The patient bends the arm at the elbow after the needle is removed.

_____

_____

15. The patient lifts a heavy object after the procedure.

_____

_____

C. Venipuncture Situations

You are responsible for performing the venipunctures in your medical office. In the space provided, explain what you would do in each of the following situations:

1. The patient asks you whether the venipuncture will hurt.

_____

_____

2. On palpating the patient's vein, you find that it feels stiff and hard.

_____

_____

3. You have attempted one venipuncture in a patient with small veins using the vacuum tube method of venipuncture; however, the vein collapsed, and you were unable to obtain blood.

_____

_____

4. The patient moves during the procedure, causing the needle to come out of his or her arm.

_____

_____

5. You have inserted the needle in the vein but notice a sudden swelling around the puncture site.

_____

_____

6. You inadvertently puncture the brachial artery after inserting the needle.

_____

_____

7. The patient begins to sweat and tells you that he or she feels warm and light-headed.

_____

_____

D. Skin Puncture

The medical assistant is performing a skin puncture on an adult patient to obtain a capillary blood specimen for a hemo-globin test. For each of the following situations, write **C** if the technique is correct and **I** if the technique is incorrect. If the technique is correct, explain the rationale for performing it that way; if incorrect, explain what might happen if the technique were performed in the incorrect manner.

_____ 1. Before making the puncture, the medical assistant asks the patient to rinse his or her hand in warm water.

_____

_____

_____ 2. The puncture is made with the patient in a standing position.

_____

_____

_____ 3. The site is allowed to dry thoroughly after it is cleansed with an antiseptic wipe.

_____

_____

_____ 4. The specimen is collected from the lateral part of the tip of the ring finger.

_____

_____

_____ 5. The puncture is made perpendicular to the lines of the fingerprint.

_____

_____

_____ 6. The depth of the puncture is 4 mm.

_____

_____

_____ 7. The first drop of blood is wiped away.

_____

_____

_____ 8. The puncture site is squeezed to obtain the blood specimen.

_____

_____

E. Crossword Puzzle: Phlebotomy

Directions: Complete the crossword puzzle using the clues provided.

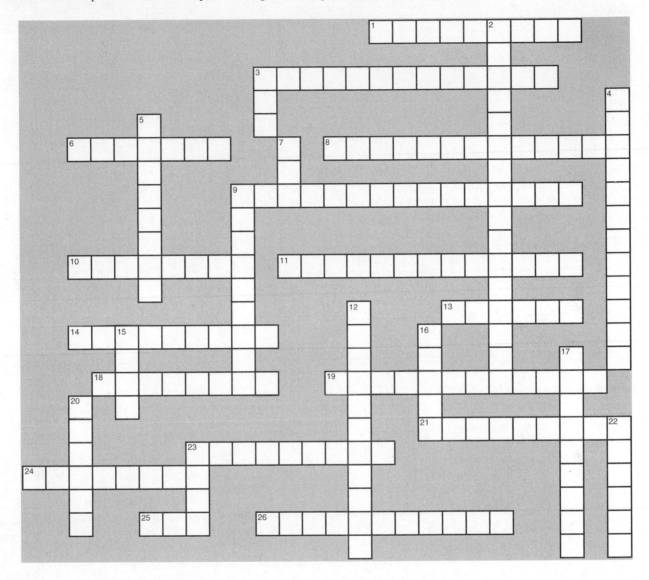

Across

1 What BP does during fainting
3 Makes RBCs clot quicker
6 Rolling vein
8 Best VP vein
9 Inflammation of bone and cartilage
10 Outdated tube problem
11 Inhibits blood clotting
13 Faint position
14 PT tube
18 EDTA tube
19 Backflow of blood
21 For small veins
23 Broken RBCs
24 Bad bruise
25 No additive tube
26 Based on size of pt's finger

Down

2 In front of the elbow
3 Select lavender tube for this test
4 Collects blood
5 First drop of capillary blood?
7 Contains a "separating" gel
9 Time limit for tourniquet
12 Do not use for skin puncture
15 Fluoride/oxalate tube
16 Don't use to palpate vein
17 WBCs and platelets
20 Fainting warning signal
22 Color of serum
23 Last choice veins

Notes

Procedure 17-1: Venipuncture—Vacuum Tube Method

Practice the procedure for collecting a venous blood specimen using the vacuum tube method. Document the procedure in the chart provided.

Procedure 17-2: Venipuncture—Butterfly Method

Practice the procedure for collecting a venous blood specimen using the butterfly method. Document the procedure in the chart provided.

Procedure 17-3: Separating Serum from Whole Blood

Separate serum from whole blood, and document the procedure in the chart provided.

Procedure 17-4: Disposable Lancet

Obtain a capillary blood specimen using a disposable semiautomatic lancet device.

Procedure 17-A: Reusable Lancet

Obtain a capillary blood specimen using a reusable semiautomatic lancet.

CHART	
Date	

Notes

Procedure 17-1: Venipuncture—Vacuum Tube Method

Name: _____ Date: _____

Evaluated by: _____ Score: _____

Performance Objective

Outcome:	Perform a venipuncture using the vacuum tube method.
Conditions:	Given the following: disposable gloves, tourniquet, antiseptic wipe, double-pointed needle, plastic holder, evacuated tubes with labels, gauze pad, adhesive bandage, biohazard sharps container, biohazard specimen bag, and a laboratory request form.
Standards:	Time: 10 minutes. Student completed procedure in _____ minutes.
	Accuracy: Satisfactory score on the Performance Evaluation Checklist.

Performance Evaluation Checklist

Trial 1	Trial 2	Point Value	Performance Standards
		•	Reviewed requirements for collecting and handling the blood specimen.
		•	Sanitized hands.
		•	Greeted the patient and introduced yourself.
		•	Identified the patient.
		•	Asked the patient whether he or she prepared properly.
			Prepared the equipment
		•	Assembled equipment.
		•	Selected the proper evacuated tubes.
		•	Checked the expiration date of the tubes.
		▷	Stated the purpose of checking the expiration date.
		•	Labeled the evacuated tubes.
		•	Completed a laboratory request form, if necessary.
		•	Screwed the plastic holder onto the Luer adapter and tightened it securely.
		•	Opened the gauze packet.
		•	Positioned the evacuated tubes in the correct order of draw.
		•	Tapped the evacuated tubes with a powdered additive below the stopper.
		▷	Stated the purpose for tapping the tubes.
		•	Placed the first tube loosely in the plastic holder.
			Prepared the patient
		•	Explained the procedure to the patient and reassured the patient.
		•	Performed a preliminary assessment of both arms.
		•	Correctly applied the tourniquet.

Chapter **17 Phlebotomy**

Trial 1	Trial 2	Point Value	Performance Standards
		•	Asked the patient to clench fist.
		▷	Stated the purpose of the tourniquet and clenched fist.
		•	Assessed the veins of both arms.
		•	Determined the best vein to use.
		•	Positioned the patient's arm correctly.
		•	Thoroughly palpated the selected vein.
		•	Did not leave the tourniquet on for more than 1 minute.
		▷	Explained why the tourniquet should not be left on for more than 1 minute.
		•	Removed the tourniquet and cleansed the puncture site.
		•	Allowed the puncture site to air dry.
		▷	Explained why the site should be allowed to air dry.
		•	Did not touch the site after cleansing.
		•	Placed supplies within comfortable reach of the nondominant hand.
		•	Reapplied the tourniquet and applied gloves.
			Performed the venipuncture
		•	Correctly positioned the safety shield and removed the cap from the needle.
		•	Properly held the venipuncture setup (bevel up) with the dominant hand.
		•	Positioned the tube with the label facing downward.
		▷	Explained why the label should face downward.
		•	Grasped the patient's arm and anchored the vein correctly.
		•	Positioned the venipuncture setup at a 15-degree angle to the arm, with the needle pointing in the same direction as the vein to be entered.
		•	Positioned the needle approximately $\frac{1}{8}$ inch below the place where the vein is to be entered.
		•	Told the patient that a small stick will be felt.
		•	With one continuous motion, entered the skin and then the vein.
		•	Stabilized the vacuum tube setup.
		▷	Stated why the vacuum tube setup should be stabilized.
		•	Pushed the tube forward slowly to the end of the holder using the flange.
		•	Allowed the evacuated tube to fill to the exhaustion of the vacuum.
		▷	Explained why the tube should be allowed to fill to the exhaustion of the vacuum.
		•	Removed the tube from the plastic holder using the flange.

Trial 1	Trial 2	Point Value	Performance Standards
		•	Immediately and gently inverted the tube 5 times if it contained a clot activator and 8 to 10 times if it contained an anticoagulant.
		•	Inserted the next tube into the holder using the flange.
		•	Continued until the last tube was filled.
		•	Removed the tourniquet and asked the patient to unclench fist.
		★	Removed the last tube from the holder.
		•	Stated why the last tube should be removed.
		▷	Placed gauze pad slightly above puncture site and withdrew the needle slowly and at the same angle as that for penetration.
		•	Immediately moved gauze over the puncture site and applied pressure.
		•	Pushed the safety shield forward with the thumb until an audible click is heard.
		•	Properly disposed of the holder and needle in a biohazard sharps container.
		•	Instructed the patient to apply pressure with the gauze pad for 1 to 2 minutes.
		▷	Stated why pressure should be applied.
		•	Applied an adhesive bandage to the puncture site.
		•	Placed the tubes in an upright position in a test tube rack.
		•	Removed gloves and sanitized hands.
		•	Documented the procedure correctly.
		•	Tested the specimen or prepared the specimen for transport according to medical office policy.
			Demonstrated the following affective behavior(s) during this procedure:
		Ⓐ	Applied critical thinking when performing patient assessment.
		Ⓐ	Showed awareness of a patient's concerns related to the procedure being performed.
		Ⓐ	Recognized the implications for failure to comply with the Centers for Disease Control and Prevention (CDC) regulations in health care settings.
		★	Completed the procedure within 10 minutes.
			Totals

CHART	
Date	

Evaluation of Student Performance

EVALUATION CRITERIA			COMMENTS
Symbol	**Category**	**Point Value**	
★	Critical Step	16 points	
•	Essential Step	6 points	
Ⓐ	Affective Competency	6 points	
▷	Theory Question	2 points	

Score calculation: 100 points

− _____ points missed

_____ Score

Satisfactory score: 85 or above

CAAHEP Competencies Achieved

Psychomotor (Skills)
☑ I. 2. b. Perform venipuncture.
☑ III. 10. Demonstrate proper disposal of biohazardous material: (a) sharps, (b) regulated waste.

Affective (Behavior)
☑ I. 1. Apply critical thinking when performing patient assessment.
☑ I. 3. Show awareness of a patient's concerns related to the procedure being performed.
☑ III. 1. Recognize the implications for failure to comply with the Centers for Disease Control and Prevention (CDC) regulations in health care settings.

ABHES Competencies Achieved

☑ 8. a. Practice standard precautions and perform disinfection/sterilization techniques.
☑ 9. c. Dispose of biohazardous materials.
☑ 9. d. (1). Collect, label and process specimens: Perform venipuncture.

Procedure 17-2: Venipuncture—Butterfly Method

Name: _____   Date: _____

Evaluated by: _____   Score: _____

Performance Objective

Outcome:	Perform a venipuncture using the butterfly method.
Conditions:	Given the following: disposable gloves, tourniquet, antiseptic wipe, winged infusion set, plastic holder, evacuated tubes with labels, gauze pad, adhesive bandage, biohazard sharps container, biohazard specimen bag, and a laboratory request form.
Standards:	Time: 10 minutes. Student completed procedure in _____ minutes.
	Accuracy: Satisfactory score on the Performance Evaluation Checklist.

Performance Evaluation Checklist

Trial 1	Trial 2	Point Value	Performance Standards
		•	Reviewed requirements for collecting and handling the blood specimen.
		•	Sanitized hands.
		•	Greeted the patient and introduced yourself.
		•	Identified the patient.
		▷	Stated why the patient must be correctly identified.
		•	Asked the patient whether he or she prepared properly.
		▷	Explained why it is important for the patient to prepare properly.
			Prepared the equipment
		•	Assembled equipment.
		•	Selected the proper evacuated tubes.
		•	Checked the expiration date of the tubes.
		•	Labeled the evacuated tubes.
		•	Completed a laboratory request form, if necessary.
		•	Removed the winged infusion set from its package.
		•	Extended the tubing to its full length and stretched it.
		▷	Explained why the tubing should be extended and stretched.
		•	Screwed the plastic holder onto the Luer adapter and tightened it securely.
		•	Opened the gauze packet.
		•	Positioned the evacuated tubes in the correct order of draw.
		•	Tapped the evacuated tubes with a powdered additive below the stopper.

Trial 1	Trial 2	Point Value	Performance Standards
		▷	Stated why tubes with powdered additives must be tapped.
		•	Placed the first tube loosely in the plastic holder with the label facing downward.
		▷	Explained why the label should be facing downward.
			Prepared the patient
		•	Explained the procedure to the patient and reassured the patient.
		•	Performed a preliminary assessment of both arms.
		•	Correctly applied the tourniquet and asked the patient to clench fist.
		•	Assessed the veins of both arms.
		•	Determined the best vein to use.
		•	Positioned the patient's arm correctly.
		▷	Stated why the arm must be positioned correctly.
		•	Thoroughly palpated the selected vein.
		▷	Stated the purpose of palpating the vein.
		•	Did not leave the tourniquet on for more than 1 minute.
		•	Removed the tourniquet and cleansed the puncture site.
		•	Allowed the puncture site to air dry.
		•	Did not touch the site after cleansing.
		•	Placed supplies within comfortable reach.
		•	Reapplied the tourniquet and applied gloves.
			Performed the venipuncture
		•	Grasped the winged infusion set correctly.
		•	Removed the protective shield.
		•	Positioned the needle with the bevel up.
		▷	Explained why the bevel should be up.
		•	Grasped the patient's arm and anchored the vein correctly.
		•	Positioned the needle at a 15-degree angle to the arm, with the needle pointing in the same direction as the vein to be entered.
		•	Positioned the needle approximately $1/8$ inch below the place where the vein is to be entered.
		•	Told the patient that a small stick will be felt.
		•	With one continuous motion, entered the skin and then the vein.
		▷	Explained why a continuous motion should be used.
		•	Decreased the angle of the needle to 5 degrees.

730

Trial 1	Trial 2	Point Value	Performance Standards
		•	Seated the needle.
		▷	Stated the purpose of seating the needle.
		•	Opened the butterfly wings and rested them flat against the skin.
		•	Kept the tube and holder in a downward position.
		•	Slowly pushed the tube forward to the end of the plastic holder.
		•	Allowed the evacuated tube to fill to the exhaustion of the vacuum.
		▷	Explained why the tube should be filled to the exhaustion of the vacuum.
		•	Removed the tube from the plastic holder.
		•	Immediately and gently inverted the evacuated tube 5 times if it contained a clot activator and 8 to 10 times if it contained an anticoagulant.
		▷	Explained why a tube with an anticoagulant must be inverted immediately.
		•	Inserted the next tube into the holder.
		•	Continued until the last tube was filled.
		★	Removed the tourniquet and asked the patient to unclench fist.
		▷	Stated why the tourniquet must be removed before the needle.
		•	Removed the last tube from the holder.
		•	Placed a gauze pad slightly above puncture site. Grasped the setup just below the wings and withdrew the needle slowly and at the same angle as that for penetration.
		•	Immediately moved the gauze over the puncture site and applied pressure.
		•	Instructed the patient to apply pressure with the gauze.
		•	Activated the safety shield on the needle.
		•	Properly disposed of the winged infusion set and plastic holder in a biohazard sharps container.
		•	Continued to apply pressure for 1 to 2 minutes.
		•	Applied an adhesive bandage.
		•	Placed the tubes in an upright position in a test tube rack.
		•	Removed gloves and sanitized hands.
		•	Documented the procedure correctly.
		•	Tested the specimen or prepared the specimen for transport according to medical office policy.
			Demonstrated the following affective behavior(s) during this procedure:
		Ⓐ	Applied critical thinking when performing patient assessment.
		Ⓐ	Showed awareness of a patient's concerns related to the procedure being performed.

Trial 1	Trial 2	Point Value	Performance Standards
		Ⓐ	Recognized the implications for failure to comply with the Centers for Disease Control and Prevention (CDC) regulations in health care settings.
		★	Completed the procedure within 10 minutes.
			Totals

CHART

Date	

Evaluation of Student Performance

EVALUATION CRITERIA			COMMENTS
Symbol	**Category**	**Point Value**	
★	Critical Step	16 points	
•	Essential Step	6 points	
Ⓐ	Affective Competency	6 points	
▷	Theory Question	2 points	

Score calculation: 100 points

− _____ points missed

_____ Score

Satisfactory score: 85 or above

CAAHEP Competencies Achieved

Psychomotor (Skills)
☑ I. 2. b. Perform venipuncture.
☑ III. 10. Demonstrate proper disposal of biohazardous material: (a) sharps, (b) regulated waste.

Affective (Behavior)
☑ I. 1. Apply critical thinking when performing patient assessment.
☑ I. 3. Show awareness of a patient's concerns related to the procedure being performed.
☑ III. 1. Recognize the implications for failure to comply with the Centers for Disease Control and Prevention (CDC) regulations in health care settings.

ABHES Competencies Achieved

☑ 8. a. Practice standard precautions and perform disinfection/sterilization techniques.
☑ 9. c. Dispose of biohazardous materials.
☑ 9. d. (1). Collect, label and process specimens: Perform venipuncture.

732

Procedure 17-3: Separating Serum from a Blood Specimen

Name: _____   Date: _____

Evaluated by: _____   Score: _____

Performance Objective

Outcome:	Separate serum from whole blood.
Conditions:	Given the following: red evacuated tube venipuncture setup, test tube rack, disposable pipet, transfer tube and label, disposable gloves, face shield or mask and eye protection device, centrifuge, and a biohazard sharps container.
Standards:	Time: 20 minutes. Student completed procedure in _____ minutes.
	Accuracy: Satisfactory score on the Performance Evaluation Checklist.

Performance Evaluation Checklist

Trial 1	Trial 2	Point Value	Performance Standards
		•	Collected the blood specimen by performing a venipuncture.
		▷	Stated why a red-stoppered tube should be used.
		•	Placed the specimen tube in an upright position for 30 to 45 minutes at room temperature while keeping a stopper on the specimen tube.
		▷	Explained why the specimen tube must be placed in an upright position.
		•	Placed the specimen tube in the centrifuge, with the stopper end upward.
		▷	Stated why the stopper must remain on the specimen tube.
		•	Balanced the specimen with the same type and weight of tube.
		▷	Stated the purpose for balancing the centrifuge.
		•	Centrifuged the specimen for 10 minutes.
		▷	Explained the purpose of centrifugation.
		•	Put on a face shield or a mask and an eye protection device and applied gloves.
		▷	Stated the purpose of wearing personal protective equipment.
		•	Removed the specimen tube from the centrifuge without disturbing the contents.
		▷	Explained what must be done if the contents of the tube are disturbed.
		•	Carefully removed the stopper from the tube.
		•	Squeezed the bulb of the pipet and placed the tip of the pipet against the side of the specimen tube approximately ¼ inch above the cell layer.
		▷	Explained why the bulb should be squeezed before inserting the pipet into serum.
		•	Released the bulb to suction serum into the pipet.
		•	Transferred serum to the transfer tube.

Trial 1	Trial 2	Point Value	Performance Standards
		•	Did not disturb the cell layer.
		•	Continued pipetting until as much serum as possible was removed.
		•	Capped the specimen tube tightly and held it up to the light to examine it for hemolysis.
		▷	Explained what should be done if hemolysis is present in the specimen.
		•	Made sure that the proper amount of serum was obtained.
		•	Properly disposed of equipment.
		•	Removed gloves and sanitized hands.
		•	Tested the specimen or prepared the specimen for transport to an outside laboratory according to medical office policy.
			Demonstrated the following affective behavior(s) during this procedure:
		Ⓐ	Showed awareness of a patient's concerns related to the procedure being performed.
		Ⓐ	Recognized the implications for failure to comply with the Centers for Disease Control and Prevention (CDC) regulations in health care settings.
		★	Completed the procedure within 20 minutes.
			Totals

Evaluation of Student Performance

EVALUATION CRITERIA			COMMENTS
Symbol	**Category**	**Point Value**	
★	Critical Step	16 points	
•	Essential Step	6 points	
Ⓐ	Affective Competency	6 points	
▷	Theory Question	2 points	

Score calculation: 100 points

− _____ points missed

_____ Score

Satisfactory score: 85 or above

CAAHEP Competencies Achieved

Psychomotor (Skills)
☑ I. 2. b. Perform venipuncture.
☑ III. 10. Demonstrate proper disposal of biohazardous material: (a) sharps, (b) regulated waste.

Affective (Behavior)
☑ I. 3. Show awareness of a patient's concerns related to the procedure being performed.
☑ III. 1. Recognize the implications for failure to comply with the Centers for Disease Control and Prevention (CDC) regulations in health care settings.

ABHES Competencies Achieved

☑ 8. a. Practice standard precautions and perform disinfection/sterilization techniques.
☑ 9. c. Dispose of biohazardous materials.
☑ 9. d. (1). Collect, label and process specimens: Perform venipuncture.

Notes

e Procedure 17-4: Skin Puncture—Disposable Semiautomatic Lancet Device

Name: _____   Date: _____

Evaluated by: _____   Score: _____

Performance Objective

Outcome:	Obtain a capillary blood specimen.
Conditions:	Given the following: disposable gloves, antiseptic wipe, CoaguChek lancet, gauze pad, and a biohazard sharps container.
Standards:	Time: 5 minutes. Student completed procedure in _____ minutes.
	Accuracy: Satisfactory score on the Performance Evaluation Checklist.

Performance Evaluation Checklist

Trial 1	Trial 2	Point Value	Performance Standards
		•	Sanitized hands.
		•	Greeted the patient and introduced yourself.
		•	Identified the patient.
		•	Asked the patient whether he or she prepared properly.
		•	Assembled equipment.
		•	Opened a sterile gauze packet.
		•	Explained the procedure to the patient and reassured the patient.
		•	Seated the patient in a chair.
		•	Extended the palmar surface of the patient's hand facing upward.
		•	Selected a puncture site.
		•	Warmed the site if needed.
		▷	Explained why the site should be warmed.
		•	Cleansed the puncture site and allowed it to air dry.
		▷	Explained why the site should be allowed to air dry.
		•	Did not touch the site after cleansing.
		•	Applied gloves.
		•	Firmly grasped the patient's finger.
		•	Positioned the lancet firmly on the fingertip slightly to the side of center.
		•	Depressed the activation button without moving the lancet or finger.
		▷	Stated why the lancet and finger should not be moved.
		•	Disposed of the lancet in a biohazard sharps container.

737

Trial 1	Trial 2	Point Value	Performance Standards
		•	Waited a few seconds to allow blood flow to begin.
		•	Wiped away the first drop of blood with a gauze pad.
		▷	Stated why the first drop of blood should be wiped away.
		•	Allowed a second large, well-rounded drop of blood to form.
		•	Did not squeeze finger to obtain blood.
		•	Collected the blood specimen on a test strip or in the appropriate microcollection device.
		•	Instructed the patient to hold a gauze pad over the puncture site with pressure.
		•	Remained with the patient until bleeding stopped.
		•	Applied an adhesive bandage if needed.
		•	Tested the blood specimen following the manufacturer's instructions.
		•	Removed gloves.
		•	Sanitized hands.
			Demonstrated the following affective behavior(s) during this procedure:
		Ⓐ	Applied critical thinking when performing patient assessment.
		Ⓐ	Showed awareness of a patient's concerns related to the procedure being performed.
		Ⓐ	Recognized the implications for failure to comply with the Centers for Disease Control and Prevention (CDC) regulations in health care settings.
		★	Completed the procedure within 5 minutes.
			Totals

Evaluation of Student Performance

EVALUATION CRITERIA			COMMENTS
Symbol	**Category**	**Point Value**	
★	Critical Step	16 points	
•	Essential Step	6 points	
Ⓐ	Affective Competency	6 points	
▷	Theory Question	2 points	

Score calculation: 100 points

− _____ points missed

_____ Score

Satisfactory score: 85 or above

Psychomotor (Skills)
☑ I. 2. c. Perform capillary puncture.
☑ III. 10. Demonstrate proper disposal of biohazardous material: (a) sharps, (b) regulated waste.

Affective (Behavior)
☑ I. 1. Apply critical thinking when performing patient assessment.
☑ I. 3. Show awareness of a patient's concerns related to the procedure being performed.
☑ III. 1. Recognize the implications for failure to comply with the Centers for Disease Control and Prevention (CDC) regulations in health care settings.

☑ 8. a. Practice standard precautions and perform disinfection/sterilization techniques.
☑ 9. c. Dispose of biohazardous materials.
☑ 9. d. (2). Collect, label, and process specimens: Perform capillary puncture.

Notes

Procedure 17-A: Skin Puncture—Reusable Semiautomatic Lancet Device

Name: _____   Date: _____

Evaluated by: _____   Score: _____

Performance Objective

Outcome:	Obtain a capillary blood specimen.
Conditions:	Given the following: disposable gloves, antiseptic wipe, Glucolet II lancet device, sterile lancet/endcap, gauze pad, and a biohazard sharps container.
Standards:	Time: 10 minutes. Student completed procedure in _____ minutes.
	Accuracy: Satisfactory score on the Performance Evaluation Checklist.

Performance Evaluation Checklist

Trial 1	Trial 2	Point Value	Performance Standards
		•	Sanitized hands.
		•	Greeted the patient and introduced yourself.
		•	Identified the patient.
		•	Asked the patient whether he or she prepared properly.
		•	Assembled equipment.
		•	Pushed the transparent barrel toward the release button until it clicked into place.
		•	Inserted the lancet/endcap onto the lancet device.
		•	Opened a sterile gauze packet.
		•	Explained the procedure to the patient and reassured the patient.
		•	Seated the patient in a chair.
		•	Extended the palmar surface of the patient's hand facing upward.
		•	Selected a puncture site.
		•	Warmed the site if needed.
		▷	Explained how the patient's finger can be warmed.
		•	Cleansed the puncture site and allowed it to air dry.
		•	Applied gloves.
		•	Twisted off the plastic post from the endcap.
		•	Firmly grasped the patient's finger.
		•	Placed the endcap firmly on the fingertip slightly to the side of center.
		•	Depressed the activation button without moving the Glucolet or finger.
		•	Wiped away the first drop of blood with a gauze pad.

Trial 1	Trial 2	Point Value	Performance Standards
		•	Allowed a second large, well-rounded drop of blood to form.
		▷	Explained why the finger should not be squeezed.
		•	Collected the blood specimen on a test strip or in the appropriate microcollection device.
		•	Instructed the patient to hold a gauze pad over the puncture site with pressure.
		•	Remained with the patient until bleeding stopped.
		•	Applied an adhesive bandage if needed.
		•	Removed the endcap from the lancet device.
		•	Discarded the endcap in a biohazard waste container.
		•	Tested the blood specimen following the manufacturer's instructions.
		•	Removed gloves.
		•	Sanitized hands.
		•	Sanitized and disinfected the Glucolet.
		•	Stored the Glucolet in its resting position.
			Demonstrated the following affective behavior(s) during this procedure:
		Ⓐ	Applied critical thinking when performing patient assessment.
		Ⓐ	Showed awareness of a patient's concerns related to the procedure being performed.
		Ⓐ	Recognized the implications for failure to comply with the Centers for Disease Control and Prevention (CDC) regulations in health care settings.
		★	Completed the procedure within 5 minutes.
			Totals

Evaluation of Student Performance

EVALUATION CRITERIA			COMMENTS
Symbol	**Category**	**Point Value**	
★	Critical Step	16 points	
•	Essential Step	6 points	
Ⓐ	Affective Competency	6 points	
▷	Theory Question	2 points	

Score calculation: 100 points

− _____ points missed

_____ Score

Satisfactory score: 85 or above

CAAHEP Competencies Achieved

Psychomotor (Skills)
- ☑ I. 2. c. Perform capillary puncture.
- ☑ III. 10. Demonstrate proper disposal of biohazardous material: (a) sharps, (b) regulated waste.

Affective (Behavior)
- ☑ I. 1. Apply critical thinking when performing patient assessment.
- ☑ I. 3. Show awareness of a patient's concerns related to the procedure being performed.
- ☑ III. 1. Recognize the implications for failure to comply with the Centers for Disease Control and Prevention (CDC) regulations in health care settings.

ABHES Competencies Achieved

- ☑ 8. a. Practice standard precautions and perform disinfection/sterilization techniques.
- ☑ 9. c. Dispose of biohazardous materials.
- ☑ 9. d. (2). Collect, label, and process specimens: Perform capillary puncture.

18 Hematology

CHAPTER ASSIGNMENTS

√ After Completing	Date Due	Study Guide Pages	STUDY GUIDE ASSIGNMENTS (CTA = Critical Thinking Activity)	Possible Points	Points You Earned
		749	📰 Pretest	10	
		750-751	Term Key Term Assessment		
		750	A. Definitions	19	
		751	B. Word Parts (Add 1 point for each key term)	18	
		751-755	📄 Evaluation of Learning questions	42	
		755-758	CTA A: Diseases	40	
		759	CTA B: Hematocrit	5	
		759	CTA C: Iron Content of Food	10	
		760-761	CTA D: Iron-Deficiency Anemia	20	
		762	CTA E: Dear Gabby	10	
			e Evolve Site: Name That Cell: Identification of Blood Cells (Record points earned)		
		763	CTA F: Crossword Puzzle	23	
			e Evolve Site: Time for a Test: Hematologic Tests (Record points earned)		
			e Evolve Site: Apply Your Knowledge questions	10	
			e Evolve Site: Video Evaluation	38	
		749	📰 Posttest	10	

			ADDITIONAL ASSIGNMENTS		
			Total points		

√ When Assigned by Your Instructor	Study Guide Pages	Practices Required	LABORATORY ASSIGNMENTS (Procedure Number and Name)	Score*
	765-767	3	**Practice for Competency** 18-A: Hemoglobin Determination Textbook reference: p. 666-667	
	769-771		**Evaluation of Competency** 18-A: Hemoglobin Determination	*
	765-767	3	**Practice for Competency** 18-1: Hematocrit Textbook reference: pp. 668-671	
	773-775		**Evaluation of Competency** 18-1: Hematocrit	*
	765-767	10	**Practice for Competency** 18-2: Preparation of a Blood Smear for a Differential Cell Count Textbook reference: pp. 674-676	
	777-778		**Evaluation of Competency** 18-2: Preparation of a Blood Smear for a Differential Cell Count	*
			ADDITIONAL ASSIGNMENTS	

Notes

Name: _____   Date: _____

True or False

_____ 1. Plasma makes up approximately 55% of the blood volume.

_____ 2. A mature erythrocyte has a biconcave shape and contains a nucleus.

_____ 3. Erythrocytes are responsible for defending the body against infection.

_____ 4. The life span of a red blood cell is 120 days.

_____ 5. The function of hemoglobin is to assist in blood clotting.

_____ 6. Leukocytosis is an abnormal increase in the number of leukocytes.

_____ 7. Another name for a thrombocyte is a platelet.

_____ 8. A low hemoglobin reading occurs with polycythemia.

_____ 9. An increase in neutrophils occurs during an acute infection.

_____ 10. The PT test measures how long it takes for an individual's blood to form a clot.

POSTTEST

True or False

_____ 1. A function of the plasma is to transport antibodies, enzymes, and hormones.

_____ 2. The red bone marrow of the sternum produces red blood cells in the adult.

_____ 3. The normal range for a red blood cell count for an adult female is 4 to 5.5 million.

_____ 4. The normal range for hemoglobin for an adult male is 12 to 16 g/dL.

_____ 5. The normal adult range for a white blood cell count is 4500 to 11,000.

_____ 6. Leukocytes do their work in the tissues.

_____ 7. Bilirubin is an orange-colored pigment that is produced through the breakdown of hemoglobin.

_____ 8. An immature form of a neutrophil is known as a seg.

_____ 9. The primary function of a neutrophil is to form antibodies.

_____ 10. The function of warfarin is to inhibit the growth of bacteria in the body.

A. Definitions

Directions: Match each key term with its definition.

_____ 1. Ameboid movement

_____ 2. Anemia

_____ 3. Anisocytosis

_____ 4. Anticoagulant

_____ 5. Bilirubin

_____ 6. Diapedesis

_____ 7. Hematology

_____ 8. Hemoglobin

_____ 9. Hemolysis

_____ 10. Hypochromic

_____ 11. Leukocytosis

_____ 12. Leukopenia

_____ 13. Microcytic

_____ 14. Macrocytic

_____ 15. Normochromic

_____ 16. Normocytic

_____ 17. Oxyhemoglobin

_____ 18. Phagocytosis

_____ 19. Polycythemia

A. An abnormal decrease in the number of white blood cells (less than 4500 per cubic millimeter of blood)

B. The breakdown of erythrocytes with the release of hemoglobin into the plasma

C. Movement used by leukocytes that permits them to propel themselves from the capillaries into the tissues

D. The ameboid movement of blood cells (especially leukocytes) through the wall of a capillary and out into the tissues

E. A disorder in which there is an increase in the red blood cell mass

F. A condition in which there is a decrease in the number of erythrocytes or in the amount of hemoglobin in the blood

G. Hemoglobin that has combined with oxygen

H. The study of blood and blood-forming tissues

I. An abnormal increase in the number of white blood cells (greater than 11,000 per cubic millimeter of blood)

J. An orange-colored bile pigment produced by the breakdown of heme from the hemoglobin molecule

K. The engulfing and destruction of foreign particles, such as bacteria, by special cells called *phagocytes*

L. The protein- and iron-containing pigment of erythrocytes that transports oxygen in the body

M. A substance that inhibits blood clotting

N. A red blood cell with a decreased concentration of hemoglobin

O. An abnormally small red blood cell

P. An abnormally large red blood cell

Q. A red blood cell with a normal concentration of hemoglobin

R. A normal-sized red blood cell

S. A variation in the size of red blood cells

B. Word Parts

Directions: Indicate the meaning of each word part in the space provided. List as many medical terms as possible that incorporate the word part in the space provided.

Word Part	Meaning of Word Part	Key Terms That Incorporate Word Part
1. anis/o		
2. cyt/o		
3. -ia		
4. -osis		
5. anti-		
6. -coagulant		
7. hemat/o		
8. -ology		
9. -lysis		
10. hypo-		
11. chrom/o		
12. -ic		
13. leuk/o		
14. -penia		
15. micro-		
16. norm/o		
17. phag/o		
18. poly-		

EVALUATION OF LEARNING

Directions: Fill in each blank with the correct answer.

1. List the tests generally included in a complete blood cell count (CBC).

_____

_____

2. What is the function of plasma?

_____

_____

3. Where are erythrocytes formed in the adult?

_____

_____

4. Describe the shape of an erythrocyte, and explain how it acquires this shape.

_____

_____

5. Describe the normal appearance of arterial and venous blood.

_____

_____

6. What is the average life span of a red blood cell?

_____

7. What is the function of leukocytes?

_____

_____

8. Where do leukocytes do their work?

_____

9. What is the function of platelets?

_____

10. What is the normal range for platelets in an adult?

_____

11. What is the normal hemoglobin range?

   a. Adult female: _____

   b. Adult male: _____

12. List five conditions that cause a decrease in the hemoglobin level.

_____

_____

_____

13. What is the purpose of the hematocrit?

_____

_____

14. What is the normal hematocrit range?

   a. Adult female: _____

   b. Adult male: _____

15. What is the normal range for the white blood count for an adult?

    _____

16. List examples of conditions that may result in leukocytosis.

    _____

    _____

17. What is the normal range for the red blood count for an adult?

    a. Adult female: _____

    b. Adult male: _____

18. List the five types of white blood cells and the normal adult range for each.

    _____

    _____

    _____

19. What is measured by each of the following red blood cell indices?

    MCV: _____

    MCII: _____

    MCHC: _____

    RDW: _____

20. What is the most common cause of microcytic anemia?

    _____

21. What are the most common causes of macrocytic anemia?

    _____

22. Hypochromia occurs with what type of conditions?

    _____

23. What are the advantages of the following methods for performing a differential cell count?

    a. Automatic method: _____

    b. Manual: _____

24. Why must the white blood cells be stained when performing a manual differential cell count?

    _____

    _____

25. The least numerous type of white blood cell is the _____

26. Why are neutrophils also known as "segs"?

_____

_____

27. What is a band?

_____

28. The largest of the white blood cells is the _____

29. What is the function of lymphocytes?

_____

_____

30. List the abbreviation for each of the following tests:

    a. Hematocrit _____

    b. Hemoglobin _____

    c. Differential cell count _____

    d. White blood cell count _____

    e. Red blood cell count _____

31. What does the PT test measure?

_____

32. What is the PT adult reference range?

_____

33. What is the purpose of performing an INR on a PT test?

_____

_____

34. What is the range for a PT/INR result of a healthy individual with a normal clotting ability?

_____

35. What is the function of warfarin?

_____

36. What are the most common conditions for which warfarin is prescribed?

_____

_____

37. What is the usual desired PT/INR range for a patient who is on warfarin therapy for a heart attack or stroke?

_____

38. What is the goal of warfarin therapy?

_____

_____

39. How often should a patient on warfarin therapy have a PT/INR test performed?

_____

40. What color-stoppered tube should be used to collect a specimen for a PT/INR test?

_____

41. Why is it important to fill the blood tube for a PT/INR test to the exhaustion of the vacuum?

_____

_____

42. What are the advantages of PT/INR home testing?

_____

_____

CRITICAL THINKING ACTIVITIES

A. Diseases

1. You and your classmates work at a large clinic. It is National Disease Awareness Week. The providers at your clinic ask you to develop informative, creative, and colorful brochures for patients about various diseases. Choose a condition from the list, and design a brochure using the blank Frequently Asked Questions (FAQ) brochure provided on the following page. Each student in the class should select a different disease. On a separate sheet of paper, write three true/false questions relating to the information in your brochure.

2. Present your brochure to the class. After all the brochures have been presented, each student should ask three questions to the entire class to see how well the class understands the diseases that were presented. (*Note:* Students can take notes during the presentations and refer to them when answering the questions.)

Conditions

1. Addison's disease

2. Amyotrophic lateral sclerosis

3. Aplastic anemia

4. Bell's palsy

5. Cirrhosis

6. Crohn's disease

7. Cushing's syndrome

8. Cystic fibrosis

9. Degenerative disc disease

10. Epilepsy

11. Hemolytic anemia

12. Hemophilia

13. Hernia

14. Hodgkin's disease

15. Hyperthyroidism

16. Hypothyroidism

17. Leukemia

18. Lupus erythematosus

19. Multiple sclerosis

20. Muscular dystrophy

21. Parkinson's disease

22. Peptic ulcer

23. Pernicious anemia

24. Polycythemia

25. Sickle-cell anemia

26. Ulcerative colitis

FAQ
ON:

Q: A:

Q: A:

Q: A:

Q: A:

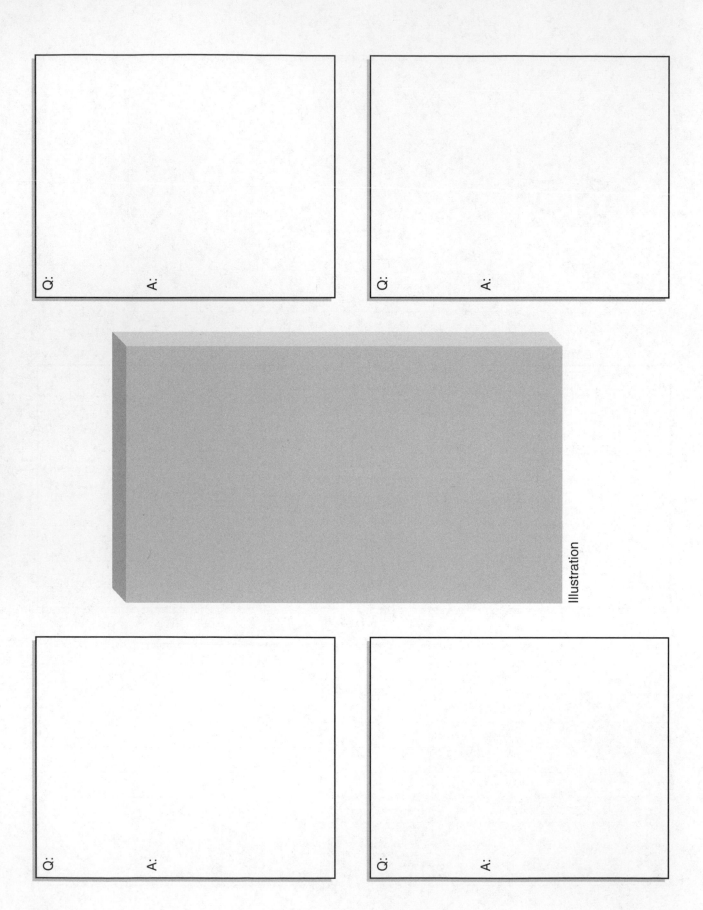

Q:

A:

Q:

A:

Illustration

Q:

A:

Q:

A:

B. Hematocrit

Label the layers of this microhematocrit capillary tube that has been centrifuged. Place an arrow at the point where you would take the hematocrit reading.

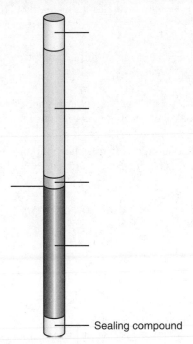

Sealing compound

C. Iron Content of Food

Consuming food that is high in iron helps to prevent iron-deficiency anemia. To become familiar with foods that are high in iron content and foods that contain little or no iron, plan the following two meals. One meal should be as high as possible in iron content, and the other meal should not contain any iron at all.

Meal 1

_____

_____

_____

_____

Meal 2

_____

_____

_____

_____

D. Iron-Deficiency Anemia

Create a profile of an individual who has iron-deficiency anemia following these guidelines:

1. Using colored pencils, crayons, or markers, draw a figure of an individual exhibiting iron-deficiency anemia. Be as creative as possible.

2. Do not use any text on your drawing other than to label items you have drawn in your picture. (A picture is worth a thousand words!)

3. Try to include all of the symptoms of iron-deficiency anemia in your drawing. The Iron-Deficiency Anemia Patient Teaching Box on pp. 668 in your textbook can be used as a reference source.

4. In the classroom, find a partner and trade drawings. Identify the symptoms of iron-deficiency anemia in your partner's drawing. With your partner, discuss what treatment is recommended and also what this person could do to prevent iron-deficiency anemia.

IRON-DEFICIENCY ANEMIA

E. Dear Gabby

Gabby is attending her class reunion and wants you to fill in for her. In the space provided, respond to the following letter.

Dear Gabby,

I am a housewife with two adorable children, ages 2 and 4. I have been feeling run down and tired lately, so I bought some vitamin pills at the drugstore. They came individually packaged in foil and plastic. They are hard to open, so I cut each package and transferred the iron pills to a little plastic baggie. When I told my mother about what I thought was a great idea, she got very upset. She told me that I could possibly be putting my children at danger. She said that iron is poisonous to children and that I should not do that. Gabby, my mom has always been overprotective. Is this just another one of her episodes?

Signed,

Curious in Kansas

_____

_____

_____

_____

_____

_____

_____

_____

_____

_____

_____

F. Crossword Puzzle: Hematology

Directions: Complete the crossword puzzle using the clues provided.

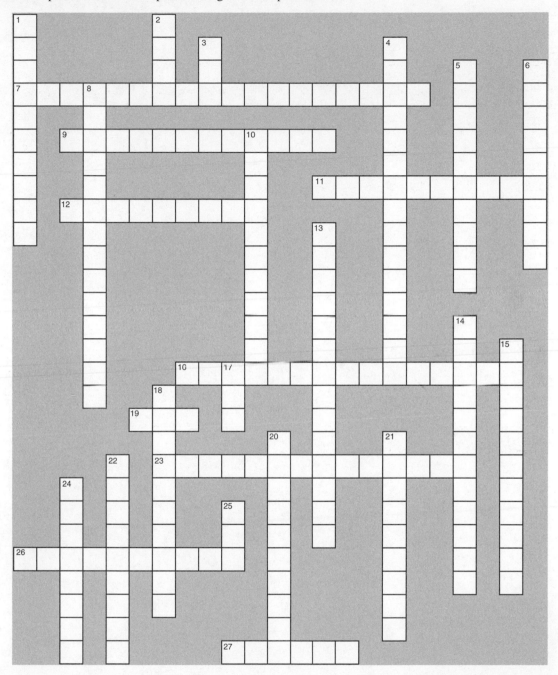

Across
- **7** Cause of blood pooling in heart
- **9** Condition of too many RBCs
- **11** Carries oxygen
- **12** Platelets and WBCs
- **16** Causes inaccurate PT/INR results
- **19** Common hematology test
- **23** Common cause of anemia
- **26** To separate blood
- **27** Liquid part of blood

Down
- **1** Study of blood
- **2** Differential WBC count abbreviation
- **3** Hemoglobin abbreviation
- **4** Blood clotting test
- **5** Most numerous WBC
- **6** Symptom of anemia
- **8** Causes black stool
- **10** Red blood cell

- **13** May affect PT/INR test results
- **14** Above 11,000 WBCs
- **15** Indication for warfarin
- **17** Aka thrombophlebitis
- **18** Calculations on CBC tests
- **20** Below 4500 WBCs
- **21** White blood cell
- **22** Color tube for PT/INR
- **24** Warfarin brand name
- **25** Hematocrit abbreviation

763

Notes

PRACTICE FOR COMPETENCY

Procedure 18-A: Hemoglobin Determination

    a. Run controls on a CLIA-waived hemoglobin analyzer, and document results on the quality control log on p. 767.

    b. Perform a hemoglobin determination on a patient using a CLIA-waived hemoglobin analyzer, and document results in the chart provided. Circle any values that fall outside the normal range.

Procedure 18-1: Hematocrit Determination

Perform a hematocrit determination in duplicate, and document results in the chart provided. Circle any values that fall outside the normal range.

Procedure 18-2: Preparation of a Blood Smear for a Differential Cell Count

Prepare a blood smear for a differential white blood cell count.

CHART	
Date	

Chapter **18 Hematology**

CHART	
Date	

QUALITY CONTROL HEMOGLOBIN LOG SHEET

Name of Meter: _____   Control Lot Number: _____

Low-Level Range: _____   Control Exp. Date: _____

High-Level Range: _____

Date	Test Cards: Lot # and Expiration	Low-Level Value	Accept	Reject	High-Level Value	Accept	Reject	Technician

Notes

e **Procedure 18-A: Hemoglobin Determination**

Name: _____   Date: _____

Evaluated by: _____   Score: _____

Performance Objective

Outcome:	Perform a hemoglobin determination.
Conditions:	Using a hemoglobin meter and operating manual and given the following: disposable gloves, antiseptic wipe, lancet, gauze pad, test cards, cod key, control solutions, quality control log, and a biohazard sharps container.
Standards:	Time: 10 minutes., Student completed procedure in _____ minutes.
	Accuracy: Satisfactory score on the Performance Evaluation Checklist.

Performance Evaluation Checklist

Trial 1	Trial 2	Point Value	Performance Standards
		•	Sanitized hands.
		•	Assembled equipment.
		•	Checked the expiration date of the test cards.
		•	Calibrated the hemoglobin meter.
		▷	Stated the purpose of calibrating the meter.
		•	Checked the expiration date of the control solution.
		•	Applied gloves and ran a low and high control.
		▷	Stated the purpose of running controls.
		•	Removed gloves and sanitized hands.
		•	Documented the control results in the quality control log.
		•	Greeted the patient and introduced yourself.
		•	Identified the patient and explained the procedure.
		•	Turned on the hemoglobin meter and checked the code number.
		•	Inserted a test card into the meter.
		•	Opened gauze packet.
		•	Cleansed the puncture site and allowed it to air-dry.
		▷	Stated what happens to the blood drop if the site is not dry.
		•	Applied gloves and performed a finger puncture.
		•	Wiped away the first drop of blood.

Trial 1	Trial 2	Point Value	Performance Standards
		•	Collected the blood specimen.
		•	Placed a gauze pad over the puncture site and applied pressure.
		•	Applied the blood specimen to the test card.
		•	Waited while the hemoglobin meter analyzed the blood specimen.
		•	Read the results on the display screen.
		▷	Stated the normal hemoglobin range for a female (12 to 16 g/dL) and a male (14 to 18 g/dL).
		•	Removed the test card from the meter.
		•	Properly disposed of the test card in a biohazard waste container.
		•	Checked the puncture site and applied an adhesive bandage, if needed.
		•	Removed gloves and sanitized hands.
		•	Documented the test results correctly.
		★	The hemoglobin documentation was identical to the reading on the digital display screen.
			Demonstrated the following affective behavior(s) during this procedure:
		Ⓐ	Explained to a patient the rationale for performance of a procedure.
		Ⓐ	Reassured a patient of the accuracy of the test results.
		★	Completed the procedure within 10 minutes.
			Totals

CHART	
Date	

Evaluation of Student Performance

EVALUATION CRITERIA			COMMENTS
Symbol	**Category**	**Point Value**	
★	Critical Step	16 points	
•	Essential Step	6 points	
Ⓐ	Affective Competency	6 points	
▷	Theory Question	2 points	

Score calculation: 100 points

             − _____ points missed

             _____ Score

Satisfactory score: 85 or above

CAAHEP Competencies Achieved

Psychomotor (Skills)
☑ I. 10. Perform a quality control measure.
☑ I. 11. a. Obtain specimens and perform CLIA-waived hematology test.
☑ II. 2. Differentiate between normal and abnormal test results.

Affective (Behavior)
☑ II. 1. Reassure a patient of the accuracy of the test results.
☑ V. 4. Explain to a patient the rationale for performance of a procedure.

ABHES Competencies Achieved

☑ 9. a. Practice quality control.
☑ 9. b. (2). Perform selected CLIA-waived tests that assist with diagnosis and treatment: hematology testing.

Procedure 18-1: Hematocrit

Name: _____   Date: _____

Evaluated by: _____   Score: _____

Performance Objective

Outcome:	Perform a hematocrit determination.
Conditions:	Given the following: microhematocrit centrifuge, disposable gloves, lancet, antiseptic wipe, gauze pad, capillary tubes, sealing compound, and a biohazard sharps container.
Standards:	Time: 10 minutes. Student completed procedure in _____ minutes.
	Accuracy: Satisfactory score on the Performance Evaluation Checklist.

Performance Evaluation Checklist

Trial 1	Trial 2	Point Value	Performance Standards
		•	Sanitized hands.
		•	Greeted the patient and introduced yourself.
		•	Identified the patient and explained the procedure.
		•	Assembled equipment.
		•	Opened the gauze packet.
		•	Cleansed the site with an antiseptic wipe and allowed it to air-dry.
		•	Applied gloves.
		•	Performed a finger puncture and discarded the lancet in a biohazard sharps container.
		•	Wiped away the first drop of blood.
		•	Massaged the finger until a large blood drop formed.
		•	Held one end of the capillary tube horizontally but slightly downward next to the free-flowing puncture.
		•	Kept the tip of the pipet in the blood but did not allow it to press against the skin of the patient's finger.
		▷	Explained why the capillary tube should be kept in the blood specimen.
		•	Filled the capillary tube (calibrated tubes filled to the calibration line; uncalibrated tubes filled approximately three-fourths full).
		▷	Explained why a tube with air bubbles is unacceptable.
		•	Filled a second capillary tube.
		▷	Stated why 2 capillary tubes must be filled.
		•	Placed a gauze pad over the puncture site and applied pressure.

Trial 1	Trial 2	Point Value	Performance Standards
		•	Sealed the dry end of each capillary tube.
		•	Checked the puncture site and applied an adhesive bandage, if needed.
		•	Placed the capillary tubes in the microhematocrit centrifuge with the sealed end facing toward the outside.
		▷	Explained why the sealed end must face toward the outside.
		•	Balanced one tube with the other tube placed opposite it.
		•	Placed the cover over the capillary tubes and locked it securely.
		•	Centrifuged the blood specimen for 3 to 5 minutes.
		▷	Explained the reason for centrifuging the blood specimen.
		•	Allowed the centrifuge to come to a complete stop.
		•	Removed the protective cover from the capillary tubes.
		•	Read the results using the appropriate reading device.
		•	Determined whether the results agreed within 4 percentage points.
		▷	Explained what to do if the results are not within 4 percentage points.
		•	Averaged the values of the two tubes together to derive the test results.
		★	The results were within ±1% of the evaluator's results.
		▷	Stated the normal hematocrit range for a female (37% to 47%) and a male (40% to 54%).
		•	Properly disposed of the capillary tubes in a biohazard sharps container.
		•	Removed gloves and sanitized hands.
		•	Documented the test results correctly.
		•	Returned equipment.
			Demonstrated the following affective behavior(s) during this procedure:
		Ⓐ	Explained to a patient the rationale for performance of a procedure.
		Ⓐ	Reassured a patient of the accuracy of the test results.
		★	Completed the procedure within 10 minutes.
			Totals

CHART

Date			

774

Evaluation of Student Performance

EVALUATION CRITERIA			COMMENTS
Symbol	**Category**	**Point Value**	
★	Critical Step	16 points	
•	Essential Step	6 points	
Ⓐ	Affective Competency	6 points	
▷	Theory Question	2 points	

Score calculation: 100 points

      − _____ points missed

      _____ Score

Satisfactory score: 85 or above

CAAHEP Competencies Achieved

Psychomotor (Skills)
☑ I. 10. Perform a quality control measure.
☑ I. 11. a. Obtain specimens and perform CLIA-waived hematology test.
☑ II. 2. Differentiate between normal and abnormal test results.

Affective (Behavior)
☑ II. 1. Reassure a patient of the accuracy of the test results.
☑ V. 4. Explain to a patient the rationale for performance of a procedure.

ABHES Competencies Achieved

☑ 9. a. Practice quality control.

☑ 9. b. (2) Perform selected CLIA-waived tests that assist with diagnosis and treatment: hematology testing.

Notes

Procedure 18-2: Preparation of a Blood Smear for a Differential Cell Count

Name:_____   Date: _____

Evaluated by: _____   Score: _____

Performance Objective

Outcome:	Prepare a blood smear for a differential white blood cell count.
Conditions:	Given the following: disposable gloves, supplies to perform a finger puncture or venipuncture, slides with a frosted edge, slide container, biohazard specimen bag, laboratory request form, and a biohazard sharps container.
Standards:	Time: 10 minutes. Student completed procedure in _____ minutes.
	Accuracy: Satisfactory score on the Performance Evaluation Checklist.

Performance Evaluation Checklist

Trial 1	Trial 2	Point Value	Performance Standards
		•	Sanitized hands.
		•	Greeted the patient and introduced yourself.
		•	Identified the patient and explained the procedure.
		•	Assembled equipment.
		•	Labeled the slides.
		•	Opened the gauze packet.
		•	Cleansed the puncture site.
		•	Applied gloves.
		•	Performed a venipuncture (using a lavender-stoppered tube) or a finger puncture.
		•	Placed a drop of blood in the middle of each slide approximately ¼ inch from the frosted edge of the slide.
		•	Held a spreader slide at a 30-degree angle to the first slide in front of the drop of blood.
		▷	Stated what occurs if the angle is more than 30 degrees or less than 30 degrees.
		•	Moved the spreader slide until it touched the drop of blood.
		•	Spread the blood thinly and evenly across slide using the spreader slide.
		•	Prepared the second blood smear.
		•	Disposed of the spreader slide in a biohazard sharps container.
		•	Laid the blood smears on a flat surface and allowed them to dry.
		▷	Explained why the blood smears should be dried immediately.
		•	The length of the smear was approximately 1½ inches.
		•	The smear was smooth and even, with no ridges, holes, lines, streaks, or clumps.
		•	The smear was not too thick or too thin.
		•	There was a feathered edge at the thin end of the smear.
		•	There was a margin on all sides of the smear.
		•	Placed the slides in a protective slide container.
		•	Placed lavender-stoppered tube and slide container in a biohazard specimen bag.

Chapter **18** **Hematology**

Trial 1	Trial 2	Point Value	Performance Standards
		•	Removed gloves and sanitized hands.
		•	Completed a laboratory request form.
		•	Placed the lab request in the outside pocket of the specimen bag.
		•	Documented the procedure correctly.
		•	Filed a copy of the lab request in the patient's medical record.
		•	Placed the specimen bag in the appropriate location for pickup by a lab courier.
		•	Documented the procedure correctly.
			Demonstrated the following affective behavior(s) during this procedure:
		Ⓐ	Explained to a patient the rationale for performance of a procedure.
		★	Completed the procedure within 10 minutes.
			Totals

CHART

Date	

Evaluation of Student Performance

EVALUATION CRITERIA			COMMENTS
Symbol	**Category**	**Point Value**	
★	Critical Step	16 points	
•	Essential Step	6 points	
Ⓐ	Affective Competency	6 points	
▷	Theory Question	2 points	

Score calculation: 100 points

− _____ points missed

_____ Score

Satisfactory score: 85 or above

CAAHEP Competencies Achieved

Psychomotor (Skills)
☑ I. 10. Perform a quality control measure.
Affective (Behavior)
☑ V. 4. Explain to a patient the rationale for performance of a procedure.

ABHES Competencies Achieved

☑ 9. a. Practice quality control
☑ 9. d. Collect, label, and process specimens

778

19 Blood Chemistry and Immunology

CHAPTER ASSIGNMENTS

√ After Completing	Date Due	Study Guide Pages	STUDY GUIDE ASSIGNMENTS (CTA = Critical Thinking Activity)	Possible Points	Points You Earned
		783	? Pretest	10	
		784	Term Key Term Assessment	17	
		784-790	Evaluation of Learning questions	55	
		790-792	CTA A: Type 2 Diabetes	40	
		793	CTA B: Oral Glucose Tolerance Test (2 points each)	10	
		793-794	CTA C: Coronary Artery Disease	20	
		795	CTA D: Cholesterol and Saturated Fat (5 points each)	15	
			e Evolve Site: The Right Chemistry: Blood Chemistry Tests (Record points earned)		
		795-796	CTA E: Rh Incompatibility (2 points each)	20	
		796	CTA F: Crossword Puzzle	25	
			e Evolve Site: Immunologic Tests (Record points earned)		
			e Evolve Site: Apply Your Knowledge questions	20	
			e Evolve Site: Video Evaluation	16	
		783	? Posttest	10	
			ADDITIONAL ASSIGNMENTS		
			Total points		

Notes

√ When Assigned By Your Instructor	Study Guide Pages	Practices Required	LABORATORY ASSIGNMENTS (Procedure Number and Name)	Score*
	797-798	3	**Practice for Competency** 19-A: Performing a Blood Chemistry Test Textbook reference: pp. 683-689	
	803-805		**Evaluation of Competency** 19-A: Performing a Blood Chemistry Test	*
	797-799	3	**Practice for Competency** 19-1: Blood Glucose Measurement Using the Accu-Chek Advantage Glucose Meter Textbook reference: pp. 698-701	
	807-809		**Evaluation of Competency** 19-1: Blood Glucose Measurement Using the Accu-Chek Advantage Glucose Meter	*
	797-801	3	**Practice for Competency** 19-B: Rapid Mononucleosis Testing (QuickVue + Mono Test) Textbook reference: pp. 706-708	
	811-813		**Evaluation of Competency** 19-B: Rapid Mononucleosis Testing (QuickVue + Mono Test)	*
			ADDITIONAL ASSIGNMENTS	

Notes

Name: _____ Date: _____

True or False

_____ 1. The function of glucose in the body is to build and repair tissue.

_____ 2. Insulin is required for normal use of glucose in the body.

_____ 3. An abnormally low level of glucose in the body is known as *hypoglycemia*.

_____ 4. The hemoglobin A_{1C} test measures the average amount of blood glucose over a 3-month period.

_____ 5. Most of the cholesterol found in the blood comes from the intake of dietary cholesterol.

_____ 6. The primary use of the cholesterol test is to screen for the presence of coronary artery disease.

_____ 7. LDL picks up cholesterol from ingested fats and the liver and carries it to the cells.

_____ 8. An antibody is a substance that is capable of combining with an antigen.

_____ 9. Mononucleosis is transmitted through coughing and sneezing.

_____ 10. Blood antigens (A, B, Rh) are located on the surface of red blood cells.

POSTTEST

True or False

_____ 1. Serum is required for most blood chemistry tests.

_____ 2. The normal range for a fasting blood glucose level is 120 to 160 mg/dL.

_____ 3. The oral glucose tolerance test is used to assist in the diagnosis of diabetes mellitus.

_____ 4. Before meals, it is recommended that the blood glucose level for a diabetic patient be 60 to 80 mg/dL.

_____ 5. The recommended hemoglobin A1C level for a patient with diabetes is 4% to 6%.

_____ 6. The buildup of plaque (resulting from high cholesterol) on the walls of arteries is known as thrombophlebitis.

_____ 7. An HDL cholesterol level greater than 50 mg/dL is a risk factor for coronary artery disease.

_____ 8. The triglyceride test requires that the patient not eat or drink for 12 hours before the test.

_____ 9. The RPR test is a screening test for syphilis.

_____ 10. The varicella virus causes infectious mononucleosis.

✎ Term KEY TERM ASSESSMENT

Directions: Match each key term with its definition.

_____ 1. Agglutination

_____ 2. Antibody

_____ 3. Antigen

_____ 4. Antiserum

_____ 5. Blood antibody

_____ 6. Blood antigen

_____ 7. Donor

_____ 8. Gene

_____ 9. Glycogen

_____ 10. HDL cholesterol

_____ 11. Hyperglycemia

_____ 12. Hypoglycemia

_____ 13. In vitro

_____ 14. In vivo

_____ 15. LDL cholesterol

_____ 16. Lipoprotein

_____ 17. Recipient

A. An abnormally high level of glucose in the blood
B. A complex molecule consisting of protein and a lipid fraction such as cholesterol
C. The form in which carbohydrate is stored in the body
D. A lipoprotein consisting of protein and cholesterol that removes excess cholesterol from the cells
E. An abnormally low level of glucose in the blood
F. A lipoprotein, consisting of protein and cholesterol, that picks up cholesterol and delivers it to the cells
G. A substance that is capable of combining with an antigen, resulting in an antigen-antibody reaction
H. Substance capable of stimulating the formation of antibodies
I. One who receives something, such as a blood transfusion, from a donor
J. Clumping of blood cells
K. A protein present on the surface of red blood cells that determines a person's blood type
L. Occurring in the living body or organism
M. A unit of heredity
N. A serum that contains antibodies
O. One who furnishes something, such as blood, tissue, or organs, to be used in another individual
P. Occurring in glass; refers to tests performed under artificial conditions, as in the laboratory
Q. A protein present in the blood plasma that is capable of combining with its corresponding blood antigen to produce an antigen-antibody reaction

📖 EVALUATION OF LEARNING

Directions: Fill in each blank with the correct answer.

1. What type of specimen is required for most blood chemistry tests?

_____

2. What is the purpose of quality control?

_____

_____

3. What is the purpose of calibrating a blood chemistry analyzer?

_____

_____

4. At a minimum, when should a calibration check be performed on a blood chemistry analyzer?

_____

5. What is the purpose of running a control on a blood chemistry analyzer?

_____

_____

6. List three reasons why a control may not produce expected results.

_____

_____

7. When running controls on a blood chemistry analyzer, what should be done if the controls do not perform as expected?

_____

8. What is the function of glucose in the body?

_____

_____

9. Explain the function of insulin in the body.

_____

_____

10. List the abbreviation for each of the following tests:

    a. Fasting blood glucose _____

    b. Two-hour postprandial blood glucose _____

    c. Oral glucose tolerance test _____

11. What type of patient preparation is required for a fasting blood glucose test?

_____

_____

12. List two reasons for performing a fasting blood glucose test.

_____

13. What is prediabetes?

_____

_____

14. What are the values recommended by the American Diabetes Association for interpreting fasting blood glucose results?

    a. Normal _____

    b. Prediabetes _____

    c. Diabetes _____

15. What type of patient preparation is required for a 2-hour postprandial blood glucose test?

_____

_____

Chapter **19 Blood Chemistry and Immunology**

16. Describe the procedure for performing a 2-hour postprandial blood glucose test.

_____

_____

17. What is the purpose of an oral glucose tolerance test?

_____

_____

18. What type of patient preparation is required for an oral glucose tolerance test?

_____

_____

19. Describe the procedure for an oral glucose tolerance test.

_____

_____

20. Define hypoglycemia and list three conditions that may cause it to occur.

_____

_____

21. Why is it important for a patient with insulin-dependent diabetes to perform self-monitoring of blood glucose (SMBG)?

_____

_____

22. What is the ideal insulin testing schedule for SMBG?

_____

_____

23. What type of damage can occur to the body from prolonged high blood glucose levels?

_____

_____

24. List three advantages of blood glucose monitoring at home.

_____

_____

_____

25. What is the recommended blood glucose level for a diabetic patient during the following times of the day?

a. Before meals _____

b. One to 2 hours after meals _____

c. At bedtime _____

26. What information is provided by a hemoglobin A$_{1C}$ test?

_____

_____

27. What is the normal A$_{1C}$ range for an individual without diabetes?

_____

28. What is the recommended A$_{1C}$ percentage for an individual with diabetes?

_____

_____

29. What are the storage requirements for blood glucose reagent test strips?

_____

_____

30. When should the calibration (coding) procedure be performed on a glucose meter?

_____

31. What is cholesterol?

_____

_____

32. List the two main sources of cholesterol in the blood.

_____

_____

33. What is atherosclerosis, and why is it a health risk?

_____

_____

34. Why is LDL cholesterol referred to as *bad cholesterol* and HDL referred to as *good cholesterol*?

_____

_____

_____

35. What does a total cholesterol test measure?

_____

_____

36. List the ranges for each of the following cholesterol categories:

a. Desirable cholesterol level _____

b. Borderline cholesterol level _____

c. High cholesterol level _____

37. At what level is HDL cholesterol considered a risk factor for coronary heart disease?

_____

_____

38. What is the primary use of the cholesterol test?

_____

_____

39. What type of patient preparation is required for a triglyceride test?

_____

_____

40. List the ranges for each of the following triglyceride categories:

a. Normal _____

b. Borderline high _____

c. High _____

d. Very high _____

41. What conditions result in elevated blood triglycerides?

_____

_____

_____

42. What is the purpose of performing a BUN?

_____

_____

43. What is the definition of immunology?

_____

_____

_____

44. List three examples of antigens.

_____

_____

45. What is the purpose of performing each of the following serologic tests?

    a. Rheumatoid factor

_____

_____

    b. Antistreptolysin test

_____

_____

    c. C-reactive protein

_____

_____

    d. ABO and Rh blood typing

_____

_____

46. How is infectious mononucleosis transmitted?

_____

_____

47. What are the symptoms of infectious mononucleosis?

_____

_____

48. What happens when a blood antigen and antibody combine?

_____

_____

49. Where are the A, B, and Rh antigens located?

_____

50. Why is agglutination of blood in vivo a threat to life?

_____

_____

51. If a person has type A blood, what antigens and antibodies are present?

_____

_____

_____

52. If a person has type B blood, what antigens and antibodies are present?

_____

_____

53. If a person has type AB blood, what antigens and antibodies are present?

_____

54. If a person has type O blood, what antigens and antibodies are present?

_____

55. What is the difference between Rh-positive and Rh-negative blood?

_____

_____

CRITICAL THINKING ACTIVITIES

A. Type 2 Diabetes

You are working for a provider specializing in internal medicine. The provider is concerned about the increased numbers of patients developing type 2 diabetes mellitus. He asks you to design a colorful, creative, and informative brochure on type 2 diabetes, using the brochure format provided on the next page. This brochure will be published and placed in the waiting room to provide patients with education on type 2 diabetes. Diabetes Internet sites can be used to complete this activity.

FAQ
ON:

Q: A:

Q: A:

Q: A:

Q: A:

Q: A:

Q: A:

Illustration

Q: A:

Q: A:

792

B. Oral Glucose Tolerance Test

Marty Wolf has arrived at your office for an oral glucose tolerance test. What should you tell her regarding the following subjects? Explain the reason for each answer.

1. Consumption of food and fluid

   _____

   _____

2. Water consumption

   _____

   _____

3. Smoking

   _____

   _____

4. Leaving the test site

   _____

   _____

5. Activity

   _____

   _____

C. Coronary Artery Disease

Create a profile of an individual who is at risk for coronary artery disease (CAD) following these guidelines:

1. Using colored pencils, crayons, or markers, draw a figure of an individual exhibiting risk factors for CAD. Be as creative as possible.

2. Do not use any text on your drawing other than to label items you have drawn in your picture. (A picture is worth a thousand words!)

3. Try to include at least eight risk factors for CAD in your drawing. The *Highlight on Heart Disease* box on p. 702 in your textbook can be used as a reference source.

4. In the classroom, find a partner and trade drawings. Identify the risk factors for CAD in your partner's drawing. With your partner, discuss what this person could do to lower his or her chances of developing coronary heart disease.

AT RISK FOR CAD

D. Cholesterol and Saturated Fat

Using a reference source, complete the following activities:

1. Create a dinner meal that is as high as possible in saturated fat and cholesterol.

_____

_____

_____

_____

_____

2. Create a dinner meal that is as low as possible in saturated fat and cholesterol.

_____

_____

_____

_____

_____

3. Choose a fast-food restaurant, and plan a meal that is as low as possible in saturated fat and cholesterol.

_____

_____

_____

_____

_____

E. Rh Incompatibility

Erythroblastosis fetalis is a blood disorder of the newborn. It usually is caused by incompatibility between the infant's blood and the mother's blood. Using a reference source, answer the following questions regarding this condition in the space provided.

1. Explain how Rh incompatibility between the mother and infant can cause this condition to occur.

_____

_____

_____

_____

2. Describe the symptoms associated with erythroblastosis fetalis.

_____

_____

_____

3. Explain the treatment used for this condition.

_____

_____

_____

795

4. How can this condition be prevented?

_____

_____

_____

F. Crossword Puzzle: Blood Chemistry and Immunology

Directions: Complete the crossword puzzle using the clues provided.

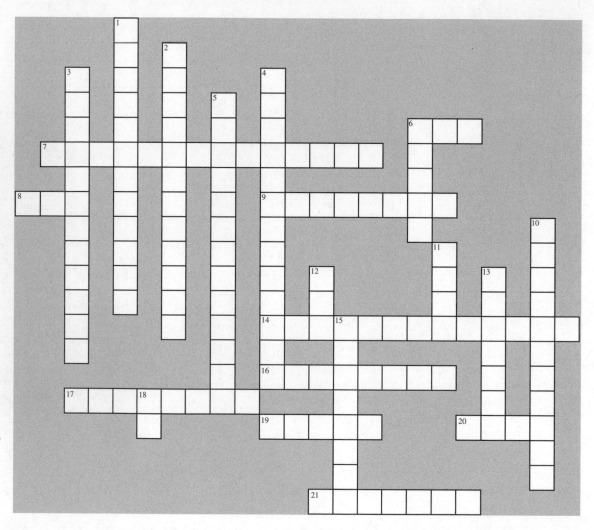

Across
- **6** Bad cholesterol
- **7** Cholesterol 200-239
- **8** Good cholesterol
- **9** Stored glucose
- **14** Kissing disease
- **16** Combines with an antigen
- **17** Increases HDL cholesterol
- **19** Keep diabetic A1c below this
- **20** Series of glucose tests
- **21** Provides energy for body

Down
- **1** No. 1 killer in the U.S.
- **2** Raises cholesterol level
- **3** Low BG
- **4** High BG
- **5** Desirable: ,150 mg/dL
- **6** Makes cholesterol
- **10** FBG: 100-125 mg/dL
- **11** Syphilis test
- **12** Detects renal disease
- **13** Risk factor for CAD
- **15** Unsaturated fat (ex)
- **18** Rheumatoid arthritis test

Procedure 19-A: Blood Chemistry Test

Perform a blood chemistry test, and document results in the chart provided. Examples of blood chemistry tests: cholesterol, triglycerides, and BUN.

Procedure 19-1: Blood Glucose Measurement

a. Run controls on a CLIA-waived glucose meter, and document results on the quality control log on page 799.

b. Perform a fasting blood glucose test, and document results in the chart provided.

Procedure 19-B: Rapid Mononucleosis Test

a. Run controls on a CLIA-waived mono test, and document results on the quality control log on page 801.

b. Perform a rapid mononucleosis test, and document results in the chart provided.

CHART	
Date	

797

CHART	
Date	

QUALITY CONTROL LOG

BLOOD GLUCOSE

NAME OF METER				CONTROLS			
Test Strips: Lot Number: _____ Exp Date: _____ Code Number: _____				**Low-Level Control:** Lot Number: _____ Exp Date: _____ Expected Range: _____ **High-Level Control:** Lot Number: _____ Exp Date: _____ Expected Range: _____			
Date	Low-Level Control	Accept	Reject	High-Level Control	Accept	Reject	Technician

Chapter **19 Blood Chemistry and Immunology**

QUALITY CONTROL LOG

MONONUCLEOSIS TEST

Date	Name of Test	Control Lot #	Control Expiration Date	External Positive Control Results	External Negative Control Results	Technician

Notes

Procedure 19-A: Performing a Blood Chemistry Test

Name: _____   Date: _____

Evaluated by: _____   Score: _____

Performance Objective

Outcome:	Perform a fasting blood glucose test.
Conditions:	Given the following: disposable gloves, an antiseptic wipe, a lancet, gauze pad, quality control log, and a biohazard sharps container. Using an automated blood chemistry analyzer and operating manual.
Standards:	Time: 10 minutes. Student completed procedure in _____ minutes.
	Accuracy: Satisfactory score on the Performance Evaluation Checklist.

Performance Evaluation Checklist

Trial 1	Trial 2	Point Value	Performance Standards
		•	Sanitized hands.
		•	Assembled equipment.
		•	Calibrated the blood chemistry analyzer.
		•	Applied gloves and ran controls.
		•	Documented results in the quality control log.
		•	Sanitized hands.
		•	Greeted the patient and introduced yourself.
		•	Identified the patient and explained the procedure.
		•	Applied gloves.
		•	Performed a finger puncture.
		•	Collected the specimen according to manufacturer's instructions.
		•	Placed a gauze pad over the puncture site and applied pressure.
		•	Inserted the specimen into the blood chemistry analyzer according to manufacturer's instructions.
		•	Operated the blood chemistry analyzer according to manufacturer's instructions.
		•	Read the results on the digital display screen.
		•	Properly disposed of used materials.
		•	Checked the puncture site and applied an adhesive bandage if needed.
		•	Removed gloves.
		•	Sanitized hands.

Trial 1	Trial 2	Point Value	Performance Standards
		•	Documented the test results correctly.
		★	The documentation was identical to the reading on the digital display screen.
			Demonstrated the following affective behavior(s) during this procedure:
		Ⓐ	Explained to a patient the rationale for performance of a procedure.
		Ⓐ	Reassured a patient of the accuracy of the test results.
		★	Completed the procedure within 10 minutes.
			Totals

CHART

Date	

Evaluation of Student Performance

EVALUATION CRITERIA			COMMENTS
Symbol	**Category**	**Point Value**	
★	Critical Step	16 points	
•	Essential Step	6 points	
Ⓐ	Affective Competency	6 points	
▷	Theory Question	2 points	

Score calculation: 100 points
− _____ points missed
_____ Score

Satisfactory score: 85 or above

CAAHEP Competencies Achieved

Psychomotor (Skills)
☑ I. 10. Perform a quality control measure.
☑ I. 11. b. Obtain specimens and perform CLIA-waived chemistry test.
☑ II. 2. Differentiate between normal and abnormal test results.
☑ II. 3. Maintain lab test results using flow sheets.

Affective (Behavior)
☑ II. 1. Reassure a patient of the accuracy of the test results.
☑ V. 4. Explain to a patient the rationale for performance of a procedure.

ABHES Competencies Achieved

☑ 9. a. Practice quality control.
☑ 9. b. (3) Perform selected CLIA-waived tests that assist with diagnosis and treatment: chemistry testing.

Notes

Procedure 19-1. Blood Glucose Measurement Using the Accu-Chek Advantage Glucose Meter

Name: _____   Date: _____

Evaluated by: _____   Score: _____

Performance Objective

Outcome:	Perform a fasting blood glucose test.
Conditions:	Given the following: disposable gloves, Accu-Chek Advantage glucose meter, reagent test strips, check strip, code key, control solutions, lancet, antiseptic wipe, gauze pad, quality control log, and a biohazard sharps container.
Standards:	Time: 10 minutes. Student completed procedure in _____ minutes.
	Accuracy: Satisfactory score on the Performance Evaluation Checklist.

Performance Evaluation Checklist

Trial 1	Trial 2	Point Value	Performance Standards
		•	Sanitized hands.
			Assembled equipment.
			...the expiration date on the container of test strips.
			...the code key.
		▷	
		•	Ran a low and ...
		▷	Stated the purpose for running controls.
		•	Documented the results in the quality control log.
		•	Sanitized hands.
		•	Greeted the patient and introduced yourself.
		•	Identified the patient and explained the procedure.
		•	Asked the patient if he or she prepared properly.
		▷	Stated the preparation required for a fasting blood glucose test.
		•	Removed a test strip from the container.
		•	Immediately replaced the lid of the container.
		▷	Explained why the lid should be replaced immediately.
		•	Gently inserted the test strip into the test strip guide.
		•	Checked that the code number matches the code number on the test s... con- tainer.
		•	Opened a gauze packet.

Chapter **19 Blood Chemistry** ... nology

Trial 1	Trial 2	Point Value	Performance Standards
		•	Cleansed the puncture site with an antiseptic wipe and allowed it to dry.
		•	Applied gloves.
		•	Performed a finger puncture.
		•	Disposed of the lancet in the biohazard sharps container.
		•	Wiped away the first drop of blood with a gauze pad.
		▷	Explained why the first drop of blood should be wiped away.
		•	Placed the patient's hand in a dependent position and gently massaged the finger until a large drop of blood formed.
		•	Applied the drop of blood to the yellow target area of the test strip.
		•	Completely filled the yellow target area with blood.
		▷	Explained what to do if the yellow area is not completely covered with blood.
		•	Placed a gauze pad over the puncture site and applied pressure.
		•	Observed the digital display of the test results.
		▷	Stated the normal range for a fasting blood glucose level (70 to 99 mg/dL).
		•	Removed the test strip from the meter and discarded it in a biohazard waste container.
		•	Turned off the meter.
		•	Checked the puncture site and applied an adhesive bandage, if needed.
		•	Removed gloves and sanitized hands.
		•	Documented the test results correctly.
		★	The documentation was identical to the reading on the digital display screen.
		•	Properly stored the glucose meter.
			Demonstrated the following affective behavior(s) during this procedure:
		Ⓐ	Explained to a patient the rationale for performance of a procedure.
		Ⓐ	Reassured a patient of the accuracy of the test results.
		★	Completed the procedure within 10 minutes.
			Totals

Evaluation of Student Performance

EVALUATION CRITERIA			COMMENTS
Symbol	**Category**	**Point Value**	
★	Critical Step	16 points	
•	Essential Step	6 points	
Ⓐ	Affective Competency	6 points	
▷	Theory Question	2 points	

Score calculation: 100 points
 −_____ points missed
_____ Score
Satisfactory score: 85 or above

CAAHEP Competencies Achieved

Psychomotor (Skills)
☑ I. 10. Perform a quality control measure.
☑ I. 11. b. Obtain specimens and perform CLIA-waived chemistry test.
☑ II. 2. Differentiate between normal and abnormal test results.
☑ II. 3. Maintain lab test results using flow sheets.

Affective (Behavior)
☑ II. 1. Reassure a patient of the accuracy of the test results.
☑ V. 4. Explain to a patient the rationale for performance of a procedure.

ABHES Competencies Achieved

☑ 9. a. Practice quality control.
☑ 9. b. (3) Perform selected CLIA-waived tests that assist with diagnosis and treatment: chemistry testing.

Notes

Procedure 19-B: Rapid Mononucleosis Testing (QuickVue+ Mono Test)

Name: _____   Date: _____

Evaluated by: _____   Score: _____

Performance Objective

Outcome:	Perform a rapid mononucleosis test.
Conditions:	Given the following: disposable gloves, the supplies needed to perform a finger puncture, a mononucleosis testing kit, and a biohazard container.
Standards:	Time: 10 minutes. Student completed procedure in _____ minutes.
	Accuracy: Satisfactory score on the Performance Evaluation Checklist.

Performance Evaluation Checklist

Trial 1	Trial 2	Point Value	Performance Standards
		•	Sanitized hands.
		•	Assembled equipment.
		•	Checked the expiration date on the testing kit.
		•	Applied gloves and ran a positive and a negative control, if necessary.
		•	Removed gloves and documented the results in the quality control log.
		•	Greeted the patient and introduced yourself.
		•	Identified the patient and explained the procedure.
		•	Cleansed the puncture site and allowed it to air dry.
		•	Applied gloves.
		•	Performed a finger puncture.
		•	Disposed of the lancet in a biohazard sharps container.
		•	Wiped away the first drop of blood.
		•	Collected the blood specimen with a capillary tube.
		•	Placed a gauze pad over the puncture site and applied pressure.
		•	Dispensed the blood specimen into the Add well on the test cassette.
		•	Added 5 drops of developing solution to the Add well.
		•	Waited 5 minutes and read the results.
		▷	Described the appearance of a positive and negative test result.
		•	Disposed of the test cassette in a biohazard waste container.
		•	Checked the puncture site and applied an adhesive bandage, if needed.

Chapter **19 Blood Chemistry and Immunology**

Trial 1	Trial 2	Point Value	Performance Standards
		•	Removed gloves.
		•	Sanitized hands.
		•	Documented the results correctly.
		•	The results were identical to the evaluator's results.
		•	Explained to a patient the rationale for performance of a procedure.
		•	Reassured a patient of the accuracy of the test results.
		•	Completed the procedure within 10 minutes.
			Totals

CHART

Date	

Evaluation of Student Performance

EVALUATION CRITERIA			COMMENTS
Symbol	**Category**	**Point Value**	
★	Critical Step	16 points	
•	Essential Step	6 points	
Ⓐ	Affective Competency	6 points	
▷	Theory Question	2 points	
Score calculation: 100 points − _____ points missed _____ Score Satisfactory score: 85 or above			

Psychomotor (Skills)

☑ I. 10. Perform a quality control measure.
☑ I. 11. d. Obtain specimens and perform CLIA-waived immunology test.
☑ II. 2. Differentiate between normal and abnormal test results.

Affective (Behavior)

☑ II. 1. Reassure a patient of the accuracy of the test results.
☑ V. 4. Explain to a patient the rationale for performance of a procedure.

ABHES Competencies Achieved

☑ 9. a. Practice quality control.
☑ 9. b. (4) Perform selected CLIA-waived tests that assist with diagnosis and treatment: immunolo   sting.

20 Medical Microbiology

CHAPTER ASSIGNMENTS

√ After Completing	Date Due	Study Guide Pages	STUDY GUIDE ASSIGNMENTS (CTA = Critical Thinking Activity)	Possible Points	Points You Earned
		819	Pretest	10	
		820	Term Key Term Assessment	13	
		820-826	Evaluation of Learning questions	62	
		827	CTA A: Stages of an Infectious Disease	20	
			Evolve Site: Microscope Identification (Record points earned)		
		828	CTA B: Sensitivity Testing	12	
		829	CTA C: Crossword Puzzle	21	
			Evolve Site: Apply Your Knowledge questions	10	
			Evolve Site: Video Evaluation	15	
		819	Posttest	10	
			ADDITIONAL ASSIGNMENTS		
			Total points		

√ When Assigned by Your Instructor	Study Guide Pages	Practices Required	LABORATORY ASSIGNMENTS (Procedure Number and Name)	Score*
	831	3	**Practice for Competency** 20-1: Using the Microscope Textbook reference: pp. 720-722	
	835-837		**Evaluation of Competency** 20-1: Using the Microscope	
	831-832	3	**Practice for Competency** 20-2: Collecting a Throat Specimen Textbook reference: p. 724-726	
	839-841		**Evaluation of Competency** 20-2: Collecting a Throat Specimen	
	831-833	3	**Practice for Competency** 20-3: CLIA-Waived Rapid Strep Testing Textbook reference: p. 730-732	
	843-845		**Evaluation of Competency** 20-3: CLIA-Waived Rapid Strep Testing	*
	831-833	3	**Practice for Competency** 20-4: Rapid Influenza Testing Textbook reference: p 732-735	
	847-850		**Evaluation of Competency** 20-4: Rapid Influenza Testing	
			ADDITIONAL ASSIGNMENTS	

Name: _____ Date: _____

True or False

_____ 1. Microbiology is the scientific study of microorganisms and their activities.

_____ 2. A disease that can be spread from one person to another is known as an infectious disease.

_____ 3. Droplet infection is the transfer of pathogens from a fine spray emitted from a person already infected with the disease.

_____ 4. Streptococci are round bacteria that grow in pairs.

_____ 5. Chickenpox is caused by a virus.

_____ 6. The coarse adjustment on a microscope is used to obtain precise focusing of an object.

_____ 7. The purpose of transport media is to provide nutrients for the multiplication of the specimen.

_____ 8. A throat specimen should be collected from the tonsillar area and posterior pharynx.

_____ 9. Strep throat is primarily transmitted through droplet infection and by sharing personal items with an infected person.

_____ 10. Antiviral medications can be used to prevent influenza.

? POSTTEST

True or False

_____ 1. Microorganisms that reside in the body but do not cause disease are known as transient flora.

_____ 2. The invasion of the body by a pathogenic microorganism is known as infection.

_____ 3. The interval of time between the invasion by a pathogen and the first symptoms of disease is known as the *prodromal period*.

_____ 4. Staphylococcal infections usually result in pus formation.

_____ 5. *Escherichia coli* normally reside in the urinary tract.

_____ 6. The high-power objective has a magnification of 40×.

_____ 7. Examination of urine sediment requires the use of the oil immersion objective.

_____ 8. A throat specimen is the preferred specimen for a rapid influenza diagnostic test.

_____ 9. A mixed culture contains two or more types of microorganisms.

_____ 10. The purpose of sensitivity testing is to identify the type of microorganism present.

Directions: Match each key term with its definition.

_____ 1. Bacilli

_____ 2. Cocci

_____ 3. Contagious

_____ 4. Culture

_____ 5. Culture medium

_____ 6. Incubate

_____ 7. Incubation period

_____ 8. Infectious disease

_____ 9. Inoculate

_____ 10. Microbiology

_____ 11. Normal flora

_____ 12. Specimen

_____ 13. Spirilla

A. A disease caused by a pathogen that produces harmful effects on its host

B. Capable of being transmitted directly or indirectly from one person to another

C. To introduce microorganisms into a culture medium for growth and multiplication

D. Bacteria that have a round shape

E. The scientific study of microorganisms and their activities

F. A mixture of nutrients in which microorganisms are grown in the laboratory

G. The interval of time between invasion by a pathogenic microorganism and the appearance of the first symptoms of the disease

H. Bacteria that have a spiral or curved shape

I. Harmless, nonpathogenic microorganisms that normally reside in many parts of the body but do not cause disease

J. Bacteria that have a rod shape

K. The propagation of a mass of microorganisms in a laboratory culture medium

L. In microbiology, the act of placing a culture in a chamber that provides optimal growth requirements for the multiplication of the organisms, such as the proper temperature, humidity, and darkness

M. A small sample or part taken from the body to show the nature of the whole

EVALUATION OF LEARNING

Directions: Fill in each blank with the correct answer.

1. What are microorganisms? _____

_____

2. What life processes are performed within a unicellular microbe? _____

_____

3. What is meant by the following phrase: "Microorganisms are ubiquitous"?

_____

_____

4. What occurs when pathogens invade the body, and what is the response of the body to the invasion?

_____

_____

5. Describe two examples of microorganisms making up the normal flora that are beneficial to the body.

_____

_____

6. What defense mechanisms are used by the body to stop the invasion of a pathogen once it has entered the body?

_____

_____

7. What is droplet infection?

_____

_____

8. How might the spread of a droplet infection be prevented?

_____

_____

9. What occurs during the incubation period?

_____

_____

10. What is the prodromal period of an infectious disease?

_____

_____

11. What is the acute period of an infectious disease?

_____

_____

12. List three infectious diseases caused by *Staphylococcus aureus.*

_____

_____

13. List three infectious diseases caused by different types of streptococci.

_____

_____

14. List three infectious diseases caused by different types of bacilli.

_____

_____

15. In what part of the body do *E. coli* bacteria normally reside? What can occur if *E. coli* enters the urinary tract?

_____

_____

16. List four infectious diseases caused by viruses.

_____

_____

Chapter **20 Medical Microbiology**

17. Explain the purpose of each of the following parts of a microscope:

Stage

_____

_____

Substage condenser

_____

_____

Diaphragm

_____

_____

Coarse adjustment

_____

_____

Fine adjustment

_____

_____

Eyepiece (ocular lens)

_____

_____

18. Describe the function of each of the following objective lenses:

Low power

_____

_____

High power

_____

_____

Oil immersion

_____

_____

19. What is the purpose of using oil with the oil-immersion objective?

_____

_____

20. List five guidelines that should be followed for proper care of the microscope.

_____

_____

_____

_____

21. List five common areas of the body from which a microbiologic specimen may be obtained.

_____

_____

22. What are extraneous microorganisms? What may occur if extraneous microorganisms enter a microbiologic specimen?

_____

_____

23. List two ways to prevent contamination of a specimen with extraneous microorganisms.

_____

_____

24. List two precautions a medical assistant should take to prevent infecting herself or himself with a microbiologic specimen.

_____

_____

25. Why should a specimen for microbial culture be processed as soon as possible after it is collected?

_____

26. When collecting a microbiologic specimen, why is it important to indicate on the laboratory request if the patient is receiving antibiotic therapy?

_____

_____

27. Describe the procedure for collecting a wound specimen.

_____

_____

28. What is the purpose of a transport medium?

_____

_____

29. How should a collection and transport system be stored?

_____

_____

823

30. What is strep throat?

_____

_____

31. What is the age range that strep throat is most likely to affect?

_____

32. What are the symptoms of strep throat?

_____

_____

33. How is strep throat transmitted from one person to another?

_____

34. What is a poststreptococcal complication?

_____

_____

35. List two poststreptococcal complications that may occur in a patient with strep throat. How can these complications be prevented?

_____

_____

36. What is the advantage of using a RADT to diagnose strep throat in the medical office?

_____

37. Describe the three different types of influenza viruses:

   a. Influenza Type A: _____

   _____

   b. Influenza Type B: _____

   _____

   _____

   c. Influenza Type C: _____

   _____

38. List two ways in which influenza can be transmitted from one person to another?

_____

_____

39. What is the incubation period for influenza? _____

40. How long is an individual infected with influenza contagious?

_____

41. How do the symptoms of influenza differ from the symptoms of a cold?

_____

42. What are the symptoms of influenza?

_____

_____

43. What factors can increase an individual's risk of developing serious complications from influenza?

_____

_____

44. What complications may occur from contracting influenza?

_____

_____

45. What is the best means for preventing an influenza infection?

_____

46. Who should receive an influenza vaccine?

_____

47. Why must a new influenza vaccine be produced each year?

_____

_____

48. What are three benefits that are derived from the influenza vaccine?

_____

_____

49. What infection control measures can be taken to prevent the transmission of influenza?

_____

_____

50. What home care measures can be taken to treat the symptoms of influenza?

_____

_____

51. How do antiviral medications work to treat influenza?

_____

_____

Chapter **20** **Medical Microbiology**

52. What is the recommendation for prescribing an antiviral medication against influenza? When is this medication most effective?

_____

_____

53. How is influenza typically diagnosed? Explain your answer.

_____

_____

54. When might a rapid influenza test be performed to diagnose influenza?

_____

55. Why is a nasopharyngeal specimen usually preferred for rapid influenza diagnostic test?

_____

56. What is the advantage of using a flocked swab to collect a nasopharyngeal specimen?

_____

57. How can the distance to insert a nasopharyngeal swab be determined?

_____

58. What is the purpose of culturing a microbiologic specimen?

_____

_____

59. What is the purpose of adding sheep's blood to an agar culture medium?

_____

_____

60. What is the name given to the type of culture that contains two or more types of microorganisms?

_____

61. What is the purpose of performing a sensitivity test on a bacterial culture?

_____

62. How are the test results interpreted when performing a disc diffusion sensitivity test?

_____

_____

_____

A. Stages of an Infectious Disease

Your provider wants you to design a poster to hang in the office that outlines the stages of an infectious disease. Complete this project using the following diagram in your study guide.

STAGES OF INFECTIOUS DISEASE

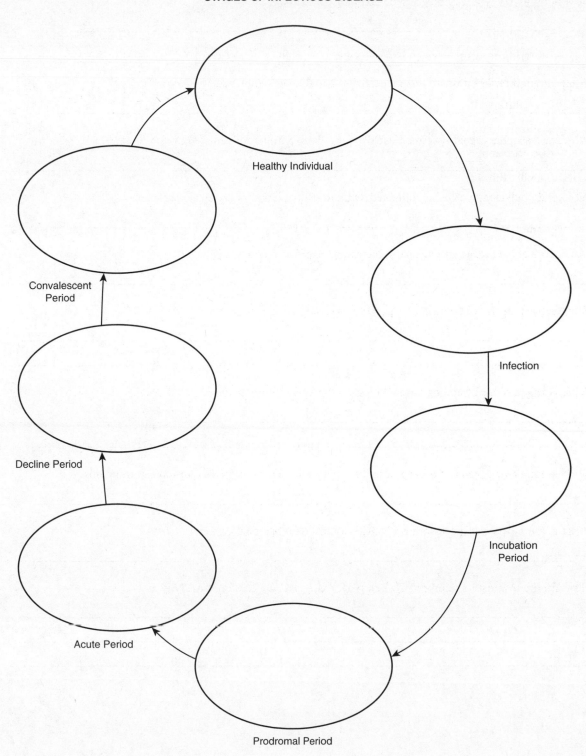

Healthy Individual

Convalescent Period

Decline Period

Acute Period

Prodromal Period

Infection

Incubation Period

B. Sensitivity Testing

Refer to Figure 20-9 of the textbook. Place a check mark next to each antibiotic that is effective against the pathogen growing on the culture medium in the Petri plate.

_____ 1. azithromycin

_____ 2. cephalothin

_____ 3. ciprofloxacin

_____ 4. cefprozil

_____ 5. clarithromycin

_____ 6. doxycycline

_____ 7. erythromycin

_____ 8. nitrofurantoin

_____ 9. norfloxacin

_____ 10. penicillin

_____ 11. sulfisoxazole

_____ 12. tetracycline

C. Crossword Puzzle: Medical Microbiology

Directions: Complete the crossword puzzle using the clues provided.

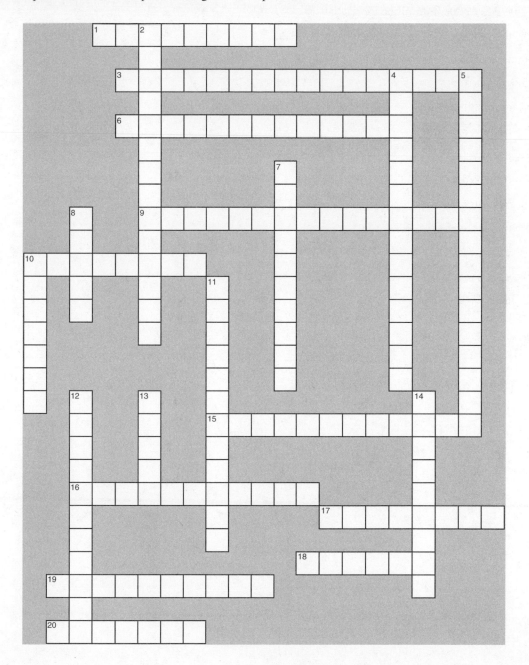

Across

1 Invasion by pathogens
3 Between invasion and first symptoms
6 Absent when present
9 Which antibiotic?
10 Sample of the body
15 Second-line natural defense mechanism
16 Treatment for strep throat
17 Disease-producing MO
18 Influenza complication
19 Can catch it!
20 Rod-shaped bacteria

Down

2 For precise focusing
4 Poststreptococcal complication
5 Way to transmit pathogens
7 It's everywhere!
8 Most prevalent influenza virus
10 Influenza preventer
11 Study of microorganisms
12 Harmless MOs residing in body
13 Round bacteria
14 Magnifies 40×

Chapter **20** **Medical Microbiology**

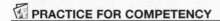

Procedure 20-1: Using the Microscope

Practice using a microscope.

Procedure 20-2: Collecting a Throat Specimen

Obtain a throat specimen using a sterile cotton swab or a collection and transport system. Document the procedure in the chart provided.

Procedure 20-3: Rapid Strep Testing

a. Run controls on a CLIA-waived rapid strep test and document results on the quality control log on page 833.
b. Perform a strep test using a CLIA-waived rapid strep testing kit, and document results in the chart provided.

Procedure 20-4: Rapid Influenza Testing

a. Run controls on a CLIA-waived rapid influenza test and document results on the quality control log on page 833.
b. Perform an influenza test using a CLIA-waived rapid influenza testing kit, and document results in the chart provided.

CHART	
Date	

Chapter **20 Medical Microbiology**

CHART	
Date	

QUALITY CONTROL LOG—STREP TEST

Date	Name of Test	Control Lot #	Control Expiration Date	External Positive Control **Results**	External Negative Control Results	Technician

QUALITY CONTROL LOG—INFLUENZA TEST

Date	Name of Test	Control Lot #	Control Expiration Date	External Positive Control Results	External Negative Control Results	Technician

Notes

Procedure 20-1: Using the Microscope

Name: _____   Date: _____

Evaluated by: _____   Score: _____

Performance Objective

Outcome:	Use a microscope.
Conditions:	Given a microscope, lens paper, specimen slide, tissue or gauze, immersion oil, xylene, and a soft cloth.
Standards:	Time: 15 minutes. Student completed procedure in _____ minutes.
	Accuracy: Satisfactory score on the Performance Evaluation Checklist.

Performance Evaluation Checklist

Trial 1	Trial 2	Point Value	Performance Standards
		•	Cleaned the ocular and objective lenses with lens paper.
		•	Turned on the light source.
		•	Rotated the nosepiece to the low-power objective.
		•	Used the coarse adjustment to provide sufficient working space for placing the slide on the stage.
		•	Placed the slide on the stage, specimen side up, and secured it.
		•	Positioned the low-power objective until it almost touched the slide using the coarse adjustment.
		•	Observed this step.
		▷	Explained why this step should be observed.
		•	Looked through the ocular lens.
		•	Brought the specimen into coarse focus using the coarse adjustment knob.
		•	Observed the specimen until it came into coarse focus.
		•	Used the fine-adjustment knob to bring the specimen into sharp, clear focus.
		•	Adjusted the light as needed using the diaphragm.
		•	Rotated the nosepiece to the high-power objective.
		•	Used the fine-adjustment knob to bring the specimen into a precise focus.
		•	Did not use the coarse-adjustment knob to focus the high-power objective.
		▷	Explained why the coarse-adjustment knob should not be used for focusing at this point.
		•	Examined the specimen as required by the test or procedure being performed.
		•	Turned off the light after use.

Trial 1	Trial 2	Point Value	Performance Standards
		•	Removed the slide from the stage.
		•	Cleaned the stage with a tissue or gauze.
		•	Properly cared for and stored the microscope.
			Using the oil-immersion objective:
		•	Rotated the nosepiece to the oil-immersion objective.
		•	Placed the objective to one side.
		•	Placed a drop of immersion oil on the slide directly over the center opening in the stage.
		•	Moved the oil-immersion objective into place.
		•	Made sure the objective did not touch the stage or slide.
		•	Used the coarse adjustment to position the oil-immersion objective.
		•	Brought the objective down until the lens touched the oil but did not come in contact with the slide.
		•	Looked through the eyepiece.
		•	Focused slowly using the coarse objective until the object was visible.
		•	Used the fine adjustment to bring the object into sharp focus.
		•	Adjusted the light as needed using the diaphragm.
		•	Examined the specimen as required by the test or procedure being performed.
		•	Turned off the light after use.
		•	Removed the slide from the stage.
		•	Cleaned the oil-immersion objective with lens paper.
		▷	Explained why the lens must be cleaned immediately.
		•	Cleaned the oil from the slide by immersing it in xylene and wiping it with a soft cloth.
		★	Completed the procedure within 15 minutes.
			Totals

Evaluation of Student Performance

EVALUATION CRITERIA			COMMENTS
Symbol	**Category**	**Point Value**	
★	Critical Step	16 points	
•	Essential Step	6 points	
Ⓐ	Affective Competency	6 points	
▷	Theory Question	2 points	

Score calculation: 100 points

− _____ points missed

_____ Score

Satisfactory score: 85 or above

CAAHEP Competencies Achieved

Psychomotor (Skills)
☑ I. 9. Assist provider with patient exam.

ABHES Competencies Achieved

☑ 8. c. Assist provider with general/physical examination.

Notes

Procedure 20-2: Collecting a Throat Specimen

Name: _____ Date: _____

Evaluated by: _____ Score: _____

Performance Objective

Outcome:	Collect a throat specimen for transport to an outside laboratory.
Conditions:	Given the following: disposable gloves, tongue depressor, sterile swab, sterile transport container, laboratory request form, biohazard specimen bag and a waste container.
Standards:	Time: 5 minutes. Student completed procedure in _____ minutes.
	Accuracy: Satisfactory score on the Performance Evaluation Checklist.

Performance Evaluation Checklist

Trial 1	Trial 2	Point Value	Performance Standards
		•	Sanitized hands.
		•	Assembled equipment.
		•	Checked the expiration date on the swab envelope.
		•	Labeled the transport container.
		•	Completed the laboratory request form.
		•	Greeted the patient and introduced yourself.
		•	Identified the patient and explained the procedure.
		•	Positioned the patient and adjusted the light.
		•	Applied gloves.
		•	Removed the sterile swab from its peel-apart package, being careful not to contaminate it.
		•	Depressed the patient's tongue with a tongue depressor.
		▷	Stated the function of the tongue depressor.
		•	Placed the swab at the back of the patient's throat and firmly rubbed it over lesions or white or inflamed areas of the tonsillar area and posterior pharynx.
		▷	Explained why the swab should be rubbed over suspicious-looking areas.
		•	Constantly rotated the swab as the specimen was being obtained.
		▷	Described why a rotating motion should be used.
		•	Did not allow the swab to touch any area other than the throat.
		▷	Explained why the swab should not be allowed to touch any areas other than the throat.
		•	Kept the patient's tongue depressed and withdrew the swab and removed the tongue depressor.

Chapter **20** **Medical Microbiology**

Trial 1	Trial 2	Point Value	Performance Standards
		•	Disposed of the tongue depressor.
		•	Properly handled and prepared the specimen for transport to an outside laboratory.
		•	Removed gloves and sanitized hands.
		•	Documented the information.
			Demonstrated the following affective behavior(s) during this procedure:
		Ⓐ	Explained to a patient the rationale for performance of a procedure.
		Ⓐ	Showed awareness of a patient's concerns related to the procedure being performed.
		★	Completed the procedure within 5 minutes.
			Totals

CHART

Date	

Evaluation of Student Performance

EVALUATION CRITERIA			COMMENTS
Symbol	**Category**	**Point Value**	
★	Critical Step	16 points	
•	Essential Step	6 points	
Ⓐ	Affective Competency	6 points	
▷	Theory Question	2 points	

Score calculation: 100 points

−   _____ points missed

_____ Score

Satisfactory score: 85 or above

Notes

Procedure 20-3: CLIA-Waived Rapid Strep Testing

Name: _____   Date: _____

Evaluated by: _____   Score: _____

Performance Objective

Outcome:	Perform a CLIA-waived rapid strep test.
Conditions:	Given the following: QuickVue rapid strep testing kit, sterile throat swab, disposable gloves, tongue depressor, external controls, manufacturer's instructions, quality control log, and a biohazard waste container.
Standards:	Time: 10 minutes. Student completed procedure in _____ minutes.
	Accuracy: Satisfactory score on the Performance Evaluation Checklist.

Performance Evaluation Checklist

Trial 1	Trial 2	Point Value	Performance Standards
		•	Sanitized hands.
		•	Assembled equipment.
		•	Checked the expiration date on the testing kit.
		•	Applied gloves and ran a positive and negative control, if needed.
		▷	Stated when controls should be run.
		•	Disposed of test cassettes and control swabs in a biohazard waste container.
		•	Removed gloves and sanitized hands.
		•	Documented results in the quality control log.
		•	Greeted the patient and introduced yourself.
		•	Identified the patient and explained the procedure.
		•	Positioned the patient and adjusted the light.
		•	Sanitized hands and applied gloves.
		•	Removed the test cassette from its foil pouch, and placed it on a clean, dry, level surface.
		•	Checked the expiration date of the sterile swab and removed the swab from its peel-apart package.
		•	Depressed the patient's tongue with the tongue depressor.
		•	Placed the swab at the back of the patient's throat and firmly rubbed it over lesions or white or inflamed areas of the tonsillar area and posterior pharynx.
		•	Constantly rotated the swab as the specimen was being obtained.
		•	Did not allow the swab to touch any area other than the throat.
		•	Kept the patient's tongue depressed and withdrew the swab.

Trial 1	Trial 2	Point Value	Performance Standards
		•	Removed the tongue depressor and discarded it.
		•	Inserted the swab completely into the swab chamber.
		•	Squeezed the extraction bottle once to break the glass ampule.
		•	Vigorously shook the extraction bottle five times.
		▷	Stated what color the solution should turn after the ampule is broken.
		•	Removed the cap of the extraction bottle and quickly filled the swab chamber to the rim.
		▷	Stated the purpose of the extraction solution.
		•	Started the timer for 5 minutes.
		•	Did not move the test cassette.
		▷	Stated what should be done if the liquid has not moved across the result window within 1 minute.
		•	Waited 5 minutes and read the results.
		▷	Described the appearance of a positive and negative result.
		▷	Described the appearance of an invalid result.
		▷	Explained what to do if an invalid result occurs.
		•	The results were identical to the evaluator's results.
		•	Disposed of the test cassette and swab in a biohazard waste container.
		•	Removed gloves and sanitized hands.
		•	Documented results in the patient's medical record.
			Demonstrated the following affective behavior(s) during this procedure:
		Ⓐ	Explained to a patient the rationale for performance of a procedure.
		Ⓐ	Showed awareness of a patient's concerns related to the procedure being performed.
		Ⓐ	Reassured a patient of the accuracy of the test results.
		★	Completed the procedure within 10 minutes.
			Totals
CHART			
Date			

Evaluation of Student Performance

EVALUATION CRITERIA			COMMENTS
Symbol	**Category**	**Point Value**	
★	Critical Step	16 points	
•	Essential Step	6 points	
Ⓐ	Affective Competency	6 points	
▷	Theory Question	2 points	

Score calculation: 100 points

    − _____ points missed

    _____ Score

Satisfactory score: 85 or above

CAAHEP Competencies Achieved

Psychomotor (Skills)
☑ I. 10. Perform a quality control measure.
☑ I. 11. e. Obtain specimens and perform CLIA-waived microbiology test.
☑ II. 2. Differentiate between normal and abnormal test results.

Affective (Behavior)
☑ I. 3. Show awareness of a patient's concerns related to the procedure being performed.
☑ II. 1. Reassure a patient of the accuracy of the test results.
☑ V. 4. Explain to a patient the rationale for performance of a procedure.

ABHES Competencies Achieved

☑ 9. a. Practice quality control.
☑ 9. b. Perform selected CLIA-waived tests that assist with diagnosis and treatment: (2) microbiology testing (6) kit testing.

Notes

Procedure 20-4: Rapid Influenza Testing

Name: _____ Date: _____

Evaluated by: _____ Score: _____

Performance Objective

Outcome:	Collect a nasopharyngeal swab specimen and perform a CLIA-waived rapid influenza diagnostic test.
Conditions:	Given the following: CLIA-waived Binax Now Influenza A and B testing kit, sterile nasopharyngeal flocked swab, disposable gloves, face mask, protective eyewear, external controls, manufacturer's instructions, quality control log, tissues, biohazard waste container.
Standards:	Time: 20 minutes. Student completed procedure in _____ minutes.
	Accuracy: Satisfactory score on the Performance Evaluation Checklist

Performance Evaluation Checklist

Trial 1	Trial 2	Point Value	Performance Standards
		•	Sanitized hands.
		•	Assembled equipment.
		•	Checked the expiration date on the testing kit.
		▷	Stated the reason for checking the expiration date.
		•	Applied gloves and ran a positive and negative control, if necessary.
		▷	Stated when controls should be run.
		•	Disposed of test devices and control swabs in a biohazard waste container.
		•	Removed gloves and sanitized hands.
		•	Documented the control results in a quality control log.
			Collected the nasopharyngeal swab specimen:
		•	Greeted the patient and introduced yourself.
		•	Identified the patient and explained the collection procedure.
		•	Explained to the patient that the collection procedure may cause coughing, sneezing, or tearing of the eyes.
		•	Positioned the patient in a sitting position.
		•	Asked the patient to blow his or her nose to remove nasal secretions.
		•	Sanitized hands and applied personal protective equipment.
		▷	Stated why personal protective equipment must be applied.
		•	Tilted the patient's head back slightly.
		▷	Stated the reason for tilting the patient's head back.

Trial 1	Trial 2	Point Value	Performance Standards
		•	Removed the cap from the extraction vial using a twisting motion.
		•	Checked the expiration date of the nasopharyngeal swab.
		•	Removed the sterile swab from its peel-apart package, being careful not to contaminate it.
		•	Estimated the distance for insertion of the swab.
		▷	Stated the reason for estimating the distance for insertion of the swab.
		•	Gently inserted the swab straight back into one nostril along the floor of the nasal passage.
		•	Slowly pushed the swab forward into the nasal passage until resistance is encountered.
		•	The depth of insertion was equal to approximately one-half of the distance from the corner of the nose to the ear lobe.
		•	Did not force the swab.
		▷	Stated what should be done if an obstruction or resistance is encountered.
		•	Rotated the swab against the mucosa of the nasopharynx between 3 and 5 times.
		▷	Stated the reason for rotating the swab.
		•	Left the swab in place for a few seconds.
		▷	Stated what can occur if an insufficient number of cells is collected.
		•	Gently removed the swab from the patient's nose with a rotating motion.
		•	Provided the patient with tissues, as required.
			Perform the Binax Now Influenza A and B Test:
		•	Inserted the swab into the extraction vial.
		•	Rinsed the swab in the extraction solution by vigorously rotating it three times without creating a lot of bubbles.
		▷	Stated the reason for vigorously rotating the swab in the solution.
		•	Removed the swab from the vial by rolling it with pressure against the inside of the vial.
		•	Properly disposed of the swab in a biohazard waste container.
		•	Removed the test device from its foil pouch and set it on a clean, dry, level surface.
		•	Filled the pipet.
		•	Checked to make sure the pipet was full and that there were no air spaces in the lower part of the pipet.
		▷	Stated what may occur if too little sample is added to the test.
		•	Slowly added the contents of the pipet to the middle of the white pad on the test strip
		•	Did not allow the pipet to touch the pad.

848

Trial 1	Trial 2	Point Value	Performance Standards
		•	Immediately peeled off the brown adhesive liner from the test device.
		•	Closed and securely sealed the test device.
		•	Waited 15 minutes and read the results.
		▷	Stated why the results should not be read before or after 15 minutes have elapsed.
		•	Interpreted the test results.
		▷	Described the appearance of negative and positive test results.
		▷	Explained what to do if an invalid result occurs.
		★	The results were identical to the evaluator's results.
		•	Disposed of the test device in a biohazard waste container.
		•	Removed personal protective equipment and sanitized hands.
		•	Documented results in the patient's medical record.
			Demonstrated the following affective behavior(s) during this procedure:
		Ⓐ	Showed awareness of a patient's concern related to the procedure being performed
		Ⓐ	Reassured a patient of the accuracy of the test results.
		Ⓐ	Explained to a patient the rationale for performance of a procedure.
		★	Completed the procedure within 20 minutes.
			Totals

CHART

Date	

Evaluation of Student Performance

EVALUATION CRITERIA			COMMENTS
Symbol	**Category**	**Point Value**	
★	Critical Step	16 points	
•	Essential Step	6 points	
Ⓐ	Affective Competency	6 points	
▷	Theory Question	2 points	

Score calculation: 100 points

− _____ points missed

_____ Score

Satisfactory score: 85 or above

CAAHEP Competencies Achieved

Psychomotor (Skills)
☑ I.10. Perform a quality control measure.
☑ I. 11.d. Obtain specimens and perform CLIA-waived immunology test.
☑ II. 2. Differentiate between normal and abnormal test results.

Affective (Behavior)
☑ I.3. Show awareness of a patient's concern related to the procedure being performed.
☑ II.1. Reassure a patient of the accuracy of the test results.
☑ V.4. Explain to a patient the rationale for performance of a procedure.

ABHES Competencies Achieved

☑ 9. a. Practice quality control.
☑ 9.b. (4) Perform selected CLIA-waived tests that assist with diagnosis and treatment: immunology testing.

21 Nutrition

CHAPTER ASSIGNMENTS

√ After Completing	Date Due	Study Guide Pages	STUDY GUIDE ASSIGNMENTS (CTA = Critical Thinking Activity)	Possible Points	Points You Earned
		855	?≡ Pretest	10	
		856-857	Term Key Term Assessment A. Definitions B. Word Parts (Add 1 point for each key term)	27 20	
		858-868	Evaluation of Learning questions	90	
		869	CTA A: Nutrition Density	8	
		869	CTA B: Sodium	10	
		870-871	CTA C: MyPlate	17	
		872	CTA D: Nutrition Facts Panel Analysis	14	
		873	CTA E: Nutrition and Disease	13	
		873	CTA F: Ingredients List	15	
		874	CTA G: Crossword Puzzle	20	
			e Evolve Site: Apply Your Knowledge Questions	10	
		855	?≡ Posttest	10	
			ADDITIONAL ASSIGNMENTS		
			Total points		

√ When Assigned By Your Instructor	Study Guide Pages	Practices Required	LABORATORY ASSIGNMENTS (Procedure Number and Name)	Score*
		3	**Practice for Competency** 21-A: Instruct a Patient According to Patient's Special Dietary Needs Textbook reference: pp. 758-767	
	875-878		✎ **Evaluation of Competency** 21-A: Instruct a Patient According to Patient's Special Dietary Needs	*

Notes

Name: _____ Date: _____

True or False

_____ 1. A food with a high nutrient density is high in calories and low in nutrients.

_____ 2. Carbohydrates provide 4 kilocalories of energy per gram.

_____ 3. Ingested glucose that is not needed for energy is stored for later use in the form of glycogen.

_____ 4. Fat transports water-soluble vitamins in the body.

_____ 5. Saturated fat is liquid at room temperature and comes primarily from plant sources.

_____ 6. The fat-soluble vitamins include A, D, E, and K.

_____ 7. Food labeling is required for most packaged foods.

_____ 8. One pound of body fat is equal to 2000 calories.

_____ 9. An individual with lactose intolerance is allergic to milk.

_____ 10. Common food allergens include milk, eggs, wheat, and peanuts.

True or False

_____ 1. An enriched food has vitamins and minerals added to it to replace those lost during the processing of that food.

_____ 2. Micronutrients include vitamins and minerals.

_____ 3. Lactose is a monosaccharide.

_____ 4. Soluble fiber helps to lower the blood cholesterol level.

_____ 5. The function of protein is to build, maintain, and repair body tissue.

_____ 6. Minor minerals are found in the body in levels of 5 grams or higher.

_____ 7. Approximately 60% to 65% of an adult's total body weight is made up of water.

_____ 8. The treatment of obesity involves a combination of nutrition therapy, a physical exercise program, and a behavior-modification plan.

_____ 9. The TLC eating plan provides recommendations for a heart-healthy diet.

_____ 10. Celiac disease may result in damage to the intestinal villi.

A. Definitions

Directions: Match each key term with its definition.

_____ 1. Antioxidant

_____ 2. Atherosclerosis

_____ 3. Bariatrics

_____ 4. Cholesterol

_____ 5. Complete protein

_____ 6. Disaccharide

_____ 7. Empty calorie food

_____ 8. Essential amino acid

_____ 9. Gluten

_____ 10. Glycogen

_____ 11. Incomplete protein

_____ 12. Kilocalorie

_____ 13. Lactose

_____ 14. Macronutrient

_____ 15. Micronutrient

_____ 16. Mineral

_____ 17. Monosaccharide

_____ 18. Nonessential amino acid

_____ 19. Nutrient

_____ 20. Nutrition

_____ 21. Nutrition therapy

_____ 22. Obesity

_____ 23. Percent daily value

_____ 24. Saturated fat

_____ 25. Triglycerides

_____ 26. Unsaturated fat

_____ 27. Vitamin

A. A food that provides calories but little or no nutrients. Also known as a low–nutrient-density food.

B. The amount of heat needed to raise the temperature of 1 kilogram of water by 1 degree Celsius. (Often referred to as a calorie.)

C. A chemical substance found in food that is needed by the body for survival and well-being.

D. The percentage of a nutrient provided by a single serving of a food item compared to how much is required for the entire day.

E. Buildup of fibrous plaques of fatty deposits and cholesterol on the inner walls of an artery that causes narrowing, obstruction, and hardening of the artery.

F. An organic compound that is required in small amounts by the body for normal growth and development.

G. A white waxy, fatlike substance that is essential for normal functioning of the body.

H. A type of protein found in certain grains such as wheat, rye, and barley.

I. The application of the science of nutrition to promote optimal health and treat illness.

J. The chemical form in which most fat exists in food, as well as in the body.

K. A molecule that inhibits the oxidation of other molecules.

L. A medical condition in which there is an excessive accumulation of body fat to the extent that it may have an adverse effect on the health and well-being of an individual.

M. A simple carbohydrate consisting of two sugar units.

N. A nutrient required in relatively large amounts by the body. Includes carbohydrates, fat, and protein.

O. A naturally occurring inorganic substance that is essential to the proper functioning of the body.

P. The branch of medicine that deals with the treatment and control of obesity and diseases associated with obesity.

Q. An amino acid that is required by the body but that cannot be manufactured by the body and must be obtained from food.

R. A protein that contains all of the essential amino acids needed by the body.

S. The study of nutrients in food, including how the body uses them and their relationship to health.

T. A simple carbohydrate consisting of one sugar unit.

U. The form in which carbohydrate is stored in the body.

V. An amino acid that is required by the body that can be synthesized by the body in sufficient quantities to meet its needs.

W. A protein that lacks one or more of the essential amino acids needed by the body.

X. A type of fat that is liquid at room temperature and comes primarily from plant sources.

Y. A disaccharide that consists of two sugar units and is found in milk and milk products.

Z. A type of fat that is solid at room temperature and comes primarily from animal sources.

AA. A nutrient required in very small amounts by the body. Includes vitamins and minerals.

Chapter **21** **Nutrition**

B. Word Parts

Directions: Indicate the meaning of each word part in the space provided. List as many medical terms as possible that incorporate the word part in the space provided.

Word Part	Meaning of Word Part	Medical Terms That Incorporate Word Part
1. anti-		
2. ox/i		
3. ather/o		
4. -sclerosis		
5. bar/o		
6. -iatrics		
7. di-		
8. -saccharide		
9. glyc/o		
10. -gen		
11. kilo-		
12. lact/o		
13. -ose		
14. macr/o		
15. micr/o		
16. mono-		
17. non-		
18. satur-		
19. tri-		
20. vit/a		

Directions: Fill in each blank with the correct answer.

1. What benefits can be derived from good nutrition?

   _____

   _____

2. List examples of tasks performed by the medical assistant that require a knowledge of basic nutritional principles.

   _____

   _____

3. Define the term *diet*.

   _____

4. What are the responsibilities of a dietitian?

   _____

5. What is the difference between an enriched food and a fortified food?

   a. Enriched food: _____

   b. Fortified food: _____

6. What is malnutrition?

   _____

   _____

7. What is nutrient density?

   _____

   _____

8. How many kilocalories per gram are provided by each of the following macronutrients?

   a. Carbohydrate: _____

   b. Fat: _____

   c. Protein: _____

9. List specific examples of body functions that require an energy source.

   _____

   _____

   _____

10. What are two functions of insulin in the body?

    _____

    _____

11. What is the difference between a simple carbohydrate and a complex carbohydrate?

a. Simple carbohydrate: _____

b. Complex carbohydrate: _____

12. What sugar units are included in the following simple carbohydrate categories?

a. Monosaccharides: _____

b. Disaccharides: _____

13. What are some examples of empty calorie foods?

_____

_____

14. What are some examples of foods that are classified as complex carbohydrates?

_____

_____

15. Why can't fiber be used as an energy source by the body?

_____

_____

16. What are the advantages of soluble fiber in the diet? What are some examples of food sources containing soluble fiber?

_____

_____

_____

17. What are the advantages of insoluble fiber in the diet? What are some examples of food sources containing insoluble fiber?

_____

_____

_____

18. What functions are performed by fat in the body?

_____

_____

19. What are some examples of foods that are high in saturated fat?

_____

_____

20. List examples of food sources that include the following type of fat?

a. Monounsaturated fat: _____

b. Polyunsaturated fat: _____

859

21. What is the purpose of adding trans fat to a food item? What are some examples of foods that may contain high levels of trans fat?

_____

_____

_____

22. What is the disadvantage of trans fat?

_____

_____

23. What is the function of cholesterol in the body? What are some examples of foods that contain cholesterol?

_____

_____

24. What may occur in an individual with a high blood cholesterol level?

_____

_____

25. Indicate the total blood cholesterol levels for each of the following categories:

a. Desirable: _____

b. Borderline high: _____

c. High: _____

26. What conditions may result in elevated triglyceride levels?

_____

_____

27. What are the functions of protein in the body? What are some rich food sources of protein?

_____

_____

_____

28. What does protein break down into through the process of digestion?

_____

29. What is the difference between an essential amino acid and a nonessential amino acid?

a. Essential amino acid: _____

b. Nonessential amino acid: _____

30. What is the difference between a complete protein and an incomplete protein? List food sources of each.

a. Complete protein: _____

Food sources: _____

b. Incomplete protein: _____

Food sources: _____

860

31. What is the difference between a water-soluble vitamin and a fat-soluble vitamin?

    a. Water-soluble vitamin: _____

    b. Fat-soluble vitamin: _____

32. What may result from an excessive consumption of fat-soluble vitamins?

_____

_____

33. What is the overall function of the B vitamins?

_____

_____

34. What are rich food sources of many of the B vitamins?

_____

_____

35. What is the function of vitamin C?

_____

_____

36. Identify diseases and conditions that may result from a deficiency of the following vitamins?

    a. B_1 (Thiamine): _____

    b. B_2 (Riboflavin): _____

    c. B_3 (Niacin): _____

    d. B_5 (Pantothenic): _____

    e. B_6 (Pyridoxine): _____

    f. B_7 (Biotin): _____

    g. B_{12} (Folic acid): _____

    h. C (Ascorbic acid): _____

37. Identify the function, food sources, and deficiency diseases and conditions of each of the following fat-soluble vitamins.

    a. Vitamin A

        Function: _____

        Food sources: _____

        Deficiency diseases/conditions: _____

        _____

    b. Vitamin D

        Function: _____

        Food sources: _____

        Deficiency diseases/conditions: _____

        _____

861

c. Vitamin E

Function: _____

Food sources: _____

Deficiency diseases/conditions: _____

_____

d. Vitamin K

Function: _____

Food sources: _____

Deficiency diseases/conditions: _____

_____

38. What effect do free radicals have on body cells? What may occur as a result of this?

_____

_____

39. What is the difference between a major mineral and a trace mineral?

a. Major mineral: _____

b. Trace mineral: _____

40. Identify the function, food sources, and deficiency diseases and conditions of each of the following major minerals.

a. Calcium

Function: _____

Food sources: _____

Deficiency diseases/conditions: _____

_____

b. Magnesium

Function: _____

Food sources: _____

Deficiency diseases/conditions: _____

_____

c. Phosphorus

Function: _____

Food sources: _____

Deficiency diseases/conditions: _____

_____

d. Potassium

Function: _____

Food sources: _____

Deficiency diseases/conditions: _____

_____

e. Chloride

Function: _____

Food sources: _____

Deficiency diseases/conditions: _____

_____

f. Sodium

Function: _____

Food sources: _____

Deficiency diseases/conditions: _____

_____

41. Identify the function, food sources, and deficiency diseases and conditions of each of the following minor minerals.

a. Iron

Function: _____

Food sources: _____

Deficiency diseases/conditions: _____

_____

b. Copper

Function: _____

Food sources: _____

Deficiency diseases/conditions: _____

_____

c. Zinc

Function: _____

Food sources: _____

Deficiency diseases/conditions: _____

_____

d. Manganese

Function: _____

Food sources: _____

Deficiency diseases/conditions: _____

_____

e. Fluoride

Function: _____

Food sources: _____

Deficiency diseases/conditions: _____

_____

f. Selenium

Function: _____

Food sources: _____

Deficiency diseases/conditions: _____

_____

g. Iodine

Function: _____

Food sources: _____

Deficiency diseases/conditions: _____

_____

h. Chromium

Function: _____

Food sources: _____

Deficiency diseases/conditions: _____

_____

42. What are the functions of water in the body?

_____

_____

_____

43. What percentage of an adult's total body weight is made up of water?

_____

44. How is water lost from the body?

_____

_____

45. What is the major objective of MyPlate and the 2015 Dietary Guidelines for Americans?

_____

_____

_____

46. What are the recommended MyPlate proportions for the following food groups?

a. Fruits and vegetables: _____

b. Protein: _____

c. Grains: _____

d. Dairy: _____

864

47. What type of food requires a food label, and what type does not require a food label?

    a. Food requiring a food label: _____

    b. Food not requiring a food label: _____

48. What are the seven basic sections of the Nutrition Facts panel?

_____

_____

_____

_____

49. What are the interpretation guidelines for the percent daily value of the following?

    a. Low nutrient level: _____

    b. Good nutrient level: _____

    c. High or rich nutrient level: _____

50. What nutrients should be limited in the diet?

_____

51. What nutrients should be obtained in adequate amounts in the diet?

_____

52. In what order are the ingredients listed on a food label (in the ingredient list)?

_____

53. What benefits are provided by the ingredient list?

_____

_____

_____

54. List some terms that are used to describe added sugar in the ingredient list?

_____

_____

55. What terms are used to describe trans fat in the ingredient list?

_____

_____

56. What types of foods typically have a short ingredient list? What types of foods typically have a lengthy ingredient list?

    a. Short ingredient list: _____

    b. Lengthy ingredient list: _____

57. What is weight management?

_____

_____

58. What is the primary cause of obesity?

_____

59. What diseases are associated with overweight and obesity?

_____

_____

60. What three components should be included in the treatment of obesity?

_____

61. What is a calorie deficit, and how does it contribute to weight loss?

_____

_____

62. How many calories make up 1 pound of body fat?

_____

63. What are the disadvantages of a fad diet?

_____

_____

64. What are the characteristics of a fad diet?

_____

_____

65. How does physical exercise contribute to weight loss?

_____

66. How many minutes per week should a healthy adult spend in moderate-intensity physical exercise?

_____

67. How does a behavior-modification plan assist in weight loss?

_____

_____

68. What may result from atherosclerosis of the coronary arteries?

_____

_____

69. According to the TLC eating plan, what is the daily recommended intake for each of the following?

a. Total fat: _____

b. Saturated fat: _____

c. Dietary fiber: _____

d. Cholesterol: _____

e. Sodium: _____

70. What are some examples of foods that are high in cholesterol?

_____

71. What can occur if hypertension is not brought under control?

_____

_____

72. How does a low-sodium diet help to lower blood pressure?

_____

_____

73. What causes type 1 diabetes?

_____

_____

74. What are the six food groups included in the diabetic exchange list system?

_____

_____

75. What is the biggest risk factor for the development of type 2 diabetes?

_____

76. What is insulin resistance?

_____

_____

77. What is lactose intolerance?

_____

78. What is the cause of lactose intolerance?

_____

79. What are the symptoms of lactose intolerance?

_____

_____

80. What is the treatment for lactose intolerance?

_____

81. What is gluten intolerance?

_____

82. What is celiac disease?

_____

83. What are the symptoms of gluten intolerance?

_____

_____

84. What are some examples of foods that:

a. Contain gluten: _____

b. Are gluten-free: _____

85. What are the most common food allergens?

_____

_____

86. What are the symptoms of a food allergy?

_____

_____

87. What is an elimination diet?

_____

_____

88. What is a rotation diet?

_____

_____

89. How does denaturation assist in treating food allergies?

_____

_____

90. How do supplemental digestive enzymes assist in treating food allergies?

_____

_____

CRITICAL THINKING ACTIVITIES

A. Nutrient Density

1. List 3 examples of snacks you consume that have a high nutrient density.

    a. _____

    b. _____

    c. _____

2. List 3 examples of snacks you consume that have a low nutrient density (empty calorie foods).

    a. _____

    b. _____

    c. _____

3. List advantages and disadvantages of high nutrient density snacks.

    _____

    _____

    _____

    _____

4. List advantages and disadvantages of empty calorie foods.

    _____

    _____

    _____

B. Sodium

Review the Nutrition Facts Panel on five packaged foods. In the space provided, list the name of the food item and the amount of sodium included in one serving. Place a checkmark next to each food item that is high in sodium.

Name of Food	Amount of Sodium
a.	
b.	
c.	
d.	
e.	

C. MyPlate

Create a breakfast, lunch, and dinner meal for yourself according to the MyPlate guidelines. Indicate your food group choices in the spaces provided in the appropriate (breakfast, lunch, or dinner) MyPlate illustration.

1. Breakfast

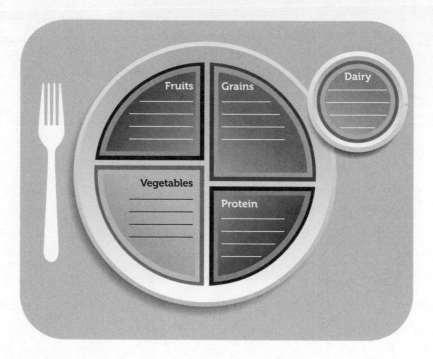

(Modified from U.S. Department of Agriculture: ChooseMyPlate, 2011, www.choosemyplate.gov.)

2. Lunch

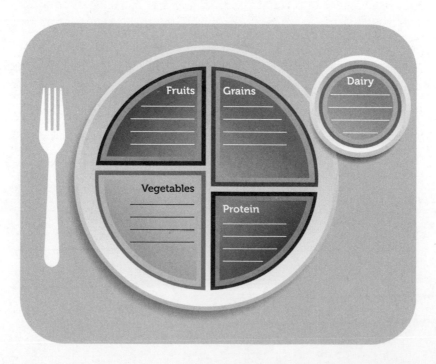

(Modified from U.S. Department of Agriculture: ChooseMyPlate, 2011, www.choosemyplate.gov.)

3. Dinner

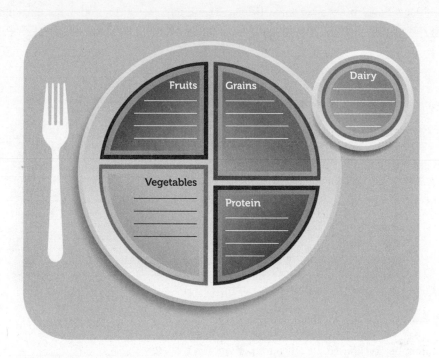

(Modified from U.S. Department of Agriculture: ChooseMyPlate, 2011, www.choosemyplate.gov.)

4. Compare each of the breakfast, lunch, and dinner MyPlate meals with the meals you typically consume. In the space provided below, discuss the similarities and differences between the meals.

_____

_____

_____

_____

_____

_____

D. Nutrition Facts Panel Analysis

Refer to the Nutrition Facts Panel in your textbook (Figure 21-10) and answer the following questions:

1. How many calories are in one serving of this food item? _____

2. How many calories in one serving of this food item come from fat? _____

3. How many servings are included in the package? _____

4. What makes up one serving of this food item? _____

5. How many total calories are in the package? _____

6. How many total grams of fat are in one serving of this food item? _____

7. What is the %DV of saturated fat in this food item? _____

8. What is the %DV of sodium in this food item? _____

9. Would this food item be considered a rich source of fiber? _____

10. Would this food item be considered a rich source of vitamin A? _____

11. Would this food item be considered a rich source of vitamin C? _____

12. Would this food item be considered a rich source of calcium? _____

13. Should an individual on a low-sodium diet avoid this food item? _____

14. Do you consider this food item a healthy food choice? Explain the rationale for your answer.

_____

_____

_____

E. Nutrition and Disease

The chart below lists the nutrients included on a nutrition facts panel. For each nutrient, indicate a disease or condition that may require a modification in consumption of that nutrient. Indicate whether the nutrient should be increased or decreased by placing a check mark in the appropriate box.

Nutrient	Disease or Condition	Increase	Decrease
1. Total fat			
2. Saturated fat			
3. Trans fat			
4. Cholesterol			
5. Sodium			
6. Total Carbohydrate			
7. Dietary Fiber			
8. Sugars			
9. Proteins			
10. Vitamin A			
11. Vitamin C			
12. Calcium			
13. Iron			

F. Ingredients List

1. Obtain an ingredient list from an unprocessed healthy food (usually has a short ingredient list), and list the ingredients of the food item below:

   _____

   _____

   _____

2. Obtain an ingredient list from a highly processed food (usually has a long ingredient list), and list the ingredients of the food item below:

   _____

   _____

   _____

   _____

3. Compare the ingredients in these two lists (unprocessed food and processed food), and discuss your findings below:

   _____

   _____

   _____

G. Crossword Puzzle: Nutrition

Directions: Complete the crossword puzzle using the clues provided.

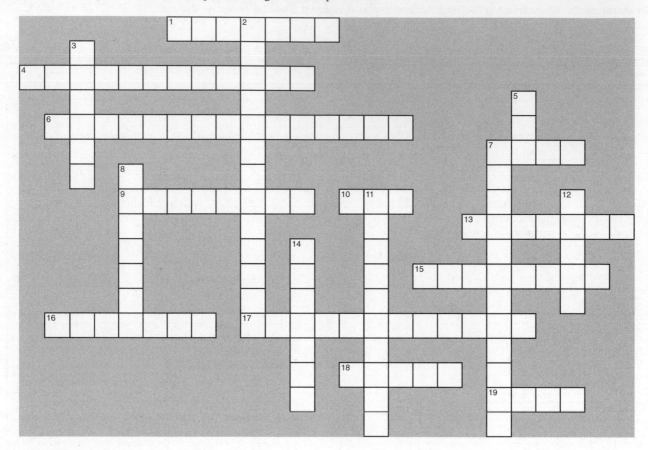

Across
1 Builds, maintains, and repairs tissue
4 Poor nutrition
6 Condition of artery plaque
7 Daily food and drink
9 Chemical substance in food needed by body
10 Provides 9 kcal/gram
13 Breaks down lactose
15 Storage product for glucose
16 Common food allergen
17 Solid fat
18 Celiac disease damages this
19 Eating plan to prevent and control hypertension

Down
2 Chemical form of fat
3 Wheat protein
5 Correlates with total body fat
7 Two sugar units
8 Enables glucose to enter a cell
11 Makes up protein
12 Makes up 60% to 65% of an adult
14 Milk sugar

Procedure 21-A: Instruct a Patient According to Patient's Special Dietary Needs

Name: _____   Date: _____

Evaluated by: _____   Score: _____

Performance Objective

Outcome:	Instruct a patient according a patient's specialized dietary needs.
Conditions:	Given the following: a scenario, a nutrition facts panel (Figure 21-10 in textbook), and an ingredients list (Figure 21-11 in textbook).
Scenario:	Based upon a thorough health history, physical examination, and laboratory test results, Dr. Cedy has determined that a patient is malnourished because of unhealthy food choices. The patient consumes approximately 2000 kcal per day and has a BMI of 24, which is within the BMI range for normal body weight. Dr. Cedy wants you to instruct the patient in reading a food label to assist the patient in making healthier food choices.
Standards:	Time: 10 minutes. Student completed procedure in _____ minutes.
	Accuracy: Satisfactory score on the Performance Evaluation Checklist.

Performance Evaluation Checklist

Trial 1	Trial 2	Point Value	Performance Standards
		•	Greeted the patient and introduced yourself.
		•	Identified the patient.
		•	Informed the patient that you will be providing instructions on reading a food label to assist the patient in making healthier food choices.
		•	Explained that the food label is required for most packaged food.
			Using Figure 21-10 in your textbook, instructed the patient on each section of the nutrition facts panel
		•	**1. Serving size:** Explained the *serving size* and *servings per package* section, including the following:
		•	a. The serving size represents the size of a single serving.
		•	b. The total number of servings in the package is included in this section.
		•	c. A packaged food frequently contains more than one serving.
		•	d. The serving size is presented in familiar units such as cups or pieces.
		•	e. The amount of calories and nutrients listed on the remainder of the label is based on one serving.
		•	f. This section allows a comparison of similar foods with the same serving size to determine which is a healthier choice.
		•	**2. Amount of calories:** Explained the *amount of calories* section, including the following:
		•	a. The amount of calories represents the total number of calories in one serving.

Trial 1	Trial 2	Point Value	Performance Standards
		•	b. The number of calories is listed on the left side, and the number of calories from fat is listed on the right side.
		•	c. It is important to pay attention to the number of calories consumed. If two servings are consumed, this doubles the amount of calories and nutrients consumed.
		•	3. **Percent daily value:** Explained the *percent daily value* section, including the following:
		•	a. Indicates the percentage of a nutrient provided by a single serving of a food item compared with how much is required for the entire day.
		•	b. Provides information on whether a nutrient in one serving contributes a little or a lot of that nutrient to the total daily diet, which helps in making informed food choices.
		•	c. The %DV is based on a 2000 kcal/day diet.
		•	d. Each nutrient is based on 100% of the recommended daily amount for that nutrient.
		•	e. Interpretation guidelines for %DV include the following: • Low nutrient level: 5% DV or less • Good nutrient level: 10% to 19% DV • High or rich nutrient level: 20% DV or more
		•	4. **Nutrients that should be limited:** Explained which nutrients are important to health but should be limited in the diet. Included the following:
		•	a. Nutrients to limit include total fat (including saturated fat and trans fat), cholesterol, and sodium.
		•	These nutrients should be limited because they contribute to health problems, such as heart disease, some cancers, and hypertension.
		•	b. Foods should be selected with a low %DV of these nutrients (5% DV or less).
		•	5. **Nutrients that should be obtained in adequate amounts:** Explained which nutrients should be obtained in adequate amounts. Included the following:
		•	a. Nutrients to obtain in adequate amounts include dietary fiber, vitamin A, vitamin C, calcium, and iron.
		•	Consuming adequate amounts of these nutrients improves health and helps reduce the risk of certain diseases and conditions.
		•	b. The patient should strive to achieve a 100% DV of these nutrients each day.
		•	c. Foods should be selected with a high %DV of these nutrients (20% DV or more).
		•	6. **Footnote with daily values:** Explained the footnote section, including the following:
		•	a. The daily values listed for total fat, saturated fat, cholesterol, and sodium are considered the maximum upper limits that should be consumed each day.

Trial 1	Trial 2	Point Value	Performance Standards
		•	b. The daily value for dietary fiber is considered the minimum level to try to reach each day.
		•	c. Relayed the DV amount for each nutrient for a 2000 kcal/day diet to the patient.
		•	**7. Additional nutrients:** Explained the *additional nutrients* section, including the following:
		•	a. Total carbohydrates consist of both simple and complex carbohydrates.
		•	b. Sugars include the simple carbohydrates.
		•	c. Dietary fiber is a complex carbohydrate.
		•	d. The remaining carbohydrate comes from starches.
		•	e. A %DV for protein is not required on a food label because most Americans consume more protein than they need.
			Using Figure 21-11 in your textbook, instructed the patient on the ingredient list
		•	Explained that the ingredients are listed in descending order of weight from highest to lowest.
		•	Stated that the first ingredient makes up the largest proportion of the food by weight than any other ingredient.
		•	Explained that the ingredient list can assist in making healthy food choices.
		•	Explained that added sugar and trans fat appear in the ingredient list under a number of different names.
		•	Provided the patient with examples of names used to describe sugar and trans fat.
		•	Explained that the ingredient list allows the consumer to scan for ingredients that may cause food allergies.
		•	Explained that unprocessed foods typically have a short and simple ingredient list.
		•	Explained that processed foods typically have a lengthy list of ingredients that include chemical terms.
		•	Answered any questions the patient had regarding food labels.
			Demonstrated the following affective behavior(s) during this procedure:
		Ⓐ	Showed awareness of patient's concerns regarding a dietary change.
		Ⓐ	Demonstrated (a) empathy, (b) active listening, (c) nonverbal communication.
		•	Charted the procedure correctly.
		★	Completed the procedure within 10 minutes.
			Totals

Trial 1	Trial 2	Point Value	Performance Standards
CHART			

Evaluation of Student Performance

EVALUATION CRITERIA			COMMENTS
Symbol	**Category**	**Point Value**	
★	Critical Step	16 points	
•	Essential Step	6 points	
Ⓐ	Affective Competency	6 points	
▷	Theory Question	2 points	

Score calculation: 100 points

−_____ points missed

_____ Score

Satisfactory score: 85 or above

2008 CAAHEP Competencies Achieved

Psychomotor (Skills)
☑ IV. 5. Instruct patients according to their needs to promote health maintenance and disease prevention.
☑ IV. 9. Document patient education.

Affective (Behavior)
☑ I. 2. Use language/verbal skills that enable patients' understanding.
☑ IV. 3. Use appropriate body language and other nonverbal skills in communicating with patients, family, and staff.

2015 CAAHEP Competencies Achieved

Psychomotor (Skills)
☑ IV. 1. Instruct a patient according to patient's special dietary needs.

Affective (Behavior)
☑ IV. 1. Show awareness of patient's concerns regarding a dietary change.
☑ V. 1. Demonstrate (a) empathy, (b) active listening, (c) nonverbal communication.

ABHES Competencies Achieved

☑ 2. d. Apply a system of diet and nutrition
  1) Explain the importance of diet and nutrition
  2) Educate patients regarding proper diet and nutrition guidelines
  3) Identify categories of patients that require special diets or diet modifications

878

22 Emergency Preparedness and Protective Practices

√ After Completing	Date Due	Study Guide Pages	STUDY GUIDE ASSIGNMENTS (CTA = Critical Thinking Activity)	Possible Points	Points You Earned
		883	?≡ Pretest	10	
		884	⚷Term Key Term Assessment	14	
		884-890	☑ Evaluation of Learning questions	60	
		890	CTA A: Disasters	20	
		891	CTA B: Personal Safety Plan	30	
		892	CTA C: Disaster Planning in the Medical Office	30	
		893	CTA D: Fire Hazards	20	
		893	CTA E: Methods of Fire Protection and Prevention	20	
		893	CTA F: Use of Fire Extinguisher	20	
		894-895	CTA G: Table-Top Fire Drill	60	
		896	CTA H: Table-top Mock Emergency Events	60	
		896	CTA I: Community Resources	9	
		897	CTA J: Crossword Puzzle	20	
			𝑒 Evolve Site: Apply Your Knowledge Questions	10	
		883	?≡ Posttest	10	
			ADDITIONAL ASSIGNMENTS		
			Total points		

Chapter **22** **Emergency Preparedness and Protective Practices**

√ When Assigned By Your Instructor	Study Guide Pages	Practices Required	LABORATORY ASSIGNMENTS (Procedure Number and Name)	Score*
	899	5	**Practice for Competency** 22-1: Demonstrating Proper Use of a Fire Extinguisher Textbook reference: pp. 784-785	
	901-902		**Evaluation of Competency** 22-1: Demonstrating Proper Use of a Fire Extinguisher	*
	899	4	**Practice for Competency** 22-2: Participating in a Mock Exposure Event Textbook reference: pp. 785-789	
	903-906		**Evaluation of Competency** 22-2: Participating in a Mock Exposure Event	*
			ADDITIONAL ASSIGNMENTS	

Notes

Name: _____   Date: _____

True or False

_____ 1. A flood is an example of a man-made disaster.

_____ 2. A positive reaction to a disaster involves the triggering of resources to meet the challenge.

_____ 3. During the alarm phase of the general adaptation syndrome (GAS), the body prepares for fight or flight.

_____ 4. During the recovery phase of the GAS, epinephrine is released into the bloodstream.

_____ 5. Hyperventilation may occur during severe anxiety.

_____ 6. Emergency exit routes must be at least 60 inches wide.

_____ 7. An oxygen tank is an example of an ignition source.

_____ 8. A fire door prevents the spread of fire from one area of a building to another.

_____ 9. The number, size, location, and type of fire extinguishers in a medical office are determined by the owner of the building.

_____ 10. The sequence of events that should be included in responding to a fire includes: rescue, activate, confine, and extinguish/evacuate.

POSTTEST

True or False

_____ 1. A man-made disaster is caused by the natural processes of the earth.

_____ 2. Stress is the body's response to threat or change.

_____ 3. Epinephrine causes a decrease in the blood pressure.

_____ 4. Anxiety is a feeling of worry or uneasiness.

_____ 5. The responsibility of an emergency evacuation coordinator is to take charge of and manage evacuation procedures.

_____ 6. A secondary exit route is the quickest and easiest way to exit a building in an emergency.

_____ 7. The elements that must exist in order for a fire to occur include a fuel source, ignition source, and carbon dioxide.

_____ 8. A flammable material catches fire easily.

_____ 9. A portable fire extinguisher can be used to fight a large fire that is out of control.

_____ 10. The batteries in a smoke detector should be changed every 6 months.

Directions: Match each key term with its definition.

_____ 1. Anxiety

_____ 2. Disaster

_____ 3. Emergency action plan

_____ 4. Emergency preparedness

_____ 5. Evacuation

_____ 6. Evacuation procedures

_____ 7. Exit route

_____ 8. Fire extinguisher

_____ 9. Fire prevention plan

_____ 10. Fire protection

_____ 11. HAZMAT

_____ 12. Man-made disaster

_____ 13. Natural disaster

_____ 14. Stress

A. The process of making plans to prevent, respond, and recover from an emergency situation

B. A feeling of worry or uneasiness, often triggered by an event that is perceived as having an uncertain outcome

C. The implementation of safety measures to reduce the unwanted effects of fire

D. A sudden event that causes damage or loss of life

E. A catastrophic event that is caused by nature or the natural process of the earth

F. A written document that describes the actions that employees should take to ensure their safety if a fire or other emergency situation occurs

G. A continuous and unobstructed path of travel from any point within a workplace to a place of safety

H. A planned systemic retreat of people to safety in an emergency situation

I. An event that causes serious damage through intentional or negligent human actions or the failure of a man-made system

J. The body's response to threat or change

K. A written document that identifies flammable and combustible materials stored in the workplace and ways to control workplace fire hazards

L. A portable device that discharges an agent designed to extinguish a fire

M. An acronym that refers to materials that pose a danger to health or the environment and that must be handled with protective equipment

N. Clear step-by-step procedures for the rapid, efficient, and safe removal of individuals from a building during an emergency

EVALUATION OF LEARNING

Directions: Fill in each blank with the correct answer.

1. Why is it important for medical offices to plan ahead for a disaster or serious emergency?

_____

_____

2. What causes a natural disaster?

_____

_____

3. What are some examples of natural disasters?

_____

_____

4. What is a man-made disaster?

_____

5. What are some examples of man-made disasters?

_____

_____

6. What does a positive reaction to a disaster involve?

_____

_____

7. When do individuals usually react negatively to a disaster?

_____

8. What characteristics of a disaster tend to cause the most serious psychological effects?

_____

_____

_____

9. What occurs during the alarm phase of the GAS?

_____

10. What changes occur in the body when epinephrine stimulates the sympathetic nervous system?

_____

_____

11. What occurs during the resistance phase of the GAS?

_____

_____

12. How long does the resistance phase last? _____

13. What are some examples of stress-related symptoms that may occur during the resistance phase?

_____

_____

14. What occurs during the recovery phase of the GAS?

_____

_____

15. What occurs during the exhaustion phase of GAS?

_____

_____

16. What is anxiety?

_____

_____

Chapter 22 Emergency Preparedness and Protective Practices

17. Why is it important to learn and practice emergency procedures?

_____

_____

18. How might severe anxiety be a problem in an emergency situation?

_____

_____

19. What are the symptoms of severe anxiety?

_____

_____

20. How should the medical assistant respond to a patient exhibiting severe anxiety?

_____

_____

21. What should the medical assistant do if an emergency occurs at his or her workplace?

_____

_____

22. What is the purpose of an emergency action plan?

_____

_____

23. What methods are typically used in the medical office to report emergency situations and/or to alert employees to the presence of an emergency situation?

_____

_____

_____

24. According to OSHA, when is it acceptable to use direct voice communication to alert employees of an emergency situation?

_____

_____

25. What is the responsibility of an emergency evacuation coordinator?

_____

_____

26. According to OSHA, what three components must be included in an emergency evacuation plan?

_____

_____

_____

27. What type of evacuation is typically required for the following?

    a. Large fire: _____

    b. Small wastebasket fire: _____

    c. Tornado: _____

28. List five guidelines (as stipulated by OSHA) that must be followed with respect to exit routes.

_____

_____

_____

29. What is the difference between a primary and secondary exit route?

    a. Primary exit route: _____

    b. Secondary exit route: _____

30. What information should be included on an evacuation floor plan?

_____

_____

_____

31. Why is it important to account for all building occupants following an emergency evacuation?

_____

_____

32. What is an evacuation warden?

_____

33. List examples of how a fire may start in the medical office.

_____

_____

34. What three elements must exist in order for a fire to occur?

_____

35. Explain the difference between a flammable and a combustible material, and list examples of each.

    a. Flammable material: _____

       Examples: _____

    b. Combustible material: _____

       Examples: _____

36. List five examples of fuel sources that may be found in the medical office.

_____

_____

37. List examples of common ignition sources.

_____

38. What effect will oxygen released from an oxygen tank have on a fire?

_____

39. What is the purpose of a fire prevention plan?

_____

_____

40. List methods of fire prevention in the medical office for each of the following categories:

a. Flammable and combustible materials:

_____

_____

b. Electrical equipment and appliances:

_____

_____

c. Inspection and maintenance:

_____

_____

41. What is the purpose of fire protection?

_____

_____

42. Explain how sprinklers are activated.

_____

43. What is the purpose of a fire door?

_____

44. What occurs when a fire alarm is activated?

_____

45. What type of testing and maintenance should be performed on battery-operated smoke detectors?

_____

46. What are some examples of fire extinguishing agents?

_____

47. What are the two primary functions of a fire extinguisher?

_____

_____

48. List the fuel sources included in the following fire classifications:

Class A: _____

Class B: _____

Class C: _____

Class D: _____

Class K: _____

49. Where are fire extinguishers usually located?

_____

50. Why is it important to properly maintain a fire extinguisher?

_____

51. What is the purpose of the tag attached to a fire extinguisher?

_____

52. Identify the steps that should be taken in operating a fire extinguisher following the PASS format.

P: _____

A: _____

S: _____

S: _____

53. Describe the steps that should be taken in responding to a fire following the RACE format.

R: _____

A: _____

C: _____

E: _____

54. What information should be included in the training of employees on the emergency action plan as required by OSHA?

_____

_____

_____

_____

55. When must the emergency action plan be reviewed with each employee?

_____

_____

_____

56. What is the purpose of an emergency practice drill?

_____

_____

57. Why is it important to conduct fire drills?

_____

_____

58. Who determines whether or not fire drills must be held at a facility?

_____

59. What is the difference between a fire drill and a disaster drill?

_____

_____

60. What role does the medical assistant serve in developing and implementing an emergency action plan?

_____

_____

CRITICAL THINKING ACTIVITIES

A. Disasters

1. Indicate a major natural disaster and a man-made disaster that have occurred in your community and/or state.

2. Provide a brief description of each disaster and the damage that resulted. (*Note:* An Internet search using the terms "Disasters in (name of your state)" will assist you in completing this activity.)

3. Natural disaster:

_____

_____

_____

_____

4. Man-made disaster:

_____

_____

_____

_____

B. Personal Safety Plan

1. Choose a natural disaster (e.g., tornado, hurricane, flood, blizzard) or man-made disaster (e.g., fire, power outage, burglary) that might occur in your locale.

2. Develop and outline a personal safety plan for responding to the disaster in your home environment. Include information on what you would do before, during, and after the disaster occurred. The following websites can assist you in locating information to complete this activity: www.redcross.org; www.fema.gov

   a. Name of disaster: _____

   b. Personal Safety Plan Response:

   Before:

   _____

   _____

   _____

   During:

   _____

   _____

   _____

   After:

   _____

   _____

   _____

C. Disaster Planning in the Medical Office

1. Choose a natural disaster or man-made disaster that might occur in your locale.

2. Outline step-by-step emergency procedures for responding to the disaster in a medical office setting using the form presented below. The following websites can assist you in locating information to complete this activity: www.redcross.org; www.fema.gov; www.osha.gov/Publications/osha3088.pdf; www.osha.gov/SLTC/emergency-preparedness

DISASTER PLANNING IN THE MEDICAL OFFICE
Name of Disaster: _____
Step-by-Step Emergency Procedure Response:
1.
2.
3.
4.
5.
6.
7.
8.
9.
10.
11.
12.

D. Fire Hazards

Perform a survey of your home to determine if there are any fire hazards. If so, list these hazards and what steps should be taken to correct them. Table 22-1 in your textbook and the following websites will assist you in completing this activity: www.fire-extinguisher101.com/hazards.html; https://www.usfa.fema.gov/prevention/

Fire Hazard: **Steps Needed to Correct:**

_____

_____

_____

_____

E. Methods of Fire Protection and Prevention

Survey the interior of a health care facility (or other type of commercial building) in your community, and indicate the fire protection and prevention methods in place at this facility. List these below:

_____

_____

_____

_____

F. Use of Fire Extinguisher

Perform an Internet search for a video of the operation of a fire extinguisher. Write a short paragraph below describing the video.

_____

_____

_____

_____

G. Table-Top Fire Drill

Participate in a table-top fire drill by completing the following:

1. Each student should create a small "paper doll" figure out of paper, cardboard, felt, and other materials (e.g., a tongue blade or a wood craft stick). The figure should be free-standing (be able to stand by itself).
2. Form a group of students and assemble around a table or other flat surface.
3. Place the evacuation floor plan (provided on page 895 of this study guide) in the center of the table.
4. Locate and review the purpose of the following using the evacuation floor plan:
   a. Primary exit route
   b. Secondary exit route
   c. Fire alarm pull stations
   d. Portable fire extinguishers
   e. Emergency exit doors
   f. Wheelchair-accessible exits
   g. Assembly areas
   h. Shelter-in-place areas
5. Choose a student (paper doll) to play the role of the emergency evacuation coordinator, which includes the following responsibilities:
   a. Calling emergency responders
   b. Identifying safe evacuation routes
   c. Ensuring that evacuation wardens are performing their duties
   d. Coordinating with emergency responders
6. Select students (paper dolls) to play the roles of patients with various types of conditions.
7. Select students (paper dolls) to play the roles of evacuation wardens. Assign various duties to these students as outlined in Table 22-1 of your textbook.
8. Place the various paper doll figures in various rooms on the evacuation floor plan.
9. Designate a fire that has erupted in one of the rooms on the floor plan.
10. Locate *Procedure 22-2: Participating in a Mock Exposure Event* in your textbook, and go to the following subheading: Conduct the Fire Drill.
11. Conduct a table-top fire drill following the step-by-step procedures listed under *Conduct the Fire Drill*. Explain the principle for performing each step in the drill after performing it.
12. Evaluate the fire drill by completing the *Fire Drill Evaluation Form* below.

		FIRE DRILL EVALUATION FORM
Date: _____		**Completed By:** _____
S	**U**	**Evaluation Criteria:**
		The fire drill was completed in an orderly, efficient, and timely manner.
		Building occupants and emergency responders were immediately alerted to the emergency situation.
		Evacuation wardens effectively completed their duties.
		Patients and visitors were escorted to the nearest exits and assembly area.
		Each building occupant was accounted for following the evacuation.
		Emergency responders were provided with appropriate information.
STRENGTHS:		
CONCERNS:		**MEANS OF IMPROVEMENT:**

EVACUATION FLOOR PLAN

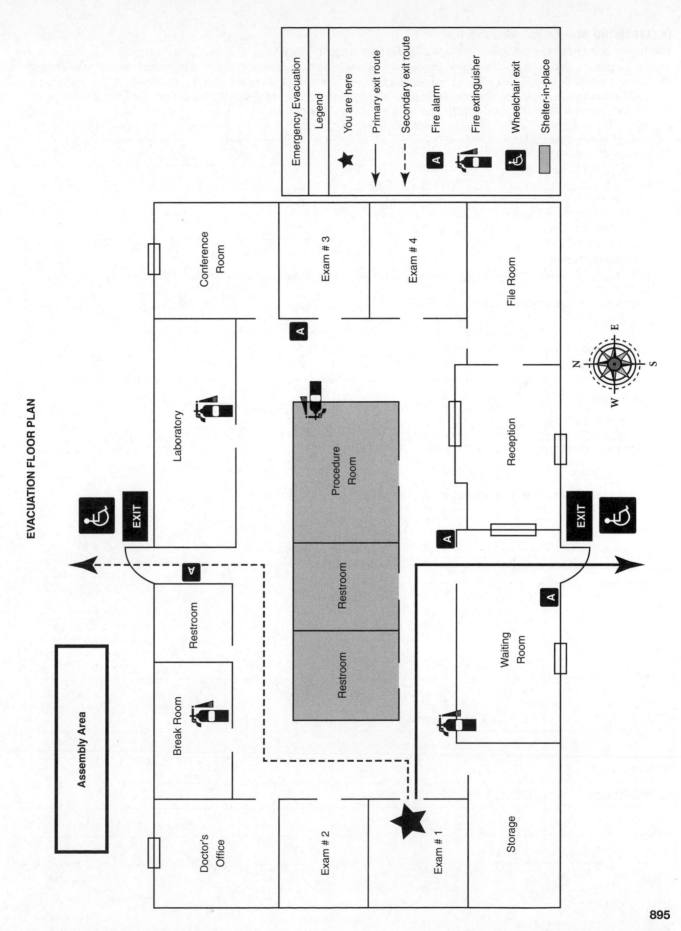

Chapter **22** **Emergency Preparedness and Protective Practices**

H. Table-Top Mock Exposure Events

Repeat the activity described above in *Critical Thinking Activity G: Table-Top Fire Drill* using a step-by-step emergency procedure plan developed by a group member as outlined in *Critical Thinking Activity C*. The group member who created the emergency plan should take the role of the evacuation coordinator. If time permits, participate in as many mock exposure events as possible, using emergency plans developed by other members of your group. Evaluate the timeliness and effectiveness of each emergency response, and document the key points below:

_____

_____

_____

_____

_____

I. Community Resources

Look up and indicate below the names and telephone numbers of the following:

1. Emergency management services (will usually be 911): _____

2. Poison control center: _____

3. Local hospital(s): _____

4. Local health department: _____

5. State health department: _____

6. State HAZMAT response team: _____

7. Local area emergency management (LEMA) office: _____

8. Local chapter of the American Red Cross: _____

9. Citizen Corps Council or Citizen Emergency Response Team (if any): _____

J. Crossword Puzzle: Emergency Preparedness and Protective Practices

Directions: Complete the crossword puzzle using the clues provided.

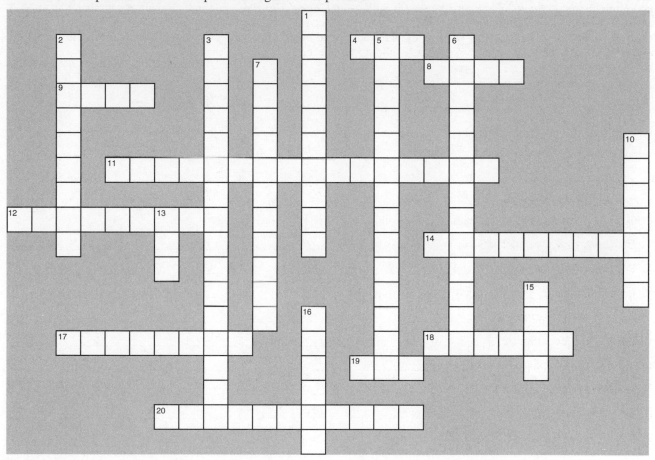

Across

4 Actions to take in an emergency
8 Man-made disaster
9 How to respond to a fire
11 Severe anxiety symptom
12 Natural disaster
14 Catches on fire easily
17 Increases blood glucose
18 Caused by threat or change
19 Reaction to stress
20 Helps to control anxiety

Down

1 Planned emergency retreat
2 Fire alerter
3 Quickest way to exit
5 Releases epinephrine
6 Alarm reaction response
7 Stimulates sympathetic NS
10 Worry or uneasiness
13 Multipurpose fire extinguisher
15 Fire extinguisher procedure
16 Fire element

Notes

Procedure 22-1: Demonstrating Proper Use of a Fire Extinguisher

Demonstrate the proper use of a fire extinguisher in a role-playing situation using a discharged fire extinguisher.

Using the information printed on the label of the fire extinguisher (or owner's manual), complete the information requested below:

1. What is the brand name of the extinguisher?

_____

2. What type of extinguishing agent is contained in the extinguisher (e.g., dry chemical, foam, carbon dioxide)?

_____

3. What types of fire classification(s) is this extinguisher capable of extinguishing?

_____

4. What type of precautions should be observed with this extinguisher?

_____

_____

5. What are the storage requirements for the fire extinguisher?

_____

_____

6. What should be done with the fire extinguisher after it has been discharged?

_____

_____

7. What type of care and maintenance is required for this extinguisher?

_____

_____

_____

Procedure 22-2: Participating in a Mock Exposure Event

a. Prepare for participating in a mock exposure (fire drill) event by first completing *Critical Thinking Activity G: Table-Top Fire Drill.*

b. Participate in a mock exposure (fire drill) event at a facility designated by your instructor.

Notes

Procedure 22-1: Demonstrating Proper Use of a Fire Extinguisher

Name: _____   Date: _____

Evaluated by: _____   Score: _____

Performance Objective

Outcome:	Demonstrate use of a fire extinguisher in a role-playing situation.
Conditions:	Given the following: portable multipurpose (ABC) fire extinguisher that has been discharged and a poster, flashing light, or other indicator to indicate the location of the fire.
Standards:	Time: 5 minutes. Student completed procedure in _____ minutes.
	Accuracy: Satisfactory score on the Performance Evaluation Checklist.

Performance Evaluation Checklist

Trial 1	Trial 2	Point Value	Performance Standards
		•	Identified a safe evacuation route before approaching the fire.
		▷	Stated the reason for identifying a safe evacuation route.
		•	Removed the fire extinguisher from its mounting device.
		•	Held the fire extinguisher upright with the nozzle pointing away from you.
		•	Stood 6 to 8 feet from the fire, keeping the back to the exit.
		▷	Explained the reason for standing at 6 to 8 feet from the fire and keeping the back to the exit.
		•	Performed a quick assessment of the fire to determine whether an attempt should be made to extinguish it with a fire extinguisher.
		▷	Stated when an attempt to extinguish a fire with a fire extinguisher should not be made.
		•	Pulled the safety pin straight out from the handle of the fire extinguisher.
		▷	Stated the purpose of the tamper-proof seal and the safety pin.
		•	Aimed the nozzle at the base of the fire (not the flames).
		▷	Stated why the nozzle should be directed at the base of the fire.
		•	Squeezed the handle slowly and continuously to release the extinguishing agent.
		▷	Stated what occurs if the pressure is released from the handle.
		•	Swept the extinguisher evenly from side to side at the base of the fire.
		▷	Stated why a sweeping motion should be used.
		•	Moved closer to the fire gradually as it began to smolder.
		•	Continued to discharge the extinguishing agent until the fire was completely out.
		▷	Stated what should be done if the fire grows larger.
		•	Backed away from the extinguished fire and continued to watch the area.

Trial 1	Trial 2	Point Value	Performance Standards
		▷	Stated the reason for continuing to watch the area.
			Demonstrated the following affective behavior(s) during this procedure:
		Ⓐ	Demonstrated self-awareness in responding to an emergency situation.
		★	Completed the procedure within 5 minutes.
			Totals

Evaluation of Student Performance

EVALUATION CRITERIA			COMMENTS
Symbol	Category	Point Value	
★	Critical Step	16 points	
•	Essential Step	6 points	
Ⓐ	Affective Competency	6 points	
▷	Theory Question	2 points	

Score calculation: 100 points

− _____ points missed

_____ Score

Satisfactory score: 85 or above

CAAHEP Competencies Achieved

Psychomotor (Skills)

☑ XII. 1. Comply with (a) safety signs, (b) symbols, (c) labels.

☑ XII. 2. b. Demonstrate proper use of fire extinguishers.

Affective (Behavior)

☑ XII. 2. Demonstrate self-awareness in responding to an emergency situation.

ABHES Competency Achieved

☑ 8. g. Recognize and respond to medical office emergencies.

Procedure 22-2: Participating in a Mock Exposure Event

Name: _____   Date: _____

Evaluated by: _____   Score: _____

Performance Objective

Outcome:	Participate in a mock exposure event.
Conditions:	Given the following: a scenario; a poster, flashing light, or other indicator to indicate the location of the fire; evacuation floor plan; employee roster; patient log-in sheet; pen; and paper.
Standards:	Time: 20 minutes. Student completed procedure in _____ minutes. Accuracy: Satisfactory score on the Performance Evaluation Checklist.

Performance Evaluation Checklist

Trial 1	Trial 2	Point Value	Performance Standards
			Predrill activities:
		•	Made a list of the names and phone numbers that may be needed in the event of a fire.
		•	Located and reviewed the purpose of the following using the evacuation floor plan: a. Primary exit route b. Secondary exit route c. Fire alarm pull stations d. Portable fire extinguishers e. Emergency exit doors f. Wheelchair-accessible exits g. Shelter-in-place areas h. Assembly areas
		•	Located and reviewed the purpose of the following: a. Sprinklers b. Smoke detectors c. Fire doors d. Exit signs
		•	Evaluated primary and secondary exit routes for the following: a. Clearly marked and well-lit b. Unobstructed and free of clutter c. Exit doors are free of decorations or signs that obscure the visibility of the exit d. Exit doors are unlocked from the inside e. Exit doors open outward f. Fire extinguishers are in place and clearly identified g. Evacuation floor plans are posted in multiple locations

Trial 1	Trial 2	Point Value	Performance Standards
		•	Assigned an emergency evacuation coordinator to perform the following: a. Calling emergency responders b. Identifying safe evacuation routes c. Ensuring that evacuation wardens are performing their duties d. Coordinating with emergency responders
		•	Compiled an employee roster.
		•	Assigned evacuation wardens.
		•	Assigned individuals to play the roles of patients.
		•	Compiled a patient log-in sheet.
			Conducted the fire drill:
		•	Rescued anyone in immediate danger of the fire.
		•	Performed the following if an individual's clothes are on fire: a. Instructed the person to stop, drop, and roll. b. Covered the person with a blanket or clothing to extinguish the flames.
		•	Activated the fire alarm.
		•	Immediately notified emergency responders.
		▷	Stated the information that should be relayed to the medical dispatcher.
		•	Closed doors and windows in the immediate area of the fire.
		▷	Stated the purpose of closing doors and windows.
		•	Extinguished the fire with a fire extinguisher if it is small and confined.
		▷	Explained what to do if the fire is too large to extinguish.
		•	Performed evacuation duties and evacuated the area immediately.
		▷	Stated why it is important to evacuate immediately.
		•	Shut down all electrical equipment and appliances in the immediate area.
		•	Before exiting a door, felt the door with the back of the hand. Performed the following if an exit door is warm: a. Did not open the door. b. Called 911 to report your location. c. Placed clothing or towels along the bottom of the door. d. Stayed calm and waited to be rescued. e. Did not break the window.
		•	Exited by the primary exit route.
		▷	Explained what to do if the primary route is blocked.
		•	Exited by stairways only.
		▷	Explained why an elevator should not be used during a fire.

904

Trial 1	Trial 2	Point Value	Performance Standards
		•	Closed doors after a room is evacuated and placed an "X" on the door.
		•	Escorted patients to the designated assembly area.
		•	Accounted for all building occupants.
		▷	Stated the reason for accounting for all building occupants.
		•	Kept building occupants together in the assembly area and did not allow them to block access to the building.
		•	Did not allow building occupants to reenter the building nor to leave until dismissed.
		•	Provided emergency responders with necessary information.
			Postdrill activities:
		•	Evaluated the effectiveness of the fire drill.
		•	Identified the strengths, concerns, and means of improvement of the fire drill.
		•	Documented the results of the fire drill.
		▷	Stated the purpose of evaluating and documenting the results of the fire drill.
			Demonstrated the following affective behavior(s) during this procedure:
		Ⓐ	Recognized the physical and emotional effects on persons involved in an emergency situation.
		Ⓐ	Demonstrated self-awareness in responding to an emergency situation.
		★	Completed the procedure within 20 minutes.
			Totals

FIRE DRILL EVALUATION FORM

Date: _____   Completed By: _____

S	U	Evaluation Criteria:
		The evacuation was completed in an orderly, efficient, and timely manner.
		Building occupants and emergency responders were immediately alerted to the situation.
		Evacuation wardens effectively completed their duties.
		Patients and visitors were escorted to the nearest exits and assembly area.
		Each building occupant was accounted for following the evacuation.
		Emergency responders were provided with appropriate information.

STRENGTHS:

CONCERNS:	MEANS OF IMPROVEMENT:

Evaluation of Student Performance

EVALUATION CRITERIA			COMMENTS
Symbol	Category	Point Value	
★	Critical Step	16 points	
•	Essential Step	6 points	
Ⓐ	Affective Competency	6 points	
▷	Theory Question	2 points	

Score calculation: 100 points
    − _____ points missed
       ____ Score

Satisfactory score: 85 or above

CAAHEP Competencies Achieved

Psychomotor (Skills)

☑ V. 9. Develop a current list of community resources related to patients' health care needs.

☑ V. 11. Report relevant information concisely and accurately.

☑ XII. 1. Comply with (a) safety signs, (b) symbols, (c) labels.

☑ XII. 2. b. Demonstrate proper use of fire extinguishers.

☑ XII. 4. Participate in a mock exposure event with documentation of specific steps.

☑ XII. 5. Evaluate the work environment to identify unsafe working conditions.

Affective (Behavior)

☑ XII. 1. Recognize the physical and emotional effects on persons involved in an emergency situation.

☑ XII. 2. Demonstrate self-awareness in responding to an emergency situation.

ABHES Competencies Achieved

☑ 4. e. Perform risk management procedures.

☑ 8. g. Recognize and respond to medical office emergencies.

☑ 8. i. Identify community resources and complementary and alternative medicine (CAM) practice.

☑ 8. j. Make adaptations for patients with special needs (psychological or physical limitations).

23 Emergency Medical Procedures and First Aid

CHAPTER ASSIGNMENTS

√ After Completing	Date Due	Study Guide Pages	STUDY GUIDE ASSIGNMENTS (CTA = Critical Thinking Activity)	Possible Points	Points You Earned
		909	Pretest	10	
		910	Term Key Term Assessment	16	
		910-915	Evaluation of Learning questions	27	
		915	CTA A: First Aid Kit	10	
		915	CTA B: EMD Information	5	
		915-916	CTA C: Emergency Care (2 points each)	6	
		916-918	CTA D: Emergency Situations (3 points each)	33	
			Evolve Site: Apply Your Knowledge Questions		
		909	Posttest	10	
			ADDITIONAL ASSIGNMENTS		
			Total points		

907

Notes

Name: _____ Date: _____

True or False

_____ 1. A specially equipped cart for holding and transporting medications, equipment, and supplies needed in an emergency is known as a crash cart.

_____ 2. Symptoms of an asthmatic attack include dyspnea and wheezing.

_____ 3. Symptoms of a heart attack include sudden weakness on one side of the body.

_____ 4. Another name for a stroke is a coronary occlusion.

_____ 5. Arterial bleeding is characterized by a slow and steady flow of blood that is dark red.

_____ 6. A laceration is an example of a closed wound.

_____ 7. Symptoms of a fracture include pain, swelling, deformity, and loss of function.

_____ 8. A sprain is a tearing of ligaments at a joint.

_____ 9. Heat stroke is a life-threatening emergency.

_____ 10. Insulin enables glucose to enter the body's cells and bc converted to energy.

⟦?⟧ **POSTTEST**

True or False

_____ 1. When providing emergency care, you should obtain information about what happened from bystanders.

_____ 2. Emphysema is a progressive lung disorder in which there is a loss of elasticity of the alveoli of the lungs.

_____ 3. Symptoms that may occur with hyperventilation include rapid and deep respirations and tachycardia.

_____ 4. The first priority for hypovolemic shock is to control bleeding.

_____ 5. Status asthmaticus is the type of shock caused by a reaction of the body to a substance to which an individual is highly allergic.

_____ 6. Another name for a nosebleed is epistaxis.

_____ 7. The type of fracture in which the broken ends of the bone are forcefully jammed together is a greenstick fracture.

_____ 8. The type of seizure in which the abnormal electrical activity is localized into very specific areas of the brain is a tonic-clonic seizure.

_____ 9. Chipmunks have a high incidence of rabies.

_____ 10. Emergency care for insulin shock is to give the patient sugar immediately.

Chapter **23** **Emergency Medical Procedures and First Aid**

Directions: Match each key term with its definition.

_____ 1. Burn

_____ 2. Crash cart

_____ 3. Crepitus

_____ 4. Dislocation

_____ 5. Emergency medical services

_____ 6. First aid

_____ 7. Fracture

_____ 8. Hypothermia

_____ 9. Poison

_____ 10. Pressure point

_____ 11. Seizure

_____ 12. Shock

_____ 13. Splint

_____ 14. Sprain

_____ 15. Strain

_____ 16. Wound

A. Network of community resources, equipment, and personnel that provides care to victims of injury or sudden illness

B. Any substance that causes illness, injury, or death if it enters the body

C. An injury to the tissues caused by exposure to thermal, chemical, electrical, or radioactive agents

D. Any device that immobilizes a body part

E. A grating sensation caused by fractured bone fragments rubbing against each other

F. A sudden episode of involuntary muscular contractions and relaxation, often accompanied by changes in sensation, behavior, and level of consciousness

G. A stretching or tearing of muscles or tendons caused by trauma

H. The immediate care that is administered to an individual who is injured or suddenly becomes ill before complete medical care can be obtained

I. A break in the continuity of an external or internal surface caused by physical means

J. A specially equipped cart for holding and transporting medications, equipment, and supplies needed for performing lifesaving procedures in an emergency

K. Any break in a bone

L. The failure of the cardiovascular system to deliver enough blood to all the vital organs of the body

M. An injury in which one end of a bone making up a joint is separated or displaced from its normal anatomic position

N. A life-threatening condition in which the temperature of the entire body falls to a dangerously low level

O. A site on the body where an artery lies close to the surface of the skin and can be compressed against an underlying bone to control bleeding

P. Trauma to a joint that causes tearing of ligaments

Directions: Fill in each blank with the correct answer.

1. What is the purpose of first aid?

_____

_____

_____

_____

2. What is the purpose of the office crash cart?

_____

_____

_____

_____

910

3. What is the difference between an EMT-basic and an EMT-paramedic?

_____

_____

_____

4. What are the responsibilities of an emergency medical dispatcher?

_____

_____

_____

5. List five OSHA Standards that should be followed when administering first aid.

_____

_____

_____

_____

6. What is the reason for performing each of the following during an emergency situation?

   a. Remaining calm and speaking in a normal tone of voice

_____

_____

   b. Making sure it is safe before approaching the patient

_____

_____

   c. Following OSHA Standards when providing emergency care

_____

_____

   d. Activating the emergency medical services

_____

_____

   e. Not moving the patient unnecessarily

_____

_____

   f. Checking the patient for a medical alert tag

_____

_____

7. What are the symptoms of asthma?

_____

_____

8. What is emphysema?

_____

_____

9. What are the symptoms of hyperventilation?

_____

_____

10. What are the symptoms of a heart attack?

_____

_____

11. What are the symptoms of a stroke?

_____

_____

12. What is the cause of the following types of shock?

   a. Hypovolemic

   _____

   _____

   b. Cardiogenic

   _____

   _____

   c. Neurogenic

   _____

   _____

   d. Anaphylactic

   _____

   _____

   e. Psychogenic

   _____

   _____

13. What are the characteristics of each of the following types of external bleeding?

   a. Capillary

   _____

   _____

   b. Venous

   _____

   _____

c. Arterial

_____

_____

14. What is the difference between an open wound and a closed wound?

_____

_____

15. What are the signs and symptoms of a fracture?

_____

_____

16. What are the characteristics of each of the following types of fractures?

a. Impacted

_____

_____

b. Greenstick

_____

_____

c. Transverse

_____

_____

d. Oblique

_____

_____

e. Comminuted

_____

_____

f. Spiral

_____

_____

17. What are the characteristics of each of the following types of burns?

a. Superficial

_____

_____

b. Partial thickness

_____

_____

Chapter 23 Emergency Medical Procedures and First Aid

c. Full thickness

_____

_____

18. What is the difference between a partial seizure and a generalized seizure?

_____

_____

19. List two examples of each of the following types of poisoning:

a. Ingested

_____

_____

b. Inhaled

_____

_____

c. Absorbed

_____

_____

d. Injected

_____

_____

20. What spiders (found in the United States) have bites that can result in serious or life-threatening reactions?

_____

_____

21. What species of snakes (found in the United States) are poisonous?

_____

_____

22. What animals tend to have a high incidence of rabies?

_____

_____

23. What factors place an individual at higher risk for developing heat- and cold-related injuries?

_____

_____

24. What areas of the body are most susceptible to frostbite?

_____

_____

25. What is the difference between type 1 diabetes and type 2 diabetes?

_____

_____

26. What is insulin shock, and what causes it to occur?

_____

_____

27. What is a diabetic coma, and what causes it to occur?

_____

CRITICAL THINKING ACTIVITIES

A. First Aid Kit

You are assembling a first aid kit. What supplies should be included in your kit? Identify one use for each of the supplies you list.

_____

_____

_____

_____

_____

_____

_____

_____

_____

B. EMD Information

Jeff Stickler suddenly develops weakness in his left arm and leg, has difficulty speaking, and has a severe headache and dizziness. You immediately call the emergency medical services (EMS). What information should you be prepared to relay to the emergency medical dispatcher (EMD)?

_____

_____

_____

C. Emergency Care

In which of the following emergency situations would you be legally permitted to administer first aid? Explain your answers.

1. A patient is unconscious and bleeding profusely.

_____

_____

915

2. You identify yourself and state your level of training and what you plan to do. You ask the patient if it is all right to administer emergency care. The patient responds by saying, "Yes, please help me."

_____

_____

3. You ask the patient if you can administer emergency care, but the patient refuses your help.

_____

_____

D. Emergency Situations

Explain what you would do in each of the following situations.

1. Holly Murphy falls while roller skating. She comes down hard on her left arm, which begins to swell and discolor. Holly guards her arm and complains of intense pain.

_____

_____

_____

_____

2. John Phillips is mowing the grass and mows over a yellow jacket nest. He is stung twice and soon starts complaining of intense itching and exhibits erythema and hives on his arms, torso, and face.

_____

_____

_____

_____

3. Steve Williams complains of severe indigestion and squeezing pain in the chest. He is short of breath and perspiring profusely.

_____

_____

_____

_____

4. Clara Miller is playing basketball and is accidentally hit in the face with the ball. Her nose begins bleeding profusely.

_____

_____

_____

_____

916

5. Debbie Carter, age 4 years, finds some children's chewable vitamins that have been left open on a table. She eats about 10 of them.

_____

_____

_____

_____

6. Rita Preston accidentally cuts her finger with a knife while preparing dinner. Her finger begins bleeding profusely.

_____

_____

_____

_____

7. Jose Perez is jogging on a cinder track. He falls and scrapes his left knee on the cinders.

_____

_____

_____

_____

8. Charlotte Lambert is getting ready to perform a piano recital for her entire church congregation. Suddenly she starts breathing very rapidly and deeply and complains that she feels light-headed and dizzy.

_____

_____

_____

_____

9. Bruce Jones is a diabetic. He is in a hurry and forgets to eat breakfast. He begins exhibiting behavior similar to that of someone who is intoxicated.

_____

_____

_____

_____

10. Debra Murray is delivering newspapers and is bitten by a strange dog. The bite causes several puncture marks and slight bleeding.

_____

_____

_____

_____

11. Tanya Howe is playing tennis on a hot and humid day and begins to feel weak and nauseous. Her skin feels cold and clammy, and she is sweating profusely and complains of dizziness.

_____

_____

_____

_____